2009
YEAR BOOK OF
**CRITICAL CARE
MEDICINE**®

The 2009 Year Book Series

Year Book of Anesthesiology and Pain Management™: Drs Chestnut, Abram, Black, Gravlee, Lee, Mathru, and Roizen

Year Book of Cardiology®: Drs Gersh, Cheitlin, Elliott, Graham, Sundt, and Waldo

Year Book of Critical Care Medicine®: Drs Dellinger, Parrillo, Balk, Bekes, Dorman, and Dries

Year Book of Dentistry®: Drs Olin, Belvedere, Davis, Henderson, Johnson, Ohrbach, Scott, Spencer, and Zakariasen

Year Book of Dermatology and Dermatologic Surgery™: Drs Thiers and Lang

Year Book of Diagnostic Radiology®: Drs Osborn, Abbara, Birdwell, Elster, Gardiner, Levy, Manaster, Oestrich, and Rosado de Christenson

Year Book of Emergency Medicine®: Drs Hamilton, Handly, Quintana, Werner, and Bruno

Year Book of Endocrinology®: Drs Mazzaferri, Bessesen, Clarke, Howard, Kennedy, Leahy, Meikle, Molitch, Rogol, and Schteingart

Year Book of Gastroenterology™: Drs Lichtenstein, Dempsey, Drebin, Jaffe, Katzka, Kochman, Makar, Morris, Osterman, Rombeau, and Shah

Year Book of Hand and Upper Limb Surgery®: Drs Chang and Steinmann.

Year Book of Medicine®: Drs Barkin, Berney, Frishman, Garrick, Loehrer, Phillips, and Khardori

Year Book of Neonatal and Perinatal Medicine®: Drs Fanaroff, Ehrenkranz, and Stevenson

Year Book of Neurology and Neurosurgery®: Drs Kim and Verma

Year Book of Obstetrics, Gynecology, and Women's Health®: Drs Dungan and Shulman

Year Book of Oncology®: Drs Loehrer, Arceci, Glatstein, Gordon, Hanna, Morrow, and Thigpen

Year Book of Ophthalmology®: Drs Rapuano, Cohen, Eagle, Flanders, Hammersmith, Myers, Nelson, Penne, Sergott, Shields, Tipperman, and Vander

Year Book of Orthopedics®: Drs Morrey, Beauchamp, Huddleston, Peterson, Swiontkowski, and Trigg

Year Book of Otolaryngology-Head and Neck Surgery®: Drs Balough, Gapany, Keefe, and Sindwani

Year Book of Pathology and Laboratory Medicine®: Drs Raab, Parwani Bejarano, and Bissell

Year Book of Pediatrics®: Dr Stockman

Year Book of Plastic and Aesthetic Surgery™: Drs Miller, Bartlett, Garner, McKinney, Ruberg, Salisbury, and Smith

Year Book of Psychiatry and Applied Mental Health®: Drs Talbott, Ballenger, Buckley, Frances, Markowitz, and Sarles

Year Book of Pulmonary Disease®: Drs Phillips, Barker, Lewis, Maurer, Tanoue, and Willsie

Year Book of Sports Medicine®: Drs Shephard, Cantu, Feldman, Jankowski, McCrory, Nieman, Pierrynowski, Rowland, and Shrier

Year Book of Surgery®: Drs Copeland, Bland, Daly, Eberlein, Fahey, Jones, Mozingo, Pruett, and Seeger

Year Book of Urology®: Drs Andriole and Coplen

Year Book of Vascular Surgery®: Dr Moneta

2009
The Year Book of CRITICAL CARE MEDICINE®

Editors-in-Chief:
R. Phillip Dellinger, MD
Professor of Medicine, Robert Wood Johnson Medical School, University of Medicine and Dentistry of New Jersey; Head, Division of Critical Care Medicine; Director, Medical/Surgical Intensive Care Unit, Cooper University Hospital, Camden, New Jersey

Joseph E. Parrillo, MD
Professor of Medicine, Robert Wood Johnson Medical School, University of Medicine and Dentistry of New Jersey; Chief, Department of Medicine, Edward D. Viner MD Chair, Department of Medicine; Director, Cooper Heart Institute, Cooper University Hospital, Camden, New Jersey

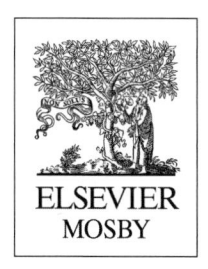

ELSEVIER
MOSBY

ELSEVIER
MOSBY

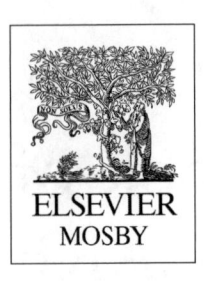

Vice President, Continuity: John A. Schrefer
Associate Developmental Editor: Yonah Korngold
Production Supervisor, Electronic Year Books: Donna M. Skelton
Electronic Article Manager: Jennifer C. Pitts
Illustrations and Permissions Coordinator: Dawn Vohsen

2009 EDITION
Copyright 2009, Mosby, Inc. All rights reserved.

No part of this publication may be reproduced, stored in a retrieval system, or transmitted, in any form or by any means, electronic, mechanical, photocopying, recording, or otherwise, without prior written permission from the publisher.

Permission to photocopy or reproduce solely for internal or personal use is permitted for libraries or other users registered with the Copyright Clearance Center, provided that the base fee of $35.00 per chapter is paid directly to the Copyright Clearance Center, 21 Congress Street, Salem, MA 01970. This consent does not extend to other kinds of copying, such as copying for general distribution, for advertising or promotional purposes, for creating new collected works, or for resale.

Printed in the United States of America
Composition by TNQ Books and Journals Pvt Ltd, India
Printing/binding by Sheridan Books, Inc.

Editorial Office:
Elsevier
Suite 1800
1600 John F. Kennedy Blvd.
Philadelphia, PA 19103-2899

International Standard Serial Number: 0734-3299
International Standard Book Number: 978-1-4160-5750-5

Associate Editors

Robert A. Balk, MD
J. Bailey Carter, MD, Professor of Medicine, Rush Medical College; Director, Division of Pulmonary and Critical Care Medicine, Rush University Medical Center, Chicago, Illinois

Carolyn Bekes, MD, MHA
Professor of Medicine, Robert Wood Johnson Medical School, University of Medicine and Dentistry of New Jersey; Senior Vice President for Academic and Medical Affairs, Cooper University Hospital, Camden, New Jersey

Todd Dorman, MD
Associate Dean and Director of Continuing Medical Education; Professor and Vice-Chair for Critical Care Services; Departments of Anesthesiology/Critical Care Medicine, Internal Medicine, Surgery, and the School of Nursing, The Johns Hopkins University, Baltimore, Maryland

David J. Dries, MSE, MD
John F. Perry, Jr. Professor, Department of Surgery, University of Minnesota; Assistant Medical Director for Surgical Care, HealthPartners Medical Group, Minneapolis, Minnesota; Director of Critical Care Services and Director of Academic Programs, Regions Hospital, St. Paul, Minnesota

Guest Editors

Guest Editor for Mechanical Ventilation
Ismail Cinel, MD, PhD
Adjunct Associate Professor of Medicine, Robert Wood Johnson Medical School, University of Medicine and Dentistry of New Jersey; Visiting Professor, Division of Critical Care Medicine, Cooper University Hospital, Camden, New Jersey

Guest Editor for Transfusion in the Critically Ill
David R. Gerber, DO
Associate Professor of Medicine, Robert Wood Johnson Medical School, University of Medicine and Dentistry of New Jersey; Associate Director, Medical/Surgical Intensive Care Unit, Cooper University Hospital, Camden, New Jersey

Guest Editor for Infection
Anand Kumar, MD
Associate Professor of Medicine, Robert Wood Johnson Medical College, University of Medicine and Dentistry of New Jersey, Camden, New Jersey; Division of Critical Care Medicine and Division of Infectious Diseases, Cooper University Hospital, Camden, New Jersey; Associate Professor of Medicine, Sections of Critical Care Medicine and Infectious Disease, University of Manitoba, Winnipeg, Canada

Guest Editor for Burns
Barbara A. Latenser, MD
Clara L. Smith Professor of Burn Treatment, Department of Surgery, University of Iowa; Director, Burn Treatment Center, University of Iowa Hospitals and Clinics, Iowa City, Iowa

Guest Editor for Postoperative Critical Care
Elizabeth A. Martinez, MD, MHS
Associate Professor of Anesthesia/Critical Care Medicine and Surgery; Medical Director, Adult Post Anesthesia Care Units, Johns Hopkins University School of Medicine, Johns Hopkins Medical Institutions, Baltimore, Maryland

Guest Editor for Neurologic Care
J. Javier Provencio, MD
Fellowship Director, Neurocritical Care Program; Associate Director for Research, Bakken Heart-Brain Institute, Cleveland Clinic Foundation, Cleveland, Ohio

Guest Editor for Critical Care Performance Improvement and ICU Administration
Christa A. Schorr, RN, BSN
Program Manager for Quality Improvement and Clinical Research Databases, Department of Medicine, Cooper University Hospital, Camden, New Jersey

Guest Editor for Emergency Medicine
Stephen Trzeciak, MD, MPH
Assistant Professor of Medicine and Emergency Medicine, Robert Wood Johnson Medical School, University of Medicine and Dentistry of New Jersey; Department of Emergency Medicine and Section of Critical Care Medicine, Cooper University Hospital, Camden, New Jersey

Guest Editor for Cardiology
Steven W. Werns, MD
Professor of Medicine, Robert Wood Johnson Medical School, University of Medicine and Dentistry of New Jersey; Director, Invasive Cardiovascular Services, Cooper University Hospital, Camden, New Jersey

Guest Editor for Sepsis
Sergio L. Zanotti-Cavazzoni, MD
Assistant Professor of Medicine, Robert Wood Johnson Medical School, University of Medicine and Dentistry of New Jersey; Associate Fellowship Director, Section of Critical Care Medicine, Cooper University Hospital, Camden, New Jersey

Contributing Editors

Amanda R. Burden, MD
Assistant Professor of Medicine, Robert Wood Johnson Medical School, University of Medicine and Dentistry of New Jersey; Co-Medical Director, Simulation Laboratory, Department of Anesthesiology, Cooper University Hospital, Camden, New Jersey

Christopher W. Deitch, MD
Assistant Professor of Medicine, Robert Wood Johnson Medical School, University of Medicine and Dentistry of New Jersey; Program Director, Gastroenterology Fellowship Program, Division of Gastroenterology, Cooper University Hospital, Camden, New Jersey

Ramya Lotano, MD
Assistant Professor of Medicine, Robert Wood Johnson Medical School, University of Medicine and Dentistry of New Jersey; Program Director, Pulmonary Critical Care Fellowship, Division of Pulmonary Critical Care, Cooper University Hospital, Camden, New Jersey

Antoinette Spevetz, MD
Associate Professor of Medicine, Robert Wood Johnson Medical School, University of Medicine and Dentistry of New Jersey; Director, Intermediate Intensive Care Unit; Associate Program Director, Internal Medicine Residency Program, Cooper University Hospital, Camden, New Jersey

Collaborative Reviewers

M. Kamran Athar, MD
Postdoctoral Fellow, Division of Critical Care Medicine, Cooper University Hospital, Camden, New Jersey

Stephen B. Heitner, MD
Postdoctoral Fellow, Division of Cardiology, Cooper University Hospital, Camden, New Jersey

Terence Lonergan, MD
Postdoctoral Fellow, Division of Critical Care Medicine, Cooper University Hospital, Camden, New Jersey

David J. Lundy, MD
Postdoctoral Shock Fellow, Department of Surgery, Cooper University Hospital, Camden, New Jersey

Rani Nanda, DO
Postdoctoral Fellow, Division of Critical Care Medicine, Cooper University Hospital, Camden, New Jersey

Nduka Okorie, MD
Postdoctoral Fellow, Division of Critical Care Medicine, Cooper University Hospital, Camden, New Jersey

Nitin Puri, MD
Postdoctoral Fellow, Division of Critical Care Medicine, Cooper University Hospital, Camden, New Jersey

Jean-Sebastien Rachoin, MD
Postdoctoral Fellow, Division of Nephrology, Cooper University Hospital, Camden, New Jersey

Brian Roberts, MD
Resident, Department of Emergency Medicine, Cooper University Hospital, Camden, New Jersey

Table of Contents

JOURNALS REPRESENTED	xvii
1. Airways/Lungs	1
Acute Lung Injury/Acute Respiratory Distress Syndrome	1
Mechanical Ventilation/Weaning	22
Airway	30
Other	34
2. Cardiovascular	41
Myocardial Infarction/Cardiogenic Shock/Cardiogenic Pulmonary Edema	41
Cardiac Arrest	55
Pulmonary Embolism/Pulmonary Artery Hypertension	62
Cardiopulmonary Resuscitation/Other	69
3. Hemodynamics and Monitoring	81
4. Burns	93
5. Infectious Disease	107
Nosocomial/Ventilator-Acquired Pneumonia	107
Miscellaneous	119
6. Postoperative Management	137
Cardiovascular Surgery	137
Other	150
7. Sepsis/Septic Shock	153
8. Metabolism/Gastrointestinal/Nutrition/Hematology-Oncology	167
9. Renal	181
10. Trauma and Overdose	189
11. Neurologic: Traumatic and Non-traumatic	211
12. Ethics/Socioeconomic/Administrative Issues	245
Quality of Life/End of Life/Outcome Prediction	245
Miscellaneous	267
13. Pharmacology/Sedation-Analgesia	279
SUBJECT INDEX	285
AUTHOR INDEX	295

Journals Represented

Journals represented in this YEAR BOOK are listed below.
Acta Anaesthesiologica Scandinavica
AJR American Journal of Roentgenology
AJNR American Journal Neuroradiology
American Journal of Cardiology
American Journal of Emergency Medicine
American Journal of Infection Control
American Journal of Medicine
American Journal of Respiratory and Critical Care Medicine
American Journal of Surgery
American Surgeon
Anaesthesia
Anaesthesia and Intensive Care
Anesthesia and Analgesia
Anesthesiology
Annals of Emergency Medicine
Annals of Internal Medicine
Annals of Otology, Rhinology & Laryngology
Annals of Surgery
Annals of Thoracic Surgery
Archives of Internal Medicine
Archives of Neurology
Archives of Surgery
British Journal of Anaesthesia
Burns
Canadian Medical Association Journal
Chest
Clinical Infectious Diseases
Clinical Radiology
Critical Care
Critical Care Medicine
Epilepsia
European Heart Journal
Heart
Hypertension
Injury
Intensive Care Medicine
Journal of Burn Care and Research
Journal of Cardiothoracic and Vascular Anesthesia
Journal of Clinical Microbiology
Journal of Neurosurgery
Journal of Surgical Research
Journal of the American Academy of Dermatology
Journal of the American College of Surgeons
Journal of the American College of Cardiology
Journal of the American Geriatrics Society
Journal of the American Medical Association
Journal of Thoracic and Cardiovascular Surgery

xviii / Journals Represented

Journal of Trauma
Lancet
Mayo Clinic Proceedings
Medical Care
Nephrology Dialysis Transplantation
Neurosurgery
New England Journal of Medicine
Pharmacotherapy
Psychologie Medicale
Stroke
Surgery
Surgical Neurology
Thrombosis and Haemostasis
World Journal of Surgery

Standard Abbreviations

The following terms are abbreviated in this edition: acquired immunodeficiency syndrome (AIDS), cardiopulmonary resuscitation (CPR), central nervous system (CNS), cerebrospinal fluid (CSF), computed tomography (CT), deoxyribonucleic acid (DNA), electrocardiography (ECG), health maintenance organization (HMO), human immunodeficiency virus (HIV), intensive care unit (ICU), intramuscular (IM), intravenous (IV), magnetic resonance (MR) imaging (MRI), and ribonucleic acid (RNA).

Note

The YEAR BOOK OF CRITICAL CARE MEDICINE® is a literature survey service providing abstracts of articles published in the professional literature. Every effort is made to assure the accuracy of the information presented in these pages. Neither the editors nor the publisher of the YEAR BOOK OF CRITICAL CARE MEDICINE® can be responsible for errors in the original materials. The editors' comments are their own opinions. Mention of specific products within this publication does not constitute endorsement.

To facilitate the use of the YEAR BOOK OF CRITICAL CARE MEDICINE® as a reference tool, all illustrations and tables included in this publication are now identified as they appear in the original article. This change is meant to help the reader recognize that any illustration or table appearing in the YEAR BOOK OF CRITICAL CARE MEDICINE® may be only one of many in the original article. For this reason, figure and table numbers will often appear to be out of sequence within the YEAR BOOK OF CRITICAL CARE MEDICINE®.

1 Airways/Lungs

Acute Lung Injury/Acute Respiratory Distress Syndrome

Cytokine Release Following Recruitment Maneuvers
Talmor D, Sarge T, Legedza A, et al (Beth Israel Deaconess Med Ctr, Boston, MA; et al)
Chest 132:1434-1439, 2007

Background.—There are reports of rigors and/or clinical deterioration following recruitment maneuvers (RMs), leading us to question whether the use of sustained high-pressure inflation could lead to/ release of inflammatory mediators.

Methods.—Prospective cohort study of 26 patients with ARDS receiving mechanical ventilation. A single RM was performed during which the mean airway pressure was increased to 40 cm H_2O and held constant for a period of 30 s. The concentration of nine cytokines (interleukin [IL]-1, IL-6, IL-8, IL-10, tumor necrosis factor [TNF]-α, Fas ligand, vascular endothelial growth factor, TNF receptor 1, TNF receptor 2) was measured longitudinally at three time points: prior to initiation of the RM, 5 min after the RM, and 60 min after the RM.

Results.—RMs were tolerated well from a hemodynamic perspective. Oxygenation improved as reflected by an increased PaO_2/fraction of inspired oxygen (FIO_2) ratio from 140 ± 49 at baseline to 190 ± 78 (mean ± SD) at 5 min after the RM ($p = 0.01$). At 60 min, the increase in PaO_2/FIO_2 ratio, to 172 ± 76, was no longer significant ($p = 0.1$). There were no important changes in the levels of any of the measured cytokines at 5 min or 60 min following RM as compared with the baseline levels.

Conclusions.—The results of our study demonstrate that recruitment maneuvers are well tolerated in patients with ARDS. Our data suggest no major hemodynamic or immunologic evidence of deterioration within the first hour of RM. In particular, cytokines, previously related to worsening lung injury and distal organ failure in patients with ARDS, are not elevated by use of an RM.

Registered at.—www.clinicaltrials.gov as NCT00127491.

▶ Recruitment maneuvers (RMs) (either sustained high inflation pressure with continuous positive airway pressure (CPAP) or intermittent large tidal volumes) clearly improve oxygenation. No clinical trials have shown differences in clinical outcome when RMs are used. RMs were dropped from the multifactorial design of the ALVEOLI trial when the improvement in oxygenation associated with RM was not sustained. This gets to the crux of the issue, which is that unless improvement in oxygenation with recruitment is followed by positive end-expiratory pressure (PEEP) setting to maintain the recruited lung open, there is no reason to anticipate benefit from recruitment. RMs are widely used, and most effectively used when associated with increase in PEEP after RM until a PEEP that maintains oxygenation benefit from recruitment can potentially be located. The 2 more important risks of recruitment are as follows: (1) hemodynamic changes and (2) barotrauma. The former is a rationale for closely monitoring blood pressure during RM with arterial line in place. The latter is a theoretical and almost certainly rare actual occurrence with recruitment.

In this article there were no major hemodynamic changes with recruitment. The authors also measured the possibility that recruitment might stimulate cytokine release as overinflation has been shown to do when sustained over significant periods of time. This is likely more of an academic issue as brief increases in cytokines (not seen in this case) would be unlikely to produce lasting significant systemic effects.

R. P. Dellinger, MD

Prone Positioning Unloads the Right Ventricle in Severe ARDS
Vieillard-Baron A, Charron C, Caille V, et al (Med Intensive Care Unit, Assistance Publique Hôpitaux de Paris, Boulogne Cedex, France)
Chest 132:1440-1446, 2007

Background.—Despite airway pressure limitation, acute cor pulmonale persists in a minority of ARDS patients. Insufficient airway pressure limitation, hypercapnia, or both may be responsible. Because prone positioning (PP) has been shown to be a safe way to reduce airway pressure and to improve alveolar ventilation, we decided to assess its effect on right ventricular (RV) pressure overload in ARDS patients.

Methods.—Between January 1998 and December 2006, we studied 42 ARDS patients treated by PP to correct severe oxygenation impairment (PaO_2/fraction of inspired oxygen ratio, <100 mm Hg). RV function was evaluated by bedside transesophageal echocardiography, before and after 18 h of prone-position ventilation. RV enlargement was measured by RV/left ventricular (LV) end-diastolic area ratio in the long axis. Septal dyskinesia was quantified by measuring short-axis systolic eccentricity of the LV.

Results.—Before PP, 21 patients (50%) had acute cor pulmonale, defined by RV enlargement associated with septal dyskinesia (group 1), whereas 21 patients had a normal RV (group 2). PP was accompanied by a significant decrease in airway pressure and $PaCO_2$. In group 1, this produced a significant decrease in mean (± SD) RV enlargement (from 0.91 ± 0.22 to 0.61 ± 0.21) after 18 h of PP (p = 0.000) and a significant reduction in mean septal dyskinesia (from 1.5 ± 0.2 to 1.1 ± 0.1) after 18 h of PP (p = 0.000).

Conclusion.—In the most severe forms of ARDS, PP was an efficient means of controlling RV pressure overload.

▶ Prone positioning, although not shown to improve survival in randomized clinical trials of acute respiratory distress syndrome (ARDS), is suggested to improve survival in patients with more severe ARDS. Unless there are contraindications or a high risk, my own personal policy is to prone patients who have been appropriately treated with the ARDSnet positive end-expiratory pressure (PEEP) setting protocol, and who remain on a fraction of inspired oxygen (FiO_2) of .8 or greater. It is generally accepted that oxygenation and compliance will improve in most patients with severe ARDS. The improvement in ventilation and perfusion matching would be expected to decrease pulmonary vascular resistance, which is known to be elevated in ARDS. This article demonstrates that the decrease in pulmonary vascular resistance is associated with improvement in right ventricular function. This is yet another benefit that could have clinical implications.

R. P. Dellinger, MD

Extrapulmonary Ventilation for Unresponsive Severe Acute Respiratory Distress Syndrome After Pulmonary Resection
Iglesias M, Martinez E, Badia JR, et al (Univ of Barcelona, Spain)
Ann Thorac Surg 85:237-244, 2008

Background.—The purpose of this study was to evaluate the feasibility of integrating an artificial, pumpless extracorporeal membrane ventilator (Novalung) to near static mechanical ventilation and its efficacy in patients with severe postresectional acute respiratory distress syndrome (ARDS) unresponsive to optimal conventional treatment.

Methods.—Indications were severe postresectional and unresponsive acute respiratory distress syndrome, hemodynamic stability, and no significant peripheral arterial occlusive disease or heparin-induced thrombocytopenia. Management included placement of the arteriovenous femoral transcutaneous interventional lung-assist membrane ventilator, lung rest at minimal mechanical ventilator settings, and optimization of systemic oxygen consumption and delivery.

Results.—Among 239 pulmonary resections performed between 2005 and 2006, 7 patients (2.9%) experienced, 4 ± 0.8 days after 5 pneumonectomies and 2 lobectomies, a severe (Murray score, 2.9 ± 0.3) acute respiratory distress syndrome unresponsive to 4 ± 2 days of conventional therapy. The interventional lung-assist membrane ventilator was left in place 4.3 ± 2.5 days, and replaced only once for massive clotting. During this time, 29% ± 0.3% or 1.4 ± 0.36 L/min of the cardiac output perfused the device, without hemodynamic impairment. Using a sweep gas flow

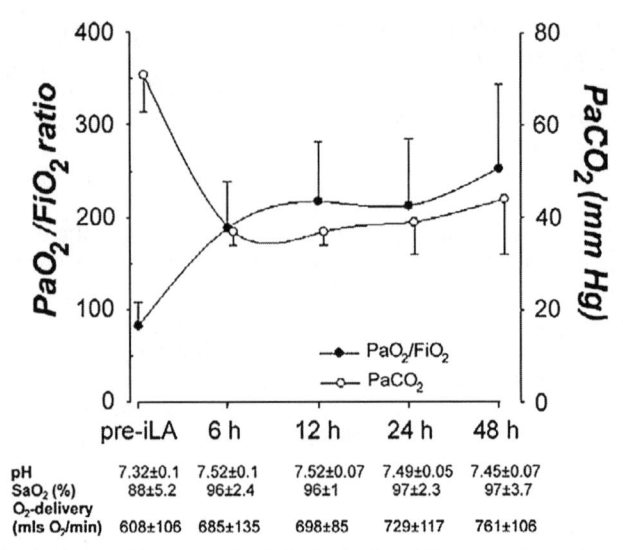

FIGURE 1.—Evolution of the oxygenation index (ratio of partial pressure of arterial oxygen [P_{AO_2}] to the fraction of inspired oxygen [F_{IO_2}]) and arterial carbon dioxide (P_{ACO_2}) as a function of time. Oxygen delivery (mL O_2/min) was calculated according to the following formula: cardiac output (L/min) × Hb (hemoglobin) concentration (g/L) × 1.31 (mL O2/g Hb) × % saturation (S_{AO_2}). (iLA = interventional assist device.) (Reprinted from Iglesias M, Martinez E, Badia JR, et al. Extrapulmonary ventilation for unresponsive severe acute respiratory distress syndrome after pulmonary resection. *Ann Thorac Surg.* 2008;85:237-244. Copyright 2008, with permission from The Society of Thoracic Surgeons.)

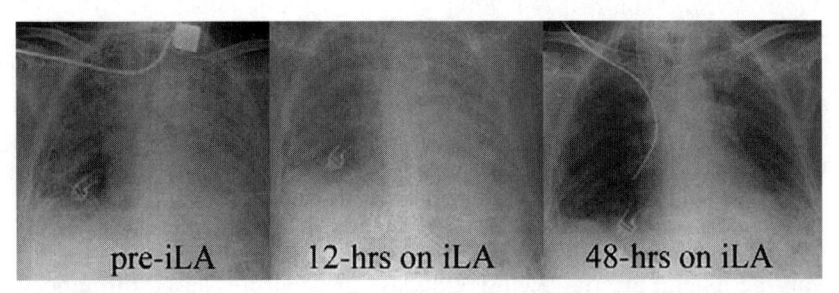

FIGURE 4.—Radiologic evolution as a function of time in a patient having had a lower lobe lobectomy and experiencing a severe unresponsive acute respiratory distress syndrome. The severity of the acute respiratory distress syndrome was calculated according to Murray and colleagues [8], as described for Figure 3. (iLA = interventional assist device.) (Reprinted from Iglesias M, Martinez E, Badia JR, et al. Extrapulmonary ventilation for unresponsive severe acute respiratory distress syndrome after pulmonary resection. *Ann Thorac Surg.* 2008;85:237-244. Copyright 2008, with permission from The Society of Thoracic Surgeons.)

of 10.7 ± 3.8 L/min, the device allowed an extracorporeal carbon dioxide removal of 255 ± 31 mL/min, lung(s) rest (tidal volume, 2.7 ± 0.8 mL/kg; respiratory rate, 6 ± 2 beats/min; fraction of inspired oxygen, 0.5 ± 0.1), early (<24 hours) significant improvement of respiratory function, and reduction of plasmatic interleukin-6 levels ($p < 0.001$) and Murray score (1.25 ± 0.1; $p < 0.003$). All but 1 patient (14%) who died of multiorgan failure were weaned from mechanical ventilation 8 ± 3 days after removal of the interventional lung-assist membrane ventilator, and all of them were discharged from the hospital.

Conclusions.—The integration of this device to near static mechanical ventilation of the residual native lung(s) is feasible and highly effective in patients with severe and unresponsive acute respiratory distress syndrome after pulmonary resection (Figs 1 and 4).

▶ Extracorporeal support for patients with acute lung injury (ALI) and acute respiratory distress syndrome (ARDS) is making a resurgence, particularly in those patients who do not tolerate or improve with lung protective ventilatory support strategies.[1] Although this is a small study of only 7 patients, it is remarkable that 6 of 7 survived. Clearly, more experience and a prospective, randomized controlled clinical trial are needed.

R. A. Balk, MD

Reference

1. Devereaux A, Christian MD, Dichter JR, et al. Summary of suggestions from the Task Force for Mass Critical Care Summit, January 26-27, 2007. *Chest*. 2008;133: 1S-7S.

Yield and safety of bedside open lung biopsy in mechanically ventilated patients with acute lung injury or acute respiratory distress syndrome
Baumann HJ, Kluge S, Balke L, et al (Univ Med Ctr Hamburg-Eppendorf, Hamburg, Germany, et al)
Surgery 143:426-433, 2008

Background.—The utility of open lung biopsy (OLB) in mechanically ventilated patients with acute lung injury (ALI) or acute respiratory distress syndrome (ARDS) of unknown origin has been questioned because of its potentially low diagnostic yield and possibly related morbidity. To quantify possible benefits and risks, and especially so for bedside lung biopsy, we reviewed retrospectively our 8-year, single unit experience with this procedure.

Methods.—Mechanically ventilated, critically ill patients with acute respiratory failure of unknown origin who underwent OLB were analyzed in a retrospective, single-center, cohort study in a medical intensive care unit in a university medical center.

Measurements and Main Results.—Twenty-seven patients were analyzed (15 female, 12 male, of mean 48 years [standard deviation, 14]), 67% of whom were immunocompromised. All patients underwent bronchoscopy and bronchoalveolar lavage before OLB. Pao$_2$/Fraction of inspired oxygen at the time of biopsy was 188 ± 109 mm Hg. Biopsies were performed in the operating room on 9 patients and at bedside on 18. A specific diagnosis was obtained in 70% of biopsies. Biopsy results led to alteration in treatment in 81% of patients. Minor complications occurred in 52% of patients and major complications in 7%. The rate of complications did not appear to differ with the location of the procedure (bedside vs operating room). No deaths were attributed to the procedure.

Conclusions.—Bedside OLB can be performed safely in selected, mechanically ventilated, critically ill patients with ALI or ARDS. Our results support the concept that lung biopsy often leads to management alterations in patients where a standardized diagnostic workup failed to yield a definitive diagnosis.

▶ The value of an open lung biopsy (OLB) in the management of patients with acute lung injury (ALI) and acute respiratory distress syndrome (ARDS) has been a topic of controversy. Typically, the decision to perform an OLB is made late in the course, when patients are often unstable, and the result is usually the histologic appearance of diffuse alveolar damage, which rarely discovers the underlying cause of the initial injury. This interesting article presents 2 unique findings. The first was a high rate of finding the specific diagnosis on the biopsy (70% of the time), and there was a change in specific therapy in 81% of the patients. The second unique observation was that the procedure was done at the patient's bedside in 67% of the patients and was felt to be reasonably safe, despite the high complication rate. These observations may prompt a renewed interest in obtaining an OLB in the management of patients with ALI and ARDS and may even cause some clinicians to explore the possibility of bedside biopsies.

R. A. Balk, MD

Positive End-Expiratory Pressure Setting in Adults With Acute Lung Injury and Acute Respiratory Distress Syndrome: A Randomized Controlled Trial
Mercat A, Richard J-CM, Vielle B, et al (Dépt de Réanimation Médicale et Médecine Hyperbare, France; Service de Réanimation Médicale et UPRES EA 38-30, CHU de Rouen; Service de Biostatistiques et Modélisation Informatique, CHU d'Angers; et al)
JAMA 299:646-655, 2008

Context.—The need for lung protection is universally accepted, but the optimal level of positive end-expiratory pressure (PEEP) in patients with acute lung injury (ALI) or acute respiratory distress syndrome remains debated.

Objective.—To compare the effect on outcome of a strategy for setting PEEP aimed at increasing alveolar recruitment while limiting hyperinflation to one aimed at minimizing alveolar distension in patients with ALI.

Design, Setting, and Patients.—A multicenter randomized controlled trial of 767 adults (mean [SD] age, 59.9 [15.4] years) with ALI conducted in 37 intensive care units in France from September 2002 to December 2005.

Intervention.—Tidal volume was set at 6 mL/kg of predicted body weight in both strategies. Patients were randomly assigned to a moderate PEEP strategy (5-9 cm H$_2$O) (minimal distension strategy; n = 382) or to a level of PEEP set to reach a plateau pressure of 28 to 30 cm H$_2$O (increased recruitment strategy; n = 385).

Main Outcome Measures.—The primary end point was mortality at 28 days. Secondary end points were hospital mortality at 60 days, ventilator-free days, and organ failure–free days at 28 days.

Results.—The 28-day mortality rate in the minimal distension group was 31.2% (n = 119) vs 27.8% (n = 107) in the increased recruitment group (relative risk, 1.12 [95% confidence interval, 0.90-1.40]; $P = .31$). The hospital mortality rate in the minimal distension group was 39.0% (n = 149) vs 35.4% (n = 136) in the increased recruitment group (relative risk, 1.10 [95% confidence interval, 0.92-1.32]; $P = .30$). The increased recruitment group compared with the minimal distension group had a higher median number of ventilator-free days (7 [interquartile range {IQR}, 0-19] vs 3 [IQR, 0-17]; $P = .04$) and organ failure–free days (6 [IQR, 0-18] vs 2 [IQR, 0-16]; $P = .04$). This strategy also was associated with higher compliance values, better oxygenation, less use of adjunctive therapies, and larger fluid requirements.

Conclusions.—A strategy for setting PEEP aimed at increasing alveolar recruitment while limiting hyperinflation did not significantly reduce mortality. However, it did improve lung function and reduced the duration of mechanical ventilation and the duration of organ failure.

Trial Registration.—clinicaltrials.gov Identifier: NCT00188058.

▶ The amount of positive end-expiratory pressure (PEEP) to use with lung-protective ventilatory support strategies for patients with acute lung injury (ALI) and acute respiratory distress syndrome (ARDS) has continued to be a source of some controversy. The controversy is fueled by those who believe that recruitment maneuvers have sustained benefit in patients with ALI and ARDS. This study, along with a study by Meade and colleagues in the same issue of JAMA, compared the use of higher levels of PEEP designed to enhance recruitment in comparison with the now established ARDS Network lung protective ventilatory support protocol.[1,2] The interesting findings in this study are demonstrated in Fig 2 in the original article. Although there was no significant difference in mortality in the overall study population, there was a trend toward improvement in the patients with ARDS who were managed with the increased recruitment (PEEP) strategy. On the other hand, the patients with ALI appeared to do better with less recruitment (PEEP). Another interesting observation was that despite no improvement in mortality, patients managed with the recruitment strategy had more rapid improvement in physiology and were able to get off the ventilator sooner. Typically, a shorter time of ventilatory support is associated with better outcomes (improved survival, less infections and other complications); however, we are not given an explanation for this lack of additional benefit. The results of these 2 trials will likely stimulate more controversy challenging the amount of PEEP to use in lung protective ventilatory support strategies and may cause additional studies to challenge the past results of the higher versus lower PEEP trial of the ARDS Network.[3]

R. A. Balk, MD

References

1. Meade MO, Cook DJ, Guyatt GH, et al. Ventilation strategy using low tidal volumes, recruitment maneuvers, and high positive end-expiratory pressure for acute lung injury and acute respiratory distress syndrome: a randomized controlled trial. *JAMA.* 2008;299:637-645.
2. Acute Respiratory Distress Syndrome Network. Ventilation with lower tidal volumes as compared with traditional tidal volumes for acute lung injury and the acute respiratory distress syndrome. *N Engl J Med.* 2000;342:1301-1308.
3. Brower RG, Lanken PN, MacIntyre N, et al. Higher versus lower positive end-expiratory pressures in patients with acute respiratory distress syndrome. *N Engl J Med.* 2004;351:327-336.

Biomarker evidence of myocardial cell injury is associated with mortality in acute respiratory distress syndrome

Bajwa EK, Boyce PD, Januzzi JL, et al (Harvard Med School, Boston, MA; et al)
Crit Care Med 35:2484-2490, 2007

Objective.—Although a number of studies have reported elevated levels of markers of myocardial necrosis among critically ill patients, the association between these markers and outcome remains poorly studied in patients with lung injury. We investigated the association of elevated troponin and creatine phosphokinase isoenzyme levels with mortality and organ failure in subjects with acute respiratory distress syndrome.

Design.—Retrospective study.

Setting.—Tertiary academic medical center.

Patients.—A total of 305 subjects with acute respiratory distress syndrome enrolled in a prospective intensive care unit cohort.

Intervention.—None.

Measurements and Main Results.—Cardiac biomarker data were available on 248 of 305 patients with acute respiratory distress syndrome (81%), of which 89 patients had at least one elevated cardiac marker level (35%). The presence of an elevated cardiac marker was associated with significantly higher mortality ($p = .01$) and was an independent predictor of mortality ($p = .02$) among patients with lower severity of illness (Acute Physiology and Chronic Health Evaluation III, <79). Patients with at least one elevated cardiac marker also had significantly more organ system derangement, including noncardiovascular organ system failures ($p = .02$).

Conclusions.—Patients with acute respiratory distress syndrome have a high prevalence of elevated cardiac markers. The presence of elevated cardiac markers is independently associated with increased 60-day mortality and increased organ failure. This association is most pronounced among patients with lower severity of illness. These results indicate that occult myocardial injury may be an important factor in acute respiratory distress syndrome morbidity and mortality. Further study of the relevant causal relationships and mechanisms is warranted.

▶ Elevated cardiac biomarkers may signify evidence of cardiac injury or simply represent a marker of significant injury that correlates with increased mortality rates and organ system dysfunction. This observation is not surprising considering the severity of the clinical impact of acute lung injury (ALI) and acute respiratory distress syndrome (ARDS). For now, I would regard this as an interesting observation and further trials are needed to determine if these markers will identify a group of ARDS patients with high risk for mortality and/or development of organ system failure. It would also be interesting to see if these cardiac biomarkers will be able to predict outcome by their response to therapy when evaluated over time.

R. A. Balk, MD

Feasibility of very high-frequency ventilation in adults with acute respiratory distress syndrome
Fessler HE, Hager DN, Brower RG (Johns Hopkins School of Medicine, Baltimore, MD)
Crit Care Med 36:1043-1048, 2008

Objective.—To assess the feasibility of using respiratory frequencies up to 15 Hz during high-frequency oscillatory ventilation (HFO) of adults with acute respiratory distress syndrome (ARDS).
Design.—Observational study.
Setting.—Medical intensive care unit at a tertiary care university hospital.
Patients.—Thirty adult patients receiving HFO at the discretion of their physicians for management of severe ARDS.
Interventions.—Clinical management algorithm for HFO that minimized delivered tidal volumes by encouraging the use of the highest frequency that allowed acceptable clearance of carbon dioxide. This contrasts with the typical use of HFO in adults, in which frequencies generally do not exceed 6 Hz.
Measurements and Main Results.—Patients were 42 ± 15 yrs old, weighed 83 ± 25 kg, and had failed conventional lung-protective ventilation due to refractory hypoxia or respiratory acidosis and high plateau airway pressures. During HFO, 25 of 30 patients maintained acceptable gas exchange at frequencies >6 Hz; 12 reached maximal frequencies of ≥10 Hz. Among patients whose maximal frequencies exceeded 6 Hz, mean maximal frequency was 9.9 ± 2.1 Hz, at a mean oscillation pressure amplitude of 81 ± 11 cm H_2O. At those settings, blood gases were pH 7.31 ± 0.06, $Paco_2$ was 58 ± 21 mm Hg, and Pao_2 was 82 ± 33 mm Hg. Survival to hospital discharge among this severely ill cohort was 37%.

Conclusions.—Most adults can maintain adequate gas exchange using HFO frequencies well above 5–6 Hz. Use of higher frequencies should minimize tidal volume and we speculate might thereby reduce ventilator-associated lung injury.

▶ In my opinion, the acute respiratory distress syndrome (ARDS) Network has established that patients with acute lung injury (ALI) and ARDS should be managed with lung-protective ventilatory support strategies to improve survival.[1] There are times when the lung-supportive ventilatory support strategy does not succeed with either oxygenation goals or the permissive hypercapnia and results in a pH that is so low, clinicians become uncomfortable in continuing with this form of ventilatory support. In this instance, we turn to alternative forms of ventilatory support. One of the alternative or salvage therapies is high-frequency oscillation. This form of ventilatory support has been beneficial for newborns with the infant respiratory distress syndrome and there are several reports detailing its use in adults with ALI and ARDS.[2,3] This report presents a small prospective evaluation of higher oscillatory frequencies in adults failing conventional lung-protective ventilatory support. The higher frequencies were chosen to minimize ventilator-induced lung injury. Although the overall mortality rate is high (63%), it should be remembered that this study population had failed conventional lung-protective ventilatory support and would be expected to have an extremely high mortality rate. Clearly, more studies are needed, but this technique may be used as a rescue therapy for selected patients with severe ALI and ARDS who are not improving with lung-protective ventilatory support.

R. A. Balk, MD

References

1. Acute Respiratory Distress Syndrome Network. Ventilation with lower tidal volumes as compared with traditional volumes for acute lung injury and the acute respiratory distress syndrome. *N Engl J Med.* 2000;342:1301-1308.
2. Derdak S, Mehta S, Stewart TE, et al. High frequency oscillatory ventilation for acute respiratory distress syndrome in adults: a randomized, controlled trial. *Am J Respir Crit Care Med.* 2002;166:801-808.
3. Mehta S, Granton J, MacDonald RJ, et al. High frequency oscillatory ventilation in adults: the Toronto experience. *Chest.* 2004;126:518-527.

Angiotensin-converting enzyme insertion/deletion polymorphism is not associated with susceptibility and outcome in sepsis and acute respiratory distress syndrome
Villar J, Flores C, Pérez-Méndez L, et al (St. Michael's Hosp, Ontario, Canada; Hosp Universitario NS de Candelaria, Spain; et al)
Intensive Care Med 34:488-495, 2008

Objective.—The insertion/deletion (I/D) of a 289 base pair *Alu* repeat sequence polymorphism in the angiotensin-converting enzyme gene (*ACE*) has been shown to predict susceptibility and outcome in the acute respiratory distress syndrome (ARDS). We hypothesized that the I/D polymorphism also confers susceptibility to sepsis and is a predisposing factor for morbidity and mortality of patients with severe sepsis.

Design and Setting.—Case-control study including 212 consecutive patients fulfilling criteria for severe sepsis admitted to a Spanish network of postsurgical and critical care units, and 364 population-based controls. Susceptibility to severe sepsis was evaluated as primary outcome; mortality in severe sepsis, susceptibility to sepsis-induced ARDS, and mortality in sepsis-induced ARDS were examined as secondary outcomes. An additive model of inheritance in which patients were classified into three genotype groups (II, ID, and DD) was used for association testing.

Measurements and Results.—Genotype and allele frequencies of I/D were distributed similarly in all septic, ARDS, and non-ARDS patients and in population-based controls. *ACE* I/D polymorphism was not associated with severe sepsis susceptibility or mortality. The *ACE* I/D polymorphism was associated neither with sepsis-induced ARDS susceptibility ($p = 0.895$) or mortality ($p = 0.950$). These results remained nonsignificant when adjusted for other covariates using multiple logistic regression analysis or Kaplan–Meier estimates of 28-day survival.

Conclusions.—Our data do not support an association of the *ACE* gene I/D polymorphism with susceptibility or mortality in severe sepsis or with sepsis-induced ARDS in Spanish patients.

▶ This article represents another study attempting to substantiate a role for angiotensin-converting enzyme (*ACE*) genetic polymorphisms in the development of the acute respiratory distress syndrome (ARDS). Past reports have suggested that these polymorphisms of the *ACE* gene on intron 16 are associated with the development and influence the outcome of patients with ARDS.[1,2] Unfortunately, these investigators were not able to find a correlation with *ACE* polymorphism and severe sepsis or the development of ARDS. This report adds to a growing list of studies that fail to substantiate a relationship between the *ACE* gene polymorphisms and the development of ARDS, pneumonia, or severe sepsis.

R. A. Balk, MD

References

1. Marshall RP, Webb S, Bellingan CJ, et al. Angiotensin converting enzyme insertion/deletion polymorphism is associated with susceptibility and outcome in acute respiratory distress syndrome. *Am J Respir Crit Care Med.* 2002;166: 646-650.
2. Jerng JS, Yu CJ, Wang HC, et al. Angiotensin-converting enzyme gene affects the outcome of acute respiratory distress syndrome. *Crit Care Med.* 2006;34: 1001-1006.

Mortality Rates for Patients With Acute Lung Injury/ARDS Have Decreased Over Time
Zambon M, Vincent J-L (Université Libre de Bruxelles, Belgium)
Chest 133:1120-1127, 2008

Background.—Over the last decade, several studies have suggested that survival rates for patients with acute lung injury (ALI) or ARDS may have improved. We performed a systematic analysis of the ALI/ARDS literature to document possible trends in mortality between 1994 and 2006.

Methods.—We used the Medline database to select studies with the key words "acute lung injury," "ARDS," "acute respiratory failure," and "mechanical ventilation." All studies that reported mortality rates for patients with ALI/ARDS defined according to the criteria of the American European Consensus Conference were selected. We excluded studies with < 30 patients and studies limited to specific subgroups of ARDS patients such as sepsis, trauma, burns, or transfusion-related ARDS.

Results.—Seventy-two studies were included in the analysis. There was a wide variation in mortality rates among the studies (15 to 72%). The overall pooled mortality rate for all studies was 43% (95% confidence interval, 40 to 46%). Metaregression analysis suggested a significant decrease in overall mortality rates of approximately 1.1%/yr over the period analyzed (1994 to 2006). The mortality reduction was also observed for hospital but not for ICU or 28-day mortality rates.

Conclusions.—In this literature review, the data are consistent with a reduction in mortality rates in general populations of patients with ALI/ARDS over the last 10 years.

▶ This study evaluated the mortality rate from 72 published reports encompassing 11 426 patients with acute lung injury (ALI) and acute respiratory distress syndrome (ARDS) to see the change in mortality rate over the 12 years. They did observe a 1.1% decrease in mortality over the 12 years of study and found an overall mortality rate over this period of 43%. Although this sounds impressive and is certainly better than an increase in mortality rate over this period of time, we must understand some of the limitations in this report. Many changes in management approach have occurred over this period of time. Some of these changes include the use of lung-protective ventilatory support strategies, a change to more conservative fluid management, the waxing and waning of the use of corticosteroids, and a more standardized approach to positive end-expiratory pressure (PEEP). In addition, sepsis and septic shock are the most common causes of ALI and ARDS and there have been significant changes in management over this period of time. These changes include new therapeutic agents such as activated protein C and the use of early goal-directed therapy and glycemic control protocols, and the introduction of new antibiotics and antimicrobial agents. Unfortunately, because of slow adoption of some treatment strategies and the delay in publication after the completion of a clinical trial, we cannot tell by the time plot whether the improvement in survival is reflective of any or all of the potential improvements in management that have occurred over this 12-year period. We can assume there is some modification of the impact of these various improvements on care because the mortality rate associated with the use of lung-protective ventilator support strategy by the ARDS network was only 31%.[1] I would encourage continued efforts to track mortality as there is a greater uptake on the use of these beneficial management approaches, so that we may see continued improvement in survival.

R. A. Balk, MD

Reference

1. Acute Respiratory Distress Syndrome Network. Ventilation with lower tidal volumes as compared with traditional volumes for acute lung injury and the Acute Respiratory Distress Syndrome. *N Engl J Med.* 2000;342:1301-1308.

Randomized Clinical Trial of Activated Protein C for the Treatment of Acute Lung Injury
Liu KD, Levitt J, Zhuo H, et al (Univ of California, San Francisco, CA; Stanford Univ, CA; Cardiovascular Res Inst, San Francisco, CA; et al)
Am J Respir Crit Care Med 178:618-623, 2008

Rationale.—Microvascular injury, inflammation, and coagulation play critical roles in the pathogenesis of acute lung injury (ALI). Plasma protein C levels are decreased in patients with acute lung injury and are associated with higher mortality and fewer ventilator-free days.

Objectives.—To test the efficacy of activated protein C (APC) as a therapy for patients with ALI.

Methods.—Eligible subjects were critically ill patients who met the American/European consensus criteria for ALI. Patients with severe sepsis and an APACHE II score of 25 or more were excluded. Participants were randomized to receive APC (24 μg/kg/h for 96 h) or placebo in a double-blind fashion within 72 hours of the onset of ALI. The primary endpoint was ventilator-free days.

Measurements and Main Results.—APC increased plasma protein C levels ($P = 0.002$) and decreased pulmonary dead space fraction ($P = 0.02$). However, there was no statistically significant difference between patients receiving placebo (n = 38) or APC (n = 37) in the number of ventilator-free days (median [25–75% interquartile range]: 19 [0–24] vs. 19 [14–22], respectively; $P = 0.78$) or in 60-day mortality (5/38 vs. 5/37 patients, respectively; $P = 1.0$). There were no differences in the number of bleeding events between the two groups.

Conclusions.—APC did not improve outcomes from ALI. The results of this trial do not support a large clinical trial of APC for ALI in the absence of severe sepsis and high disease severity.

TABLE 2.—Clinical Outcomes by Group

	Placebo ($n = 38$)	APC ($n = 37$)	P Value
Ventilator-free days, median (IQR)	19 (0–24)	19 (14–22)	0.78
Death by Day 60, n (%)	5 (13.5)	5 (13.5)	1.00
Ventilator-free days among survivors, median (IQR)	21 (5–25)	20 (16–23)	0.36
Organ failure–free days, median (IQR)	23 (14–27)	23 (16–27)	0.46
Cardiovascular failure, median (IQR)	25 (20–28)	26 (23–28)	0.30
Coagulation failure, median (IQR)	28 (28–28)	28 (28–28)	0.57
Renal failure, median (IQR)	28 (18.5–28)	28 (28–28)	0.41
Hepatic failure, median (IQR)	28 (27–28)	28 (28–28)	0.36

Definition of abbreviations: APC = activated protein C; IQR = interquartile range.
(Reprinted from Liu KD, Levitt J, Zhuo H, et al. Randomized clinical trial of activated protein C for the treatment of acute lung injury. *Am J Respir Crit Care Med.* 2008;178:618-623. Official Journal of the American Thoracic Society. Copyright of the American Thoracic Society.)

Clinical trial registered with www.clinicaltrials.gov (NCT 00112164) (Table 2).

▶ The use of activated protein C (APC) in severe sepsis and septic shock is currently involved in a prospective, multicenter, double-blind, placebo-controlled clinical trial to confirm its survival benefit for patients with severe disease as judged by multiorgan failure or high severity of illness. This trial evaluated the use of APC in acute lung injury, another clinical state that includes an inflammatory response and activation of the coagulation system. A key point of this trial was the exclusion of patients with sepsis and an Acute Physiology and Chronic Health Evaluation II (APACHE II) score ≥25, because these patients meet the package insert indications for the use of APC. As in the Recombinant Human Activated Protein C Worldwide Evaluation in Severe Sepsis (PROWESS) trial, the study was stopped early; however, this time it was for futility. The lack of efficacy in a low severity of illness population (as judged by the low mortality rate in both groups) is not a surprise. It is likely that we will need to see the results of the confirmatory APC trial before there is enthusiasm to evaluate the compound in other critical illnesses. On the positive front, the lack of a significant difference in adverse events or bleeding adds more support for the safety of APC when used in the proper population.

R. A. Balk, MD

Extracorporeal membrane oxygenation support improves survival of patients with severe Hantavirus cardiopulmonary syndrome
Dietl CA, Wernly JA, Pett SB, et al (Univ of New Mexico Health Sciences Ctr, Albuquerque, NM)
J Thorac Cardiovasc Surg 135:579-584, 2008

Objective.—The purposes of this study are to evaluate the outcome of extracorporeal membrane oxygenation support in a subgroup of patients with Hantavirus cardiopulmonary syndrome who had a predicted mortality of 100% and to assess the complications associated with this treatment modality and with different cannulation techniques.

Methods.—Thirty-eight patients with severe Hantavirus cardiopulmonary syndrome were supported with extracorporeal membrane oxygenation between April 1994 and June 2006. Cannulation of the femoral vessels was performed on an emergency basis by a percutaneous approach in 15 (39.5%) and by an open technique in 23 (60.5%) patients. Duration of extracorporeal membrane oxygenation averaged 132 hours (range: 5–276 hours).

Results.—Complications from percutaneous cannulation occurred in 4 (26.6%) of 15 patients: retroperitoneal hematoma in 2 (13.3%) and lower extremity ischemia in 2 (13.3%) patients, which resolved after insertion of a distal perfusion cannula. Complications from open femoral cannulation occurred in 8 (34.8%) of 23 patients: severe bleeding in 7 (30.4%) patients and lower extremity ischemia in 1 (4.3%) patient who required a leg amputation. The overall survival was 60.5% (23/38 patients). Six (40%) of the 15 patients cannulated percutaneously and 9 (39.1%) of 23 patients who had open cannulation died. All survivors recovered completely and were discharged from the hospital after a mean hospital stay of 20.8 days (range: 10–39 days).

Conclusions.—Almost two thirds of the patients with severe Hantavirus cardiopulmonary syndrome who were supported with extracorporeal circulation survived and recovered completely. The complications associated with both types of femoral cannulation may be attributed to the fact that all patients were in shock or in full cardiac arrest, and the procedure had to be done expeditiously. Earlier institution of extracorporeal membrane oxygenation may decrease the complication rates and improve the overall survival.

▶ Although the use of historical controls is not definitive evidence of cause and effect, it is possible that extracorporeal membrane oxygenation (ECMO) does produce better outcomes in severe *Hantavirus* cardiopulmonary syndrome (CPS). Institutions that become regional referral centers for management of severe CPS would be anticipated to improve their care over time. This might be a confounder in studies of ECMO support based on historical controls. Because this population of patients tend to be young (previously normal cardiac and pulmonary function), this is also another reason to be more aggressive and consider ECMO.

R. P. Dellinger, MD

Prone Positioning and Acute Respiratory Distress Syndrome After Cardiac Surgery: A Feasibility Study

Maillet J-M, Thierry S, Brodaty D, et al (Centre Cardiologique du Nord, Saint-Denis Cedex, France)
J Cardiothorac Vasc Anesth 22:414-417, 2008

Objective.—To determine the feasibility, safety, and efficacy on PaO_2/F_IO_2 ratio of prone positioning (PP) for acute respiratory distress syndrome (ARDS) after cardiac surgery.

Design.—Retrospective review of information entered prospectively in the authors' database.

Setting.—A private community nonteaching hospital.

Participants.—Sixteen patients who developed ARDS after cardiac surgery from January 2004 through June 2005.

Interventions.—PP to improve oxygenation.

Measurements and Main Results.—After a median duration of 18 (range, 14-27) hours in PP, PaO_2/F_IO_2 improved in 14 (87.5%) patients. For the entire population, median PaO_2/F_IO_2 rose from 87 (range, 56-161) before PP to 194 (range, 94-460; $p < 0.05$) after it. After supine repositioning (SR), PaO_2/F_IO_2 declined to 146 (range, 72-320; not significant). PaO_2/F_IO_2 at the end of PP and 1 day after SR were comparable, respectively, 194 (range, 94-460) and 184 (range, 105-342). No severe complication was associated with PP, but 5 patients developed pressure sores and 2 others had superficial sternal wound infections. Intensive care unit mortality of 37.5% reflected the number of organ failure(s); there were no deaths with 2 failures, and 60% with ≥ 3 organ failures died ($p = 0.03$). Mortality rates were comparable regardless of whether patients were PaO_2/F_IO_2 responders or their $PaCO_2$ decreased by ≥ 1 mmHg.

Conclusion.—PP to treat ARDS after cardiac surgery is feasible, safe, and can efficiently improve oxygenation. Measures to prevent pressure sores are mandatory.

▶ Severe acute respiratory distress syndrome (ARDS) is occasionally seen following cardiopulmonary bypass. Previously, there was little data on response of these patients to prone positioning, likely because of the concern with the sternal wound. This study nicely demonstrates that proning these patients produces not only the expected improvement in oxygenation and decrease in $PaCO_2$ but also, in addition, minimal problems with the sternal wound site. The same is likely true for patients who develop severe ARDS in the early post-laparotomy period. I recently had a patient with the severest of ARDS who had had emergent surgery for intra-abdominal abscess. This patient was proned within 12 hours of the surgical procedure with a very good response to proning, eventual survival, and no problems with the laparotomy wound site. Certainly more data are needed to ascertain the precise percentage of patients who will develop significant wound problems and how it might be predicted or avoided.

R. P. Dellinger, MD

Ventilation Strategy Using Low Tidal Volumes, Recruitment Maneuvers, and High Positive End-Expiratory Pressure for Acute Lung Injury and Acute Respiratory Distress Syndrome: A Randomized Controlled Trial

Meade MO, Cook DJ, Guyatt GH, et al (McMaster Univ, Hamilton, Ontario, Canada; et al)
JAMA 299:637-645, 2008

Context.—Low-tidal-volume ventilation reduces mortality in critically ill patients with acute lung injury and acute respiratory distress syndrome. Instituting additional strategies to open collapsed lung tissue may further reduce mortality.

Objective.—To compare an established low-tidal-volume ventilation strategy with an experimental strategy based on the original "open-lung approach," combining low tidal volume, lung recruitment maneuvers, and high positive end-expiratory pressure.

Design and Setting.—Randomized controlled trial with concealed allocation and blinded data analysis conducted between August 2000 and March 2006 in 30 intensive care units in Canada, Australia, and Saudi Arabia.

Patients.—Nine hundred eighty-three consecutive patients with acute lung injury and a ratio of arterial oxygen tension to inspired oxygen fraction not exceeding 250.

Interventions.—The control strategy included target tidal volumes of 6 mL/kg of predicted body weight, plateau airway pressures not exceeding 30 cm H_2O, and conventional levels of positive end-expiratory pressure (n = 508). The experimental strategy included target tidal volumes of 6 mL/kg of predicted body weight, plateau pressures not exceeding 40 cm H_2O, recruitment maneuvers, and higher positive end-expiratory pressures (n = 475).

Main Outcome Measure.—All-cause hospital mortality.

Results.—Eighty-five percent of the 983 study patients met criteria for acute respiratory distress syndrome at enrollment. Tidal volumes remained similar in the 2 groups, and mean positive end-expiratory pressures were 14.6 (SD, 3.4) cm H_2O in the experimental group vs 9.8 (SD, 2.7) cm H_2O among controls during the first 72 hours ($P < .001$). All-cause hospital mortality rates were 36.4% and 40.4%, respectively (relative risk [RR], 0.90; 95% confidence interval [CI], 0.77-1.05; $P = .19$). Barotrauma rates were 11.2% and 9.1% (RR, 1.21; 95% CI, 0.83-1.75; $P = .33$). The experimental group had lower rates of refractory hypoxemia (4.6% vs 10.2%; RR, 0.54; 95% CI, 0.34-0.86; $P = .01$), death with refractory hypoxemia (4.2% vs 8.9%; RR, 0.56; 95%CI, 0.34-0.93; $P = .03$), and previously defined eligible use of rescue therapies (5.1% vs 9.3%; RR, 0.61; 95% CI, 0.38-0.99; $P = .045$).

Conclusions.—For patients with acute lung injury and acute respiratory distress syndrome, a multifaceted protocolized ventilation strategy designed to recruit and open the lung resulted in no significant difference in all-cause hospital mortality or barotrauma compared with an established low-tidal-volume protocolized ventilation strategy. This "open-lung" strategy did appear to improve secondary end points related to hypoxemia and use of rescue therapies.

Trial Registration.—clinicaltrials.gov Identifier: NCT00182195.

▶ This study uses a somewhat different approach to try to answer the question of whether use of high positive end-expiratory pressure (PEEP) in acute lung injury improve outcome. The previous Assessment of Low tidal Volume and increased End-expiratory volume to Obviate Lung Injury (ALVEOLI) trial failed to show a benefit of higher PEEP strategy when compared with traditional ARDSnet PEEP table strategy. My interpretation of these trials is that in summation they confirm that general use of high PEEP strategies, independent of some measure of judging beneficial effect in an individual patient, is doomed to failure. This is because overinflation with higher PEEP without opening up more lung will produce a net negative effect. Therefore, the general use of a higher PEEP strategy means some patients benefit and some patients' status worsens. The study that begs to be done is to randomize patients to traditional PEEP therapy or recruitment plus PEEP therapy titrated up only as long as there is improvement in compliance.

R. P. Dellinger, MD

The relationship between arterial Po_2 and mixed venous Po_2 in response to changes in positive end-expiratory pressure in ventilated patients
Groeneveld ABJ, Schneider AJ (VU Univ Med Ctr, 1081 HV Amsterdam, The Netherlands)
Anaesthesia 63:488-494, 2008

The response of arterial Po_2 (P_aO_2) to airway pressure has been used as a measure of recruitment in mechanically ventilated patients. We hypothesised that mixed venous Po_2 ($P_{mv}O_2$) directly affects P_aO_2. Sixteen patients with acute lung injury (ALI, lung injury score ≥ 1) on volume-controlled mechanical ventilation (F_IO_2 0.40) were studied. Positive end-expiratory pressure (PEEP) was increased and decreased. Incremental PEEP increased median values of P_aO_2, diminished venous admixture (Q_{va}/Q_t) and cardiac index, but maintained arterial Pco_2 and tissue O_2 uptake. These changes were reversed during decremental PEEP. However P_aO_2 did not increase in 37% of PEEP steps and changes in P_aO_2 correlated to those in $P_{mv}O_2$ ($r_s = 0.45$, $p < 0.001$). Changes in $P_{mv}O_2$ contributed to changes in Q_{va}/Q_t in determining changes in P_aO_2 ($p < 0.05$). $P_{mv}O_2$ may be an independent determinant of P_aO_2 during mechanical ventilation for ALI, so that dosing PEEP to recruit the lung should not be guided by arterial blood oxygenation alone. Arterial hypoxaemia with increasing PEEP may improve by reducing PEEP (or increasing tissue O_2 delivery), when the fall in $P_{mv}O_2$ is greater than about 0.133 kPa.

▶ Ascertaining "beneficial effect" of positive end-expiratory pressure (PEEP) in mechanically ventilated patients with acute lung injury (ALI) is clearly more complicated than improvement in oxygenation. There are many variables interacting when PEEP is applied. These include the following: (1) PEEP-induced increase in lung open for oxygen exchange, (2) any PEEP effect on cardiac output (decreased), and (3) any effect of decreased cardiac output on mixed venous O_2 (a decrease). A decrease in cardiac output is associated with increase in P_aO_2 in patients with ALI. It is therefore possible that a PEEP-induced decrease in cardiac output would improve P_aO_2 without opening more lung. A decrease in cardiac output would also be expected to decrease mixed venous O_2, and therefore could mask a PEEP-induced lung opening benefit. Interaction of these variables would argue for not using mixed venous O_2 to measure a net effect of opening of previously closed lung, outweighing overdistension as PEEP is titrated. Compliance measurement is perhaps ideal.

R. P. Dellinger, MD

Risk Factors for ARDS in Patients Receiving Mechanical Ventilation for > 48 h

Jia X, Malhotra A, Saeed M, et al (Massachusetts Inst of Technology, Cambridge, MA)
Chest 133:853-861, 2008

Background.—Low tidal volume (VT) ventilation for ARDS is a well-accepted concept. However, controversy persists regarding the optimal ventilator settings for patients without ARDS receiving mechanical ventilation. This study tested the hypothesis that ventilator settings influence the development of new ARDS.

Methods.—Retrospective analysis of patients from the Multi Parameter Intelligent Monitoring of Intensive Care-II project database who received mechanical ventilation for ≥ 48 h between 2001 and 2005.

Results.—A total of 2,583 patients required > 48 h of ventilation. Of 789 patients who did not have ARDS at hospital admission, ARDS developed in 152 patients (19%). Univariate analysis revealed high peak inspiratory pressure (odds ratio [OR], 1.53 per SD; 95% confidence interval [CI], 1.28 to 1.84), increasing positive end-expiratory pressure (OR, 1.35 per SD; 95% CI, 1.15 to 1.58), and VT (OR, 1.36 per SD; 95% CI, 1.12 to 1.64) to be significant risk factors. Major nonventilator risk factors for ARDS included sepsis, low pH, elevated lactate, low albumin, transfusion of packed RBCs, transfusion of plasma, high net fluid balance, and low respiratory compliance. Multivariable logistic regression showed that peak pressure (OR, 1.31 per SD; 95% CI, 1.08 to 1.59), high net fluid balance (OR, 1.3 per SD; 95% CI, 1.09 to 1.56), transfusion of plasma (OR, 1.26 per SD; 95% CI, 1.07 to 1.49), sepsis (OR, 1.57; 95% CI, 1.00 to 2.45), and VT (OR, 1.29 per SD; 95% CI, 1.02 to 1.52) were significantly associated with the development of ARDS.

Conclusions.—The associations between the development of ARDS and clinical interventions, including high airway pressures, high VT, positive fluid balance, and transfusion of blood products, suggests that ARDS may be a preventable complication in some cases.

▶ This retrospective trial has provided some provocative data suggesting that the use of large tidal volumes may predispose mechanically ventilated patients to develop acute respiratory distress syndrome (ARDS). The use of lung-protective ventilatory support strategies has been well accepted as the standard of care for the management of patients with known acute lung injury or ARDS, but there is little data at this time to suggest that using high tidal volumes with or without the use of appropriate amounts of positive end-expiratory pressure (PEEP) may predispose a patient to the development of ARDS. This trial, and in particular this finding, are only generating an interesting hypothesis. It will be important to systematically approach this question with a well-designed, multicenter, prospective, and controlled clinical trial to adequately provide an answer. Until such a trial provides an answer, we should be cautious using excessively large tidal volumes, but the evidence for the tidal volume leading to lung injury (ARDS) in humans is still lacking.

R. A. Balk, MD

Barriers to low tidal volume ventilation in acute respiratory distress syndrome: Survey development, validation, and results
Dennison CR, Mendez-Tellez PA, Wang W, et al (Johns Hopkins Univ, Baltimore, MD)
Crit Care Med 35:2747-2754, 2007

Objective.—To evaluate perceived attitudes, knowledge, and behaviors regarding the use of low tidal volume ventilation in acute respiratory distress syndrome among physicians, nurses, and respiratory therapists in intensive care units.
Design.—Cross-sectional, self-administered survey.
Setting.—Large Acute Respiratory Distress Syndrome Network teaching hospital in Baltimore, MD.
Participants.—Attending, fellow, and resident physicians; staff nurses; and respiratory therapists in three intensive care units.
Interventions.—A survey was designed to assess barriers related to clinicians' perceived attitudes, knowledge, and behaviors related to low tidal volume ventilation in acute respiratory distress syndrome and intensive care unit organization-related barriers. Survey development was guided by a published framework of barriers to clinician adherence to practice guidelines; individual items were derived through literature review and refined through pilot testing. Content validity, face validity, and ease of use were verified by local clinicians. Psychometric properties were assessed and regression analyses were conducted to examine differences in perceptions and knowledge level by provider discipline and training level.

Measurements and Main Results.—There were 291 completed surveys with a response rate of 84%. Validity and acceptable psychometric properties were demonstrated. Barriers related to clinician attitudes, behaviors, and intensive care unit organization were significantly higher among nurses and respiratory therapists vs. physicians. Knowledge-related barriers also were significantly higher among nurses vs. physicians and respiratory therapists. Barriers were lower and knowledge test scores higher among fellows and attending physicians vs. residents. Similarly, barriers were lower and knowledge test scores higher among nurses with >10 yrs of experience vs. <10 yrs of experience.

Conclusions.—Important organizational and clinician barriers, including knowledge deficits, regarding low tidal volume ventilation were reported, particularly among nurses and resident physicians. Addressing these barriers may be important for increasing implementation of low tidal volume ventilation.

▶ Bridging the gap to overcome barriers and foster change requires a plan to establish administrative and staff buy-in, knowledge transfer, measurement, and evaluation. Assessing potential obstacles upfront is imperative and should include people, environmental, and equipment issues impeding translation of guideline recommendations into clinical practice.

The authors present results from a single-center survey conducted in 3 ICUs, 1 medical and 2 surgical. The goal was to evaluate barriers to implementing low tidal ventilation in acute respiratory distress syndrome using a framework based on previous work to determine why physicians do not adhere to clinical practice guidelines.

The authors reported that approximately 50% of their patients receive low tidal volume ventilation with only the medical ICU having a protocol in place. It is not surprising that knowledge deficits were unveiled in this survey for residents because of the reported variation in practice between the ICUs. Additionally, the nurses reportedly had significantly higher knowledge-related barriers that may be related to the fact that other members of the team were taking responsibility for the ventilator. In this study, the order is placed by the physician and carried out by the respiratory therapist (RT), which may more or less leave nurses out of the loop.

Knowledge transfer and guideline implementation are challenging in a single ICU. The universal use of guidelines in a hospital with several ICUs is hard, but may gain success through establishment of a Multidisciplinary Critical Care Guidelines Team. This group may include physicians, nurses, RTs, and pharmacists from the various ICUs, establishing critical care standards rather than single unit-based protocols. Development of shared protocols between units can facilitate consistency for clinicians and promote guideline adherence across multiple ICUs in one hospital or hospital system.

C. A. Schorr, RN, MSN

Mechanical Ventilation/Weaning

Changes in B-type natriuretic peptide improve weaning outcome predicted by spontaneous breathing trial

Chien J-Y, Lin M-S, Huang Y-CT, et al (Natl Taiwan Univ Hosp Yun-Lin Branch, Douliu; Duke Univ Med Ctr, Durham, NC; et al)
Crit Care Med 36:1421-1426, 2008

Objective.—Despite the use of spontaneous breathing trial (SBT), predicting weaning success remains a major clinical challenge. Because cardiovascular dysfunction could be a major underlying mechanism of weaning failure, we evaluated the role of the levels of B-type natriuretic peptide (BNP), a marker for cardiovascular function, in patients who passed a 2-hr SBT.

Design, Setting, and Patients.—Fifty-two patients recovering from acute respiratory failure were enrolled as the testing group to determine the predictive value of BNP. The predictive value of BNP was validated in a second independent cohort of 49 patients. Then, we combined both groups of patients to conduct the final analysis.

Measurements and Results.—In the testing group of 52 patients, 41 passed SBT and were extubated. Of these patients, 33 patients (80%) were extubated successfully (extubation success) while eight patients (20%) were reintubated within 48 hrs (extubation failure). There were no differences in the baseline BNP levels, but the extubation failure group had significantly greater increases in BNP at the end of SBT than the extubation success groups (32.7%, 25th–75th percentile $= 25.7\%$–50.8% vs. 0.69%, -8.8%–10.72%, $p < .001$). The area under the receiver operating characteristic curves for the BNP change was 0.93 and an increase of BNP <20% during SBT had the best combination of sensitivity, specificity, positive and negative predictive values, and diagnostic accuracy for predicting extubation success (91%, 88%, 97%, 70%, and 91%). This threshold value of BNP change was then validated in an independent cohort. Combining BNP with SBT as extubation criteria increased the extubation success rate to 95% from 78% using SBT alone ($p = .035$).

Conclusion.—Measuring the percentage change in the BNP level during a SBT may help improve the predictive value of SBT on weaning outcome (Fig 2).

▶ The ability to predict which patients can breathe without ventilatory assistance is an inaccurate science. Reintubation rates for critically ill patients were approximately 14% and the reasons why patients fail extubation remain unclear.[1] It has been proposed that subclinical cardiac dysfunction may be unmasked during spontaneous breathing trials (SBT).[2] Chien et al explore this topic by using changes in brain natriuretic peptide (BNP) to more precisely predict which patients will fail extubation. The concept of their study is not new, but their results are significantly different from the previous work. Mekontso-Dessap et al,[3] in their study, noted that baseline BNPs rather than

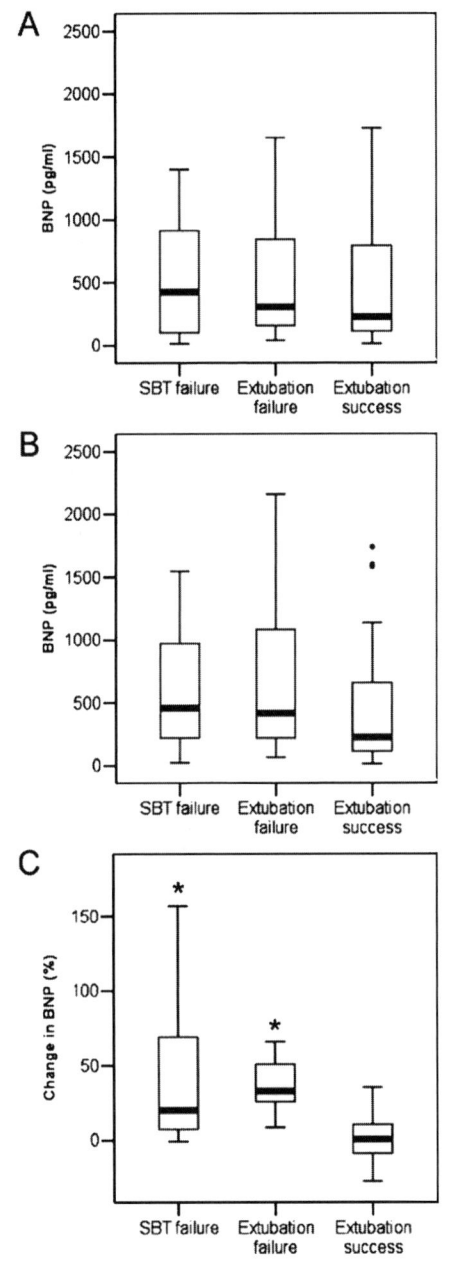

FIGURE 2.—The B-type natriuretic peptide (*BNP*) levels at the beginning of 2-hr spontaneous breathing trial (*SBT*) (*A*), at the end of 2-hr SBTs (*B*), and the percentage changes in the BNP levels during 2-hr SBTs (*C*) in the SBT failure (n = 11), extubation failure (n = 8), and extubation success (n = 33) patients of the testing group. *: $p < 0.05$ vs. extubation success group. (Reprinted from Chien J-Y, Lin M-S, Huang Y-CT, et al. Changes in B-type natriuretic peptide improve weaning outcome predicted by spontaneous breathing trial. *Crit Care Med*. 2008;36:1421-1426, with permission from the Society of Critical Care Medicine.)

the change in BNP over an hour was predictive of which patients would fail extubation. Chien et al found that measuring the change in BNP during the SBT may help to improve the predictive value of the SBT (Fig 2). However, the authors cited the increased length of ventilator support before weaning and longer duration of SBT in their patients, which accounted for their results that differ from previous studies. The authors' research was prospective, but has significant limitations. Most patients in the study carry the diagnoses of pneumonia and COPD. The absence of patients with acute respiratory distress syndrome (ARDS) and neuromuscular disorders renders the data less applicable to general medical-surgical patients. BNP is often elevated in the critically ill without cardiac dysfunction and can be elevated in patients with renal dysfunction. Moreover, the question remains whether failure to wean is entirely due to exacerbation of cardiac dysfunction. Part of the discomfort in generalizing the results would be the notion that unmasking of incipient or subclinical congestive heart failure with a 2-hour SBT is the only way to distinguish between patients ready to be extubated versus those requiring continued mechanical ventilation. The relatively high rates of extubation in the study are noteworthy. The authors' findings of increased predictive value of the SBT when combined with a greater than 20% changes in BNP necessitate larger studies on BNP in weaning trials. Practitioners would be grateful to have another tool to help predict which patients would fail extubation due to the morbidity and mortality associated with failure.

N. Puri, MD
C. Bekes, MD

References

1. Esteban A, Alia I, Tobin MJ, et al. Effect of spontaneous breathing trial duration on outcome of attempts to discontinue mechanical ventilation. Spanish Lung Failure Collaborative Group. *Am J Respir Crit Care Med*. 1999;159:512-518.
2. Lemaire F, Teboul JL, Cinotti L, et al. Acute left ventricular dysfunction during unsuccessful weaning from mechanical ventilation. *Anesthesiology*. 1988;69:171-179.
3. Mekontso-Dessap A, de Prost N, Girou E, et al. B-type natriuretic peptide and weaning from mechanical ventilation. *Intensive Care Med*. 2006;32:1529-1536.

Are daily routine chest radiographs useful in critically ill, mechanically ventilated patients? A randomized study
Clec'h C, Simon P, Hamdi A, et al (Hôpital Avicenne, Bobigny, France; Hôpital Avicenne, Bobigny Cedex, France)
Intensive Care Med 34:264-270, 2008

Objective.—Whether chest radiographs (CXRs) in mechanically ventilated patients should be routinely obtained or only when an abnormality is anticipated remains debated. We aimed to compare the diagnostic, therapeutic and outcome efficacy of a restrictive prescription of CXRs with that of a routine prescription, focusing on delayed diagnoses and treatments potentially related to the restrictive prescription.

Design.—Randomized controlled trial.
Setting.—Intensive care unit of the Avicenne Teaching Hospital, Bobigny, France.
Patients and Participants.—All consecutive patients mechanically ventilated for ≥ 48 h between January and June 2006.
Interventions.—Patients were randomly assigned to have daily routine CXRs (routine prescription group) or clinically indicated CXRs (restrictive prescription group).
Measurements and Results.—For each CXR, a questionnaire was completed addressing the reason for the CXR, the new findings, and any subsequent therapeutic intervention. The endpoints were the rates of new findings, the rates of new findings that prompted therapeutic intervention, the rate of delayed diagnoses, and mortality. Eighty-four patients were included in the routine prescription group and 81 in the restrictive prescription group. The rates of new findings and the rates of new findings that prompted therapeutic intervention in the restrictive prescription group and in the routine prescription group were 66% vs. 7.2% ($p < 0.0001$), and 56.4% vs. 5.5% ($p < 0.0001$) respectively. The rate of delayed diagnoses in the restrictive prescription group was 0.7%. Mortality was similar.
Conclusions.—Restrictive use of CXRs in mechanically ventilated patients was associated with better diagnostic and therapeutic efficacies without impairing outcome.

▶ For decades there has been a controversy concerning the value of a daily chest x-ray in the care of an intubated patient. The overall value of this test must balance the risks and benefits and should take into account the cost of the exam. Where ICU tests and procedures are concerned, a portable chest x-ray is relatively cheap. Unfortunately, the quality of the film and our ability to appreciate subtle changes in infiltrates, effusions, lines, and tubes is often suboptimum. There is always the danger that lines and tubes become altered during the process of taking of the x-ray. An important inclusion criteria for this study was that the patients subjected to the 2 different chest x-ray ordering strategies had all been intubated and ventilated for at least 48 hours. In this study, there was no difference in new findings or in the need for therapeutic intervention between the restrictive and the routine chest x-ray groups. There was no difference in outcome between the 2 monitoring strategies, suggesting that any delay in detecting a new finding on chest x-ray was not associated with any harm that influenced eventual outcome. This is comforting information and may give the clinician support to evaluate the more restrictive chest x-ray monitoring strategy in United States patients who have been ventilated for more than 48 hours. However, I would like to see additional data to confirm this observation before we all adopt this strategy.

R. A. Balk, MD

Impact of passive humidification on clinical outcomes of mechanically ventilated patients: A meta-analysis of randomized controlled trials
Siempos II, Vardakas KZ, Kopterides P, et al (Alfa Inst of Biomedical Sciences (AIBS), Athens, Greece)
Crit Care Med 35:2843-2851, 2007

Objective.—Previous meta-analyses reported advantages of passive (i.e., heat and moisture exchangers, or HMEs) compared with active (i.e., heated humidifiers, or HHs) humidifiers in reducing the incidence of ventilator-associated pneumonia, but they did not examine the effect of these devices on mortality, length of intensive care unit stay, and duration of mechanical ventilation. In addition, relevant data were recently published.

Design.—Meta-analysis of randomized controlled trials comparing HMEs with HHs for the management of mechanically ventilated patients to determine the impact of these devices on clinical outcomes of such patients.

Methods.—We searched PubMed and the Cochrane Central Register of Controlled Trials as well as reference lists from publications, with no language restrictions. We estimated pooled odds ratios (ORs) and 95% confidence intervals (CIs), using a random effects model.

Results.—Thirteen randomized controlled trials, studying 2,580 patients, were included. There was no difference in incidence of ventilator-associated pneumonia among patients managed with HMEs and HHs (OR 0.85, 95% CI 0.62–1.16). There was no difference between the compared groups regarding mortality (OR 0.98, 95% CI 0.80–1.20), length of intensive care unit stay (weighted mean differences, −0.68 days, 95% CI −3.65 to 2.30), duration of mechanical ventilation (weighted mean differences, 0.11 days, 95% CI −0.90 to 1.12), or episodes of airway occlusion (OR 2.26, 95% CI 0.55–9.28). HMEs were cheaper than HHs in each of the randomized controlled trials.

Conclusion.—The available evidence does not support the preferential performance of either passive or active humidifiers in mechanical ventilation patients in terms of ventilator-associated pneumonia incidence, mortality, or morbidity.

▶ Warming and humidifying the gases delivered to patients under invasive mechanical ventilation protects the respiratory tract mucosa and prevents ventilator-associated pneumonia (VAP). Although the passive operation and feasibility of heat and moisture exchangers (HMEs) have popularized in recent years, controversy exists about their advantage over heated humidifiers (HHs) for the prevention of VAP. Thirteen randomized controlled trials (RCTs), including more than 2500 patients, were evaluated for the comparative impact of passive and active humidification on various clinically important outcomes in patients undergoing mechanical ventilation. The findings supported the guidelines published recently by the American Thoracic Society of America and those by the Centers for Disease Control and Prevention, which concluded that no recommendation could be established for the preferential use of either HMEs or HHs to prevent VAP.

The value of any meta-analysis in the field of VAP prevention is inevitably limited by the fact that the populations studied and the criteria used for the definition of VAP were not identical in the included RCTs. There were also differences between the HMEs used regarding brand, type, and frequency of change. Routine care (eg, use of weaning protocols that presumably affect duration of mechanical ventilation and thereby, incidence of VAP) and cointerventions for VAP prevention in the selected RCTs may not be identical. However, to address this limitation, the authors used a conservative statistical random effects model to pool the available data. It is clear that none of the humidifiers should be regarded as the gold standard for gas conditioning, but HMEs could be considered a cost-saving method of providing humidification to patients undergoing mechanical ventilation.

I. Cinel, MD

Efficacy and safety of a paired sedation and ventilator weaning protocol for mechanically ventilated patients in intensive care (Awakening and Breathing Controlled trial): a randomised controlled trial

Girard TD, Kress JP, Fuchs BD, et al (Univ School of Medicine, Nashville, TN; Univ of Chicago, IL; Univ of Pennsylvania School of Medicine, Philadelphia, PA; et al)
Lancet 371:126-134, 2008

Background.—Approaches to removal of sedation and mechanical ventilation for critically ill patients vary widely. Our aim was to assess a protocol that paired spontaneous awakening trials (SATs)—ie, daily interruption of sedatives—with spontaneous breathing trials (SBTs).

Methods.—In four tertiary-care hospitals, we randomly assigned 336 mechanically ventilated patients in intensive care to management with a daily SAT followed by an SBT (intervention group; n=168) or with sedation per usual care plus a daily SBT (control group; n=168). The primary endpoint was time breathing without assistance. Data were analysed by intention to treat. This study is registered with ClinicalTrials.gov, number NCT00097630.

Findings.—One patient in the intervention group did not begin their assigned treatment protocol because of withdrawal of consent and thus was excluded from analyses and lost to follow-up. Seven patients in the control group discontinued their assigned protocol, and two of these patients were lost to follow-up. Patients in the intervention group spent more days breathing without assistance during the 28-day study period than did those in the control group (14·7 days *vs* 11·6 days; mean difference 3·1 days, 95% CI 0·7 to 5·6; p=0·02) and were discharged from intensive care (median time in intensive care 9·1 days *vs* 12·9 days; p=0·01) and the hospital earlier (median time in the hospital 14·9 days *vs* 19·2 days; p=0·04). More patients in the intervention group self-extubated than in the control group (16 patients *vs* six patients; 6·0% difference, 95% CI 0·6% to 11·8%; p=0·03), but the number of patients who required reintubation after self-extubation was similar (five patients *vs* three patients; 1·2% difference, 95% CI −5·2% to 2·5%; p=0·47), as were total reintubation rates (13·8% *vs* 12·5%; 1·3% difference, 95% CI ·8·6% to 6·1%; p=0·73). At any instant during the year after enrolment, patients in the intervention group were less likely to die than were patients in the control group (HR 0·68, 95% CI 0·50 to 0·92; p=0·01). For every seven patients treated with the intervention, one life was saved (number needed to treat was 7·4, 95% CI 4·2 to 35·5).

Interpretation.—Our results suggest that a wake up and breathe protocol that pairs daily spontaneous awakening trials (ie, interruption of sedatives) with daily spontaneous breathing trials results in better outcomes for mechanically ventilated patients in intensive care than current standard approaches and should become routine practice.

▶ I remember, before the recognition by critical care practitioners, the frequent occurrence of marked oversedation and fat deposition of continuous infusion benzodiazepines (BZDPs) in ICU patients. When BZDPs were discontinued in these patients, it often took days and days for the patient to arouse because of the marked oversedation. This occurs because BZDPs are fat soluble, and after discontinuation will leech out of the fat maintaining blood levels for long periods when they have been overadministered. I am not surprised that the approach taken by these authors of combining spontaneous awakening trials and withholding of sedation with spontaneous breathing trials (SBTs) to judge ability for extubation produces significantly greater appropriate extubations than SBTs alone. Every unit should have as part of best practice a spontaneous awakening trial before a daily SBT.

R. P. Dellinger, MD

Chest physiotherapy prolongs duration of ventilation in the critically ill ventilated for more than 48 hours
Templeton M, Palazzo MGA (Charing Cross Hosp, London, UK)
Intensive Care Med 33:1938-1945, 2007

Objective.—This study aimed to determine the impact of providing chest physiotherapy after routine clinical assessment on the duration of mechanical ventilation, outcome and intensive care length of stay.

Design and Setting.—Single-centre, single-blind, prospective, randomised, controlled trial in a university hospital general intensive care unit.

Patients and Participants.—180 patients requiring mechanical ventilation for more than 48 h.

Interventions.—Patients randomly allocated, one group receiving physiotherapy as deemed appropriate by physiotherapists after routine daily assessments and another group acting as controls were limited to receiving decubitus care and tracheal suctioning.

TABLE 3.—Outcome Measures

	Physiotherapy ($n = 87$)	Controls ($n = 85$)	Probability ($p =$)
Median time (50% patients within each group) to become ventilator-free based on Kaplan–Meier curve (days; range)	15 (3–82)	11 (3–76)	0.045
Distribution of patients in the first 86 of 172 patients (50%) to become ventilator-free (n; unit survivors)	35 (17)	51 (28)	
Median time days (range in parentheses) for patients among the first 50% of the cohort to become ventilator-free. This includes patients who died on a ventilator	6 (3–9)	5 (3–9)	
Median length of ICU stay among the unit survivors in first 50% of the cohort to become ventilator-free (days; range)	7 (5–18)	9 (5–29)	
Median length of ICU stay among unit non-survivors among the first 50% of cohort to become ventilator-free (days; range)	6 (3–38)	7 (4–61)	
Median length of ICU stay for all patients (days; range)	13 (3–82)	12 (4–76)	0.78
Median length of ICU stay of all ICU survivors (days; range)	14 (5–51)	12 (5–47)	0.35
Median length of ICU stay for all ICU non-survivors (days; range)	11 (3–82)	13 (4–76)	0.6
Patients requiring re-ventilation for respiratory insufficiency at any time after initially becoming ventilator-free (%; number in parentheses)	12.6 (11)	14.1 (12)	0.99
Median time to become re-ventilated (days; range)	1 (1–9)	3.5 (1–6)	0.13
ICU mortality (%; number in parentheses)	46.0 (40)	49.4 (42)	0.76
Median time to ICU death (days; range)	11 (3–82)	13 (4–76)	0.59
Hospital mortality (%; number in parentheses)	52.9 (46)	54.1 (46)	0.88
Median time to hospital death (days; n; range)	12 (46, 3–197)	13 (46, 4–76)	0.76
Ventilator-associated pneumonia (%; number in parentheses)	35 (40.2)	25 (29.4)	0.13
Patients needing additional (rescue) therapy over and above routine at any time while ventilated (n; percentage within group)	45 (51.7)	37 (43.5)	0.28
Total events requiring additional (rescue) therapy during period of ventilation (total routine physiotherapy assessments/treatments during same period); rescue therapy as percentage of routine physiotherapy	68 (2384); 2.8%	51 (2227); 2.3%	

(Reprinted from Templeton M, Palazzo MGA. Chest physiotherapy prolongs duration of ventilation in the critically ill ventilated for more than 48 hours. *Intensive Care Med.* 2007;33:1938-1945, with kind permission from Springer Science+Business Media: *Intensive Care Medicine*.)

Measurements and Results.—Primary endpoints were initial time to become ventilator-free, secondary endpoints included intensive care unit (ICU) and hospital mortality and ICU length of stay. Kaplan–Meier analysis censored for death revealed a significant prolongation of median time to become ventilator-free among patients receiving physiotherapy ($p = 0.047$). The time taken for 50% of patients (median time) to become ventilator-free was 15 and 11 days, respectively, for physiotherapy and control groups. There were no differences between groups in ICU or hospital mortality rates, or length of ICU stay. The number of patients needing re-ventilation for respiratory reasons was similar in both groups (Table 3).

▶ Airway clearance techniques and chest physiotherapy are major components of pulmonary management for patients with cystic fibrosis and bronchiectasis. Currently, chest physiotherapy is not routinely used in the management of ventilated patients in the United States unless they have a diagnosis of cystic fibrosis, bronchiectasis, or have a suspected mucous plug leading to atelectasis. Often, critically ill patients will not tolerate the physical process of chest physiotherapy because of their underlying severity of illness or coagulopathy. This study yielded an interesting finding with a delay in ventilator weaning associated with the performance of chest physiotherapy. Despite the delay in ventilator weaning, the length of stay in the ICU and hospital as well as mortality rate was similar between the 2 groups. This observation also leads to confusion, because I would expect a process that prolongs mechanical ventilatory support to be associated with a longer length of stay and an increase in morbidity and/or mortality rates. For now, I would continue to reserve chest physiotherapy for those patients with cystic fibrosis or bronchiectasis with significant sputum production.

R. A. Balk, MD

Airway

Duration of adrenal inhibition following a single dose of etomidate in critically ill patients
Vinclair M, Broux C, Faure P, et al (Albert Michallon Hosp, Grenoble, France; et al)
Intensive Care Med 34:714-719, 2008

Objective.—To determine the incidence and duration of adrenal inhibition induced by a single dose of etomidate in critically ill patients.
Design.—Prospective, observational cohort study.
Setting.—Three intensive care units in a university hospital.
Patients.—Forty critically ill patients without sepsis who received a single dose of etomidate for facilitating endotracheal intubation.
Measurements and Main Results.—Serial serum cortisol and 11β-deoxycortisol samples were taken at baseline and 60 min after corticotropin stimulation test (250 μg 1–24 ACTH) at 12, 24, 48, and 72 h after etomidate administration. Etomidate-related adrenal inhibition was

defined by the combination of a rise in cortisol less than 250 nmol/l (9 μg/dl) after ACTH stimulation and an excessive accumulation of serum 11β-deoxycortisol concentrations at baseline. At 12 h after etomidate administration, 32/40 (80%) patients fulfilled the diagnosis criteria for etomidate-related adrenal insufficiency. This incidence was significantly lower at 48 h (9%) and 72 h (7%). The cortisol to 11β-deoxycortisol ratio (F/S ratio), reflecting the intensity of the 11β-hydroxylase enzyme blockade, improved significantly over time.

Conclusions.—A single bolus infusion of etomidate resulted in wide adrenal inhibition in critically ill patients. However, this alteration was reversible by 48 h following the drug administration. The empirical use of steroid supplementation for 48 h following a single dose of etomidate in ICU patients without septic shock should thus be considered. Concomitant serum cortisol and 11β-deoxycortisol dosages are needed to provide evidence for adrenal insufficiency induced by etomidate in critically ill patients.

▶ There has been much discussion and debate about the role of etomidate as an agent to facilitate endotracheal intubation. A single bolus of etomidate is now recognized as having the potential to produce short-term inhibition of adrenal cortisol release. The clinical significance of this is less clear. Exogenous steroids have been shown to shorten the time period of septic shock in patients not receiving etomidate. There is a natural concern about suppressing cortisol release in patients with septic shock and likely other shock states also. The authors recommend 48 hours of empiric steroid supplementation after etomidate in ICU patients with or without shock. It is difficult to say this is a bad idea, because this dosing and time period of steroids would not be considered under any circumstance to produce any negative effect. It is less, however, clear that this is clinically needed in the overwhelming majority of patients. Etomidate remains a very good intubation facilitating drug as it does not totally negate patient respiratory reserve.

R. P. Dellinger, MD

Tracheostomy: current practice on timing, correction of coagulation disorders and peri-operative management – a postal survey in the Netherlands
Veelo DP, Dongelmans DA, Phoa KN, et al (Univ of Amsterdam, the Netherlands; et al)
Acta Anaesthesiol Scand 51:1231-1236, 2007

Background.—Several factors may delay tracheostomy. As many critically ill patients either suffer from coagulation abnormalities or are being treated with anticoagulants, fear of bleeding complications during the procedure may also delay tracheostomy. It is unknown whether such (usually mild) coagulation abnormalities are corrected first and to what extent. The purpose of this study was to ascertain current practice of tracheostomy in the Netherlands with regard to timing, pre-operative correction of coagulation disorders and peri-/intra-operative measures.

Methods.—In October 2005, a questionnaire was sent to the medical directors of all non-pediatric ICUs with ≥5 beds suitable for mechanical ventilation in the Netherlands.

Results.—A response was obtained from 44 (64%) out of 69 ICUs included in the survey. Seventy-five percent of patients receive tracheostomy within 2 days after the decision to proceed with a tracheostomy. Reasons indicated as frequent causes for delay were most often logistical factors. A heterogeneous attitude exists regarding values of coagulation parameters acceptable to perform tracheostomy. Fifty percent of the respondents have no guideline on correction of coagulation disorders or anticoagulant therapy before tracheostomy. Antimicrobial prophylaxis is almost never administered before tracheostomy. Forty-eight percent mentioned always using endoscopic guidance and 66% of ICUs only perform chest radiography on indication.

Conclusions.—There is a high variation in peri- and intra-operative practice of tracheostomy in the Netherlands. Especially on the subject of coagulation and tracheostomy there are different opinions and protocols are often lacking.

▶ As they say, you never know what really happens until you actually look and carefully evaluate. The use of a survey may be a less powerful tool to actually evaluate what is taking place at an institution, but this study had almost two-thirds of the surveyed ICUs respond with a completed survey. They found that there is quite a bit of variation in the approach to performing a tracheostomy and the goals for correction of bleeding abnormalities between the responding centers. They also noted that the use of endoscopic guidance for percutaneous procedures was more likely to occur at teaching hospitals. As is true with most issues, the most common reasons for delaying the procedure, once agreed on, were logistic, related to availability of the personnel and/or operating room. Bedside percutaneous tracheostomy would help minimize some of these logistic issues, but this is still dependent on a number of factors. As we all occasionally struggle to overcome some of these logistic barriers to get needed procedures for our patients, it is comforting to know that we are not alone, but this doesn't relieve the frustration.

R. A. Balk, MD

Monitoring Tracheal Tube Cuff Pressures in the Intensive Care Unit: A Comparison of Digital Palpation and Manometry
Morris LG, Zoumalan RA, Roccaforte JD, et al (New York Univ School of Medicine, NY)
Ann Otol Rhinol Laryngol 116:639-642, 2007

Objectives.—Tracheal tube cuff overinflation is a recognized risk factor for tracheal injury and stenosis. International studies report a 55% to 62%

incidence of cuff overinflation among intensive care unit (ICU) patients. However, there are no data on tracheotomy tubes, and no recent data from ICUs in the United States. It is unknown whether routine cuff pressure measurement is beneficial. We sought to determine the incidence of cuff overinflation in the contemporary American ICU.

Methods.—We performed an Institutional Review Board–approved, prospective, observational study of endotracheal and tracheotomy tubes at 2 tertiary-care academic hospitals that monitor cuff pressure differently. At hospital A, cuff pressures are assessed by palpation; at hospital B, cuff pressures are measured via manometry. We audited cuff pressures in an unannounced fashion at these hospitals, using a handheld aneroid manometer. Cuffs were considered overinflated above 25 cm H_2O.

Results.—We enrolled 115 patients: 63 at hospital A and 52 at hospital B. Overall, 44 patients (38%) were found to have overinflated cuffs. The incidence of overinflation was identical at the 2 hospitals (38%; p = .99). Of the endotracheal tubes, 43% were overinflated, as were 32% of the tracheotomy tubes (p = .24).

Conclusions.—Despite increasing awareness among intensivists and respiratory therapists, the incidence of tracheal tube overinflation remains high, with both endotracheal and tracheotomy tubes. Our finding that the use of manometry to assess cuff pressures did not reduce the incidence of overinflation suggests that a more vigilant management protocol may be necessary.

▶ In most ICUs it is routine to serially monitor endotracheal and tracheostomy tube balloon cuff pressures to avoid causing tracheal wall damage that may lead to tracheomalacia or tracheal stenosis. Using a "just seal" or a "minimal leak" determination of adequate inflation pressure is not sufficient to avoid compromising tracheal mucosal perfusion and injury. This study monitored the cuff pressure with an aneroid monometer and found that a significant number of patients had elevated cuff pressures despite a monitoring protocol. Unfortunately, this study did not include a long-term follow-up component to see if the elevated cuff pressure resulted in any harm. The study does emphasize that even with widespread use of high-volume, low-pressure endotracheal and tracheostomy tubes combined with a program of frequent cuff pressure monitoring, there were still a significant number of elevated tracheal cuff pressures and the potential for airway injury. This study also serves to educate all of us who work in the ICU environment that unless we continuously survey and evaluate our practices, we may not really know what happens in our unit.

R. A. Balk, MD

Other

On-demand Rather than Daily-routine Chest Radiography Prescription May Change Neither the Number Nor the Impact of Chest Computed Tomography and Ultrasound Studies in a Multidisciplinary Intensive Care Unit
Kröner A, Binnekade JM, Graat ME, et al (Univ of Amsterdam, The Netherlands)
Anesthesiology 108:40-45, 2008

Background.—Elimination of daily-routine chest radiographs (CXRs) may influence chest computed tomography (CT) and ultrasound practice in critically ill patients.

Methods.—This was a retrospective cohort study including all patients admitted to a university-affiliated intensive care unit during two consecutive periods of 5 months, one before and one after elimination of daily-routine CXR. Chest CT and ultrasound studies were identified retrospectively by using the radiology department information system. Indications for and the diagnostic/therapeutic yield of chest CT and ultrasound studies were collected.

Results.—Elimination of daily-routine CXR resulted in a decrease of CXRs per patient day from 1.1 ± 0.3 to 0.6 ± 0.4 ($P < 0.05$). Elimination did not affect duration of stay or mortality rates. Neither the number of chest CT studies nor the ratio of chest CT studies per patient day changed with the intervention: Before elimination of daily-routine CXR, 52 chest CT studies were obtained from 747 patients; after elimination, 54 CT studies were obtained from 743 patients. Similarly, chest ultrasound practice was not affected by the change of CXR strategy: Before and after elimination, 21 and 27 chest ultrasound studies were performed, respectively. Also, timing of chest CT and ultrasound studies was not different between the two study periods. During the two periods, 40 of 106 chest CT studies (38%) and 18 of 48 chest ultrasound studies (38%) resulted in a change in therapy. The combined therapeutic yield of chest CT and ultrasound studies did not change with elimination of daily-routine CXR.

Conclusions.—Elimination of daily-routine CXRs may not affect chest CT and ultrasound practice in a multidisciplinary intensive care unit.

▶ The chest x-ray has been historically known to be one of the most commonly requested radiographic examinations and an integral supplement to the physical examination in the critically ill patient.[1] Recent literature from Europe has demonstrated that the on-demand rather than daily chest x-rays are more cost-effective with minimum impact on patient care.[2,3]

The authors designed a retrospective cohort study including all patients admitted to a university-affiliated intensive care unit over the time period before and after daily chest radiographs (CXRs) were eliminated. This was done to assess the impact on the frequency of chest computed tomography (CT) and ultrasound ordering based on abnormalities found on on-demand chest x-rays.[4] The use of bedside ultrasound is gaining wide popularity[5] and may prove to become the standard of care. It may potentially replace the daily routine CXRs in the intensive care setting in the future in the United States.

A multicenter randomized controlled clinical trial to establish such practice guidelines would be invaluable in environments with high medicolegal liability.

R. Lotano, MD
C. Bekes, MD

References

1. Hill JR, Horner PE, Primack SL. ICU imaging. *Clin Chest Med.* 2008;29:59-76.
2. Hejblum G, Ioos V, Vibert JF, et al. A web-based Delphi study on the indications of chest radiographs for patients in ICUs. *Chest.* 2008;133:1107-1112.
3. Mets O, Spronk PE, Binnekade J, Stoker J, de Mol BA, Schultz MJ, et al. Elimination of daily routine chest radiographs does not change on-demand radiography practice in post-cardiothoracic surgery patients. *J Thorac Cardiovasc Surg.* 2007;134:139-144.
4. Kröner A, Binnekade JM, Graat ME, et al. On-demand rather than daily-routine chest radiography prescription may change neither the number nor the impact of chest computed tomography and ultrasound studies in a multidisciplinary intensive care unit. *Anesthesiology.* 2008;108:40-45.
5. Lichtenstein DA. [Whole-body ultrasound in the ICU. A visual approach to the critically ill]. *Bull Acad Natl Med.* 2007;191:495-516.

A Web-Based Delphi Study on the Indications of Chest Radiographs for Patients in ICUs

Hejblum G, Ioos V, Vibert J-F, et al (Hôpital Saint Antoine, Assistance Publique-Hôpitaux de Paris, France; et al)
Chest 133:1107-1112, 2008

Background.—Strategies for ordering bedside chest radiographs (CXRs) have substantial logistic and financial consequences in the ICU. Many of the indications for CXRs in the ICU are controversial, such as the ordering of daily routine CXRs for intubated patients. The opinions of intensivists about ordering CXRs have not been reported. Comparing these opinions to established guidelines and identifying situations where opinions diverge in the absence of guidelines are of considerable interest.

Methods.—We asked 190 intensivists from 34 ICUs in the area of Paris, France, to anonymously complete a 29-item questionnaire about their opinions regarding the ordering of CXRs; each item described a clinical scenario. Of the 29 scenarios, 10 dealt with the placement of medical devices, 8 with the presence of medical devices, and 11 with other clinical situations. The study was based on a Delphi process deployed over the Internet through an original software application. Three Delphi rounds were run between January and March 2006, using the same questionnaire. Detailed feedback for the answers given during the previous round was supplied to each intensivist solicited for updating his answers.

Results.—Eighty-two intensivists from 32 ICUs completed the study. A consensus emerged that routine CXRs were necessary for eight scenarios and unnecessary for two scenarios. The study also shed light on items without a consensus. In particular, 75% of intensivists (58% on the first round) did not support obtaining daily routine CXRs in intubated patients.

Conclusion.—The study underlines situations in which intensivists do not support the guidelines and outlines recommendations likely to be followed in clinical practice.

▶ The advantage of radiography in an intensive care unit (ICU) is to provide safety, especially in teaching hospital settings where trainees are involved. The roentgenograms also provide medicolegal documentation in an event of adverse outcome.

With the lack of extensively published evidence, intensivists in the United States would likely not feel comfortable withholding or decreasing the frequency of what is considered "standard of care."[1,2,3] However, the availability of bedside ultrasound,[4,5] may change this practice.

In the study by Hejblum et al[6] 190 French intensivists were asked to respond to 29 clinical case scenarios. Most French intensivists who participated in the study felt they would eliminate routine chest radiograph (CXR) in the ICU.

The Delphi technique provides an excellent means to capture expert knowledge and judgment. Developed at the RAND corporation in the 1960s, the approach was designed as a forecasting method, and has since been adapted for use in determining expert consensus in a wide variety of disciplines, including medicine, education, environmental planning, and information technology. Delphi most often uses a panel of experts who do not meet face to face, yet participate in an interactive group process. This is achieved by using a series of questionnaires, called "Delphi Rounds," each of which, after the first, include summary information about the entire panel's response to the previous round.

It has been demonstrated that endotracheal intubation performed by experienced physicians rarely led to acutely malpositioned endotracheal tubes.[7] Other authors have shown that changing from routine to an on-demand strategy could result in a reduction of 36% of chest X-rays at considerable savings.

A future study to include intensivists in teaching and nonteaching hospitals in the United States should be considered. This would be easy to achieve electronically on the World Wide Web.

R. Lotano, MD
C. Bekes, MD

References

1. Hill JR, Horner PE, Primack SL. ICU imaging. *Clin Chest Med.* 2008;29:59-76.
2. Aquino L, Mak MD, Poonam V, et al. American college of radiology expert panel on thoracic imaging. ACR appropriateness criteria: routine chest radiograph, http://www.acr.org/SecondaryMainMenuCategories/quality_safety/app_criteria/pdf/ExpertPanelonThoracicImaging/RoutineChestRadiographDoc7.aspx; 2006. Accessed August 18, 2008.

3. Rubinowitz AN, Siegel MD, Tocino I. Thoracic imaging in the ICU. *Crit Care Clin.* 2007;23:539-573.
4. Guillory RK, Gunter OL. Ultrasound in the surgical intensive care unit. *Curr Opin Crit Care.* 2008;14:415-422.
5. Lichtenstein DA. [Whole-body ultrasound in the ICU. A visual approach to the critically ill]. *Bull Acad Natl Med.* 2007;191:495-516.
6. Hejblum G, Ioos V, Vibert JF, et al. A web-based Delphi study on the indications of chest radiographs for patients in ICUs. *Chest.* 2008;133:1107-1112.
7. Lotano R, Gerber D, Aseron C, Santarelli R, Pratter M. Utility of postintubation chest radiographs in the intensive care unit. *Crit Care.* 2000;4:50-53.

Relevance of Lung Ultrasound in the Diagnosis of Acute Respiratory Failure: The BLUE Protocol

Lichtenstein DA, Mezière GA (Service de Réanimation Médicale, Paris-Ouest; Service de Réanimation Polyvalente, Paris-Ouest, France)
Chest 134:117-125, 2008

Background.—This study assesses the potential of lung ultrasonography to diagnose acute respiratory failure.

Methods.—This observational study was conducted in university-affiliated teaching-hospital ICUs. We performed ultrasonography on consecutive patients admitted to the ICU with acute respiratory failure, comparing lung ultrasonography results on initial presentation with the final diagnosis by the ICU team. Uncertain diagnoses and rare causes (frequency < 2%) were excluded. We included 260 dyspneic patients with a definite diagnosis. Three items were assessed: artifacts (horizontal A lines or vertical B lines indicating interstitial syndrome), lung sliding, and alveolar consolidation and/or pleural effusion. Combined with venous analysis, these items were grouped to assess ultrasound profiles.

Results.—Predominant A lines plus lung sliding indicated asthma (n = 34) or COPD (n = 49) with 89% sensitivity and 97% specificity. Multiple anterior diffuse B lines with lung sliding indicated pulmonary edema (n = 64) with 97% sensitivity and 95% specificity. A normal anterior profile plus deep venous thrombosis indicated pulmonary embolism (n = 21) with 81% sensitivity and 99% specificity. Anterior absent lung sliding plus A lines plus lung point indicated pneumothorax (n = 9) with 81% sensitivity and 100% specificity. Anterior alveolar consolidations, anterior diffuse B lines with abolished lung sliding, anterior asymmetric interstitial patterns, posterior consolidations or effusions without anterior diffuse B lines indicated pneumonia (n = 83) with 89% sensitivity and 94% specificity. The use of these profiles would have provided correct diagnoses in 90.5% of cases.

Conclusions.—Lung ultrasound can help the clinician make a rapid diagnosis in patients with acute respiratory failure, thus meeting the priority objective of saving time.

▶ Ultrasound (US) is being used with greater frequency to facilitate procedures in the intensive care unit. This use of US provides an increased margin of safety for the performance of the procedures. In addition, noninvasive techniques such as echocardiography and Doppler US to evaluate the heart and vascular system are well entrenched in our management armamentarium. Now we can look forward to using US of the chest to determine the underlying clinical problem. Obviously, we will all need to see more studies to substantiate this new technique and see how it stands up with all technicians, not just the highly skilled individuals who conducted this study. I anticipate we will see even greater use of US and other noninvasive diagnostic techniques in the near future.

R. A. Balk, MD

Characteristics and long-term outcome of acute exacerbations in chronic obstructive pulmonary disease: an analysis of cases in the Swedish Intensive Care Registry during 2002–2006
Berkius J, Nolin T, Mårdh C, et al (Västervik Hosp, Västervik, Sweden; Central Hosp, Kristianstad, Sweden; et al)
Acta Anaesthesiol Scand 52:759-765, 2008

Background.—Chronic obstructive pulmonary disease (COPD) represents a major and growing health problem. The purpose of this work was to examine characteristics, resource use and long-term survival in patients with an acute exacerbation of COPD that were admitted to Swedish intensive care units (ICU).

Methods.—Patient characteristics at admission, length of stay (LOS), resource use and outcome were collected for admissions due to COPD during 2002–2006 in the database of the Swedish Intensive Care Registry. Vital status was secured for 99.6% of the patients. Kaplan–Meier survival estimates were computed for index admissions only.

Results.—We identified 1009 patients with 1199 admissions due to COPD (1.3% of all intensive care admissions). The mean (SD) age was 70.2 (9.1) years and the proportion of women were 61.5%. Mean (SD) Acute Physiology and Chronic Health Evaluation II probability of hospital death was 0.31 (0.19). Median LOS was 28 (interquartile range 52) h. The number of readmissions was 190 during the 5-year study. Older patients had fewer readmissions (OR 0.96, 95% CI: 0.95–0.98/year increase in age). ICU mortality was 7.3% (87 of 1199 admissions) and 30-day mortality was 26.0% (262 of 1009 index admissions). Median survival was 14.5 months and 31% of patients survived 3 years after the index admission.

Conclusions.—Short (30 days) and long-term survival is poor in acute COPD. Readmissions are frequent reflecting the severity of this chronic illness. Patients are less likely to be readmitted with increasing age which may be due to withholding of further intensive care (Fig 2).

▶ Chronic obstructive pulmonary disease (COPD) is now the 4th leading cause of death in the United States and is a significant consumer of health dollars and resources. This study demonstrates a relatively low intensive care unit (ICU)

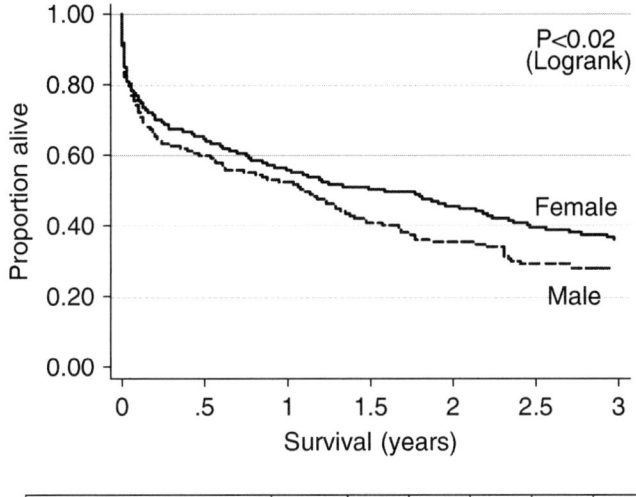

Time (yrs)	0	0.5	1.0	1.5	2.0	2.5	3.0
Patients at risk	1009	550	389	248	166	102	69

FIGURE 2.—Kaplan–Meier survival estimates by gender. (Reprinted from Berkius J, Nolin T, Mårdh C, et al. Characteristics and long-term outcome of acute exacerbations in chronic obstructive pulmonary disease: an analysis of cases in the Swedish Intensive Care Registry during 2002–2006. *Acta Anaesthesiol Scand*. 2008;52:759-765, with permission from Wiley-Blackwell Publishers.)

mortality rate associated with an acute exacerbation. However, the study also emphasizes the high 30-day and longer mortality rate. The authors felt that the reason for the high long-term mortality rate as compared with the ICU survival rate was the likelihood that these patients did not return to the hospital for care or get readmitted to the ICU when they had subsequent exacerbation episodes. Although these data may not reflect the situation in the United States, they do emphasize the significant long-term mortality rate, particularly in men, associated with an acute exacerbation of COPD.

R. A. Balk, MD

2 Cardiovascular

Myocardial Infarction/Cardiogenic Shock/Cardiogenic Pulmonary Edema

A Citywide Protocol for Primary PCI in ST-Segment Elevation Myocardial Infarction
Le May MR, So DY, Dionne R, et al (Univ of Ottawa Heart Inst, ON, Canada; Ottawa Base Hosp Program, ON, Canada; et al)
N Engl J Med 358:231-240, 2008

Background.—If primary percutaneous coronary intervention (PCI) is performed promptly, the procedure is superior to fibrinolysis in restoring flow to the infarct-related artery in patients with ST-segment elevation myocardial infarction. The benchmark for a timely PCI intervention has become a door-to-balloon time of less than 90 minutes. Whether regional strategies can be developed to achieve this goal is uncertain.

Methods.—We developed an integrated-metropolitan-a rea approach in which all patients with ST-segment elevation myocardial infarction were referred to a specialized center for primary PCI. We sought to determine whether there was a difference in door-to-balloon times between patients who were referred directly from the field by paramedics trained in the interpretation of electrocardiograms and patients who were referred by emergency department physicians.

Results.—Between May 1, 2005, and April 30, 2006, a total of 344 consecutive patients with ST-segment elevation myocardial infarction were referred for primary PCI: 135 directly from the field and 209 from emergency departments. Primary PCI was performed in 93.6% of patients. The median door-to-balloon time was shorter in patients referred from the field (69 minutes; interquartile range, 43 to 87) than in patients needing interhospital transfer (123 minutes; interquartile range, 101 to 153; P<0.001). Door-to-balloon times of less than 90 minutes were achieved in 79.7% of patients who were transferred from the field and in 11.9% of those transferred from emergency departments (P<0.001).

Conclusions.—Guideline door-to-balloon-times were more often achieved when trained paramedics independently triaged and transported patients directly to a designated primary PCI center than when patients were referred from emergency departments.

▶ A meta-analysis of randomized clinical trials that compared primary percutaneous coronary intervention (PCI) with fibrinolytic therapy for ST-segment elevation myocardial infarction (STEMI) found that the rates of short-term death, nonfatal reinfarction, stroke, and the combined endpoint of death were lower for PCI.[1] The time interval between patient presentation to a medical facility and PCI, the so-called door-to-balloon time, is an important determinant of the mortality after STEMI.[2] Also, several analyses have concluded that the advantage of PCI over fibrinolytic therapy diminishes as the door-to balloon time increases.[3,4] Therefore, current guidelines recommend that door-to-balloon time should not exceed 90 minutes, but among a cohort of 4278 patients who underwent interhospital transfer for primary PCI, the median total door-to-balloon time was 180 minutes.[5] PCI was performed within 90 minutes only for 4.2% of the patients.[5] Thus, strategies that reduce door-to-balloon time have been identified and advocated.[6]

Two strategies that have been reported to reduce time to treatment and improve clinical outcome are prehospital diagnosis and triage by paramedics.[7] The report by LeMay et al[8] incorporated this strategy in a protocol that was designed to reduce the door-to-balloon time among patients with STEMI in Ottawa, Canada. The key elements of the protocol were ECG interpretation in the field by advanced paramedics who independently triaged and transported patients with STEMI to a designated primary PCI center rather than the nearest emergency department. Among 135 patients who were transferred directly to the PCI center, door-to-balloon times < 90 minutes were achieved in 79.7% of patients compared with 11.9% among 209 patients who were transferred to the PCI center from the emergency departments of other hospitals.

A recent conference focused on the development of care systems for STEMI patients.[9] The results of the Ottawa study provide strong support for the argument that the trauma-system model of coordinated regional care should be applied to the care of patients with STEMI.[10] Nallamothu et al[11] published a study of the driving times and distances to hospitals with PCI capability in the United States. The analysis concluded that 79% of the adult United States population lived within 60 minutes of a PCI hospital in 2000. Also, for the population whose closest facility did not have PCI capability the additional time required to reach a PCI hospital was < 30 minutes among 74% of the adult population. Thus, the protocol that was implemented in Ottawa should be widely applicable to the medical care system in the United States.

S. W. Werns, MD

References

1. Keeley EC, Boura JA, Grimes CL. Primary angioplasty versus intravenous thrombolytic therapy for acute myocardial infarction: a quantitative review of 23 randomised trials. *Lancet.* 2003;361:13-20.
2. McNamara RL, Wang Y, Herrin J, et al. Effect of door-to-balloon time on mortality in patients with ST-segment elevation myocardial infarction. *J Am Coll Cardiol.* 2006;47:2180-2186.

3. Nallamothu BK, Bates ER. Percutaneous coronary intervention versus fibrinolytic therapy in acute myocardial infarction: is timing (almost) everything? *Am J Cardiol.* 2003;92:824-826.
4. Asseburg C, Vergel YB, Palmer S, et al. Assessing the effectiveness of primary angioplasty compared with thrombolysis and its relationship to time delay: a Bayesian evidence synthesis. *Heart.* 2007;93:1244-1250.
5. Nallamothu BK, Bates ER, Herrin J, Wang Y, Bradley EH, Krumholz HM. Times to treatment in transfer patients undergoing primary percutaneous coronary intervention in the United States: National Registry of Myocardial Infarction (NRMI)-3/4 analysis. *Circulation.* 2005;111:761-767.
6. Bradley EH, Herrin J, Wang Y, et al. Strategies for reducing the door-to-balloon time in acute myocardial infarction. *N Engl J Med.* 2006;355:2308-2320.
7. van 't Hof AW, Rasoul S, van de Wetering H, et al. Feasibility and benefit of pre-hospital diagnosis, triage, and therapy by paramedics only in patients who are candidates for primary angioplasty for acute myocardial infarction. *Am Heart J.* 2006;151:1255.e1-1255.e5.
8. Le May MR, So DY, Dionne R, et al. A citywide protocol for primary PCI in ST-segment elevation myocardial infarction. *N Engl J Med.* 2008;358:231-240.
9. Jacobs AK, Antman EM, Faxon DP, Gregory T, Solis P. Development of systems of care for ST-elevation myocardial infarction patients: executive summary. *Circulation.* 2007;116:217-230.
10. Jacobs AK. Regional systems of care for patients with ST-elevation myocardial infarction: being at the right place at the right time. *Circulation.* 2007;116: 689-692.
11. Nallamothu BK, Bates ER, Wang Y, Bradley EH, Krumholz HM. Driving times and distances to hospitals with percutaneous coronary intervention in the United States: implications for prehospital triage of patients with ST-elevation myocardial infarction. *Circulation.* 2006;113:1189-1195.

Effects of fondaparinux in patients with ST-segment elevation acute myocardial infarction not receiving reperfusion treatment

Oldgren J, Wallentin L, Afzal R, et al (Uppsala Univ Hosp, Sweden; McMaster Univ and Hamilton Health Sciences, ON, Canada; et al)
Eur Heart J 29:315-323, 2008

Aims.—At least one quarter of ST-segment elevation myocardial infarction (STEMI) patients do not receive reperfusion therapy, and these patients are at high risk for new ischaemic events. We evaluated fondaparinux treatment vs. usual care, i.e. placebo or unfractionated (UF) heparin, in a pre-specified subgroup of 2867 (out of 12 092) patients not receiving reperfusion treatment in the OASIS-6 trial.

Methods.—In all, 1458 patients were randomized to fondaparinux 2.5 mg once daily subcutaneously up to 8 days and 1409 patients to usual care (control). Randomization was stratified by indication for UF heparin (stratum II, $n = 1226$) or not (stratum I, $n = 1641$) based on the investigator's judgment.

Results.—The proportion of patients who suffered death or myocardial re-infarction at 30 days (primary outcome) was 12.2% in the fondaparinux vs. 15.1% in the control group, hazard ratio (HR) 0.80; 95% confidence interval (CI) 0.65–0.98. There was no increase in severe bleedings, HR 0.82; CI 0.44–1.55, or strokes, HR 0.62; CI 0.29–1.33. Consequently, the composite of death, myocardial re-infarction, or severe bleeding was significantly reduced at 30 days, HR 0.81; CI 0.67–0.99. Reductions in death or myocardial re-infarction at 30 days were consistent in stratum I with fondaparinux vs. placebo, HR 0.88; 95% CI 0.65–1.19, and in stratum II with fondaparinux vs. UF heparin infusion for 24–48 h ($n = 806$), HR 0.74; CI 95% 0.57–0.97, $P = 0.41$ for heterogeneity.

Conclusion.—In STEMI patients not receiving reperfusion treatment, fondaparinux reduces the composite of death or myocardial re-infarction without an increase in severe bleedings or strokes as compared to placebo or UF heparin.

▶ Patients with ST-segment elevation myocardial infarction (STEMI) who have contraindications to fibrinolytic therapy may undergo percutaneous coronary intervention (PCI) or may not receive reperfusion therapy. Among 10 954 patients with ST-segment elevation or left bundle-branch block who presented within 12 hours of symptom onset and were enrolled in an international registry, 33% of patients who were eligible to receive reperfusion therapy did not receive a fibrinolytic agent or undergo PCI.[1]

The rationale for anticoagulant therapy in patients with STEMI includes promotion of infarct artery patency, prevention of deep vein thrombosis, pulmonary embolism, left ventricular mural thrombus, and cerebral embolism. Relatively few clinical trials have evaluated the efficacy of anticoagulant agents in patients with STEMI who did not undergo reperfusion therapy. Cohen et al[2] conducted a randomized, multicenter trial that compared enoxaparin with unfractionated heparin and tirofiban with placebo in 1224 patients with STEMI who were ineligible for reperfusion. The incidence of the primary efficacy endpoint, the 30-day combined incidence of death, reinfarction, or recurrent angina, was 15.7% for enoxaparin versus 17.3% for unfractionated heparin (UFH) (odds ratio 0.89; 95% CI 0.66-1.21). There was no evidence of a beneficial effect of tirofiban.

OASIS-6 was a randomized, double-blind trial that compared usual care (UFH or placebo) with subcutaneous fondaparinux, a synthetic pentasaccharide that binds antithrombin and inhibits factor Xa, in patients with STEMI.[3] Among the total enrollment of 12 092 patients, 2867 patients who did not receive reperfusion therapy were randomized to fondaparinux or usual care (control). Compared with the usual care group, treatment with fondaparinux was associated with a 20% reduction in the composite endpoint of death or reinfarction at 30 days.[4]

Based on the results of the OASIS-6 study, the 2007 update of the American College of Cardiology/American Heart Association 2004 Guidelines for the Management of Patients with STEMI include a Class IIa recommendation (level of evidence B) for administration of fondaparinux to patients with STEMI who do not undergo reperfusion therapy.[5]

S. W. Werns, MD

References

1. Eagle KA, Nallamothu BK, Mehta RH, et al. Trends in acute reperfusion therapy for ST-segment elevation myocardial infarction from 1999 to 2006: we are getting better but we have got a long way to go. *Eur Heart J.* 2008;29:609-617.

2. Cohen M, Gensini GF, Maritz F, et al. The safety and efficacy of subcutaneous enoxaparin versus intravenous unfractionated heparin and tirofiban versus placebo in the treatment of acute ST-segment elevation myocardial infarction patients ineligible for reperfusion (TETAMI): a randomized trial. *J Am Coll Cardiol.* 2003;42:1348-1356.
3. Yusuf S, Mehta SR, Chrolavicius S, et al. Effects of fondaparinux on mortality and reinfarction in patients with acute ST-segment elevation myocardial infarction: the OASIS-6 randomized trial. *Jama.* 2006;295:1519-1530.
4. Oldgren J, Wallentin L, Afzal R, et al. Effects of fondaparinux in patients with ST-segment elevation acute myocardial infarction not receiving reperfusion treatment. *Eur Heart J.* 2008;29:315-323.
5. Antman EM, Hand M, Armstrong PW, et al. 2007 focused update of the ACC/AHA 2004 guidelines for the management of patients with ST-elevation myocardial infarction: a report of the American College of Cardiology/American Heart Association Task Force on Practice Guidelines. *J Am Coll Cardiol.* 2008; 51:210-247.

Continuous positive airway pressure vs. proportional assist ventilation for noninvasive ventilation in acute cardiogenic pulmonary edema

Rusterholtz T, Bollaert P-E, Feissel M, et al (Ctr Hospitalier et Universitaire, Service de Réanimation Médicale, Strasbourg, France; Ctr Hospitalier et Universitaire, Service de Réanimation Médicale, Nancy Cedex, France; Ctr Hospitalier de Belfort-Montbéliard, Service de Réanimation Médicale et des Maladies Infectieuses, Belfort, France)
Intensive Care Med 34:840-846, 2008

Objective.—To compare continuous positive airway pressure (CPAP) and proportional assist ventilation (PAV) as modes of noninvasive ventilatory support in patients with severe cardiogenic pulmonary edema.

Design and setting.—A prospective multicenter randomized study in the medical ICUs of three teaching hospitals.

Patients.—Thirty-six adult patients with cardiogenic pulmonary edema (CPA) with unresolving dyspnea, respiratory rate above 30/min and/or SpO_2 above 90% with O_2 higher than 10 l/min despite conventional therapy with furosemide and nitrates.

Interventions.—Patients were randomized to undergo either CPAP (with PEEP 10 cmH$_2$O) or PAV (with PEEP 5–6 cmH$_2$O) noninvasive ventilation through a full face mask and the same ventilator.

Measurements and Results.—The main outcome measure was the failure rate as defined by the onset of predefined intubation criteria, severe arrythmias or patient's refusal. On inclusion CPAP ($n = 19$) and PAV ($n = 17$) groups were similar with regard to age, sex ratio, type of heart disease, SAPS II, physiological parameters (mean arterial pressure, heart rate, blood gases), amount of infused nitrates and furosemide. Failure was observed in 7 (37%) CPAP and 7 (41%) PAV patients. Among these, 4 (21%) CPAP and 5 (29%) PAV patients required endotracheal intubation. Changes in physiological parameters were similar in the two groups. Myocardial infarction and ICU mortality rates were strictly similar in the two groups.

TABLE 3.—Patients Outcomes According to Study Endpoints. (*PAV*, Proportional Assist Ventilation; *CPAP*, Continuous Positive Airway Pressure)

	PAV (*n* = 17)	CPAP (*n* = 19)	*p*
Failures	7 (41%)	6 (31%)	0.99
Intubation criteria	5 (29%)	5 (26%)	
Patient refusal	2 (12%)	0	
Circulatory arrest	0	1 (5%)	
Endotracheal intubation	5 (29%)	4 (21%)	0.71
Time on NIV for failure, median (min; range)	105 (30–420)	52 (30–165)	0.82
Time on NIV for success, median (min; range)	127 (60–240)	145 (60–690)	0.85
Myocardial infarction	6 (35%)	7 (37%)	0.99
On admission[a]	3 (18%)	3 (16%)	
Within the first 6 h[b]	3 (18%)	4 (21%)	
ICU mortality	4 (23%)	4 (21%)	0.99
Length of ICU stay, median (days; range)	1 (0–39)	1 (0–33)	0.78

[a]Confirmed by significant enzymatic changes on sample drawn on admission
[b]Confirmed only by significant enzymatic changes on sample drawn 6 h after admission (normal enzymes on admission)
(Reprinted from Rusterholtz T, Bollaert P-E, Feissel M, et al. Continuous positive airway pressure vs. proportional assist ventilation for noninvasive ventilation in acute cardiogenic pulmonary edema. *Intensive Care Med.* 2008;34:840-846, with kind permission from Springer Science+Business Media, Copyright 2008.)

Conclusions.—In the present study PAV was not superior to CPAP for noninvasive ventilation in severe cardiogenic pulmonary edema with regard to either efficacy and tolerance (Table 3).

▶ The use of noninvasive ventilation has been shown to help reverse the oxygenation abnormalities of acute cardiogenic pulmonary edema faster than standard medical therapy and has been shown to produce similar improvements in short-term mortality rates.[1] The best form of noninvasive ventilatory support is still under evaluation. This study compared the use of proportional assist ventilation with the more commonly used masked continuous positive airway pressure (CPAP) in the management of acute cardiogenic pulmonary edema. Although the study was small, it was well done and found similar outcomes as detailed in Table 3. CPAP is certainly easier to use and most physicians are knowledgeable and comfortable with its use. For now, this noninvasive ventilatory support mode should be the preferred method of support, until there is data that another form of support yields better outcomes.

R. A. Balk, MD

Reference

1. Gray A, Goodacre S, Newby DE, et al. Noninvasive ventilation in acute cardiogenic pulmonary edema. *N Engl J Med.* 2008;359:142-151.

Noninvasive Ventilation in Acute Cardiogenic Pulmonary Edema
Gray A, Goodacre S, Newby DE (Univ of Sheffield, UK; Univ of Edinburgh, UK)
N Engl J Med 359:142-151, 2008

Background.—Noninvasive ventilation (continuous positive airway pressure [CPAP] or noninvasive intermittent positive-pressure ventilation [NIPPV]) appears to be of benefit in the immediate treatment of patients with acute cardiogenic pulmonary edema and may reduce mortality. We conducted a study to determine whether noninvasive ventilation reduces mortality and whether there are important differences in outcome associated with the method of treatment (CPAP or NIPPV).

Methods.—In a multicenter, open, prospective, randomized, controlled trial, patients were assigned to standard oxygen therapy, CPAP (5 to 15 cm of water), or NIPPV (inspiratory pressure, 8 to 20 cm of water; expiratory pressure, 4 to 10 cm of water). The primary end point for the comparison between noninvasive ventilation and standard oxygen therapy was death within 7 days after the initiation of treatment, and the primary end point for the comparison between NIPPV and CPAP was death or intubation within 7 days.

Results.—A total of 1069 patients (mean [±SD] age, 77.7±9.7 years; female sex, 56.9%) were assigned to standard oxygen therapy (367 patients), CPAP (346 patients), or NIPPV (356 patients). There was no significant difference in 7-day mortality between patients receiving standard oxygen therapy (9.8%) and those undergoing noninvasive ventilation (9.5%, P=0.87). There was no significant difference in the combined end point of death or intubation within 7 days between the two groups of patients undergoing noninvasive ventilation (11.7% for CPAP and 11.1% for NIPPV, P=0.81). As compared with standard oxygen therapy, noninvasive ventilation was associated with greater mean improvements at 1 hour after the beginning of treatment in patient-reported dyspnea (treatment difference, 0.7 on a visual-analogue scale ranging from 1 to 10; 95% confidence interval [CI], 0.2 to 1.3; P=0.008), heart rate (treatment difference, 4 beats per minute; 95% CI, 1 to 6; P=0.004), acidosis (treatment difference, pH 0.03; 95% CI, 0.02 to 0.04; P<0.001), and hypercapnia (treatment difference, 0.7 kPa [5.2 mm Hg]; 95% CI, 0.4 to 0.9; P<0.001). There were no treatment-related adverse events.

Conclusions.—In patients with acute cardiogenic pulmonary edema, noninvasive ventilation induces a more rapid improvement in respiratory distress and metabolic disturbance than does standard oxygen therapy but has no effect on short-term mortality. (Current Controlled Trials number, ISRCTN07448447.)

▶ This well-designed, multicenter, prospective, randomized trial evaluated standard medical therapy against 2 forms of positive pressure continuous positive airway pressure (CPAP) and noninvasive positive pressure ventilatory support ventilation in the management of acute cardiogenic pulmonary edema. There has been some concern that the use of noninvasive positive pressure ventilatory support might lead to more myocardial injury than standard medical management. These results found similar short-term mortality results, despite a more rapid improvement in oxygenation and metabolic improvement with noninvasive ventilatory support. There were no differences in adverse events supporting the safety of the 2 ventilatory strategies compared with the standard treatment. Based on this study, intensivists should feel comfortable using either CPAP or noninvasive positive pressure ventilatory support to rapidly improve oxygenation parameters, reduce dyspnea, and improve gas exchange in patients with acute cardiogenic pulmonary edema.

R. A. Balk, MD

Timing of Immunoreactive B-Type Natriuretic Peptide Levels and Treatment Delay in Acute Decompensated Heart Failure: An ADHERE (Acute Decompensated Heart Failure National Registry) Analysis

Maisel AS, Peacock WF, McMullin N, et al (Univ of California, San Diego; The Cleveland Clinic, OH; et al)
J Am Coll Cardiol 52:534-540, 2008

Objectives.—We undertook this analysis to determine whether there is a relationship between the time to measurement of immunoreactive B-type natriuretic peptide (iBNP) and early intervention for acutely decompensated heart failure (ADHF) and whether these variables are associated with morbidity and mortality in ADHF patients.

Background.—Although natriuretic peptides (NPs) can aid emergency department (ED) physicians in the diagnosis of ADHF, the relationship between the time to measurement of NP levels and time to treatment is not clear. In addition, the impact of time to treatment on clinical outcomes has not been demonstrated.

Methods.—Patients from ADHERE (Acute Decompensated Heart Failure National Registry) who were admitted to the ED and who received intravenous diuretics were included. Recordings of iBNP levels and the timing of intravenous diuretic therapy were documented. Patients were divided by quartiles of time to treatment and iBNP levels, creating 16 categories.

Results.—In 58,465 ADHF episodes from 209 hospitals, patients with the longest average time to iBNP draw also had the longest time to treatment. Mean ED time increased with increased time-to-treatment quartiles. Rales on initial examination were associated with early recognition of HF and earlier institution of therapy. The later the treatment took place, the fewer patients were asymptomatic at the time of hospital discharge. Within the time-to-treatment quartiles, mortality increased with increasing iBNP. Treatment delay was independently, but modestly, associated with increased in-hospital mortality with a risk-adjusted odds ratio 1.021, 95% confidence interval 1.010 to 1.033, and $p < 0.0001$, per every 4-h delay.

Conclusions.—In the ED setting, delayed measurement of iBNP levels and delay in treatment for ADHF were strongly associated. These delays were linked with modestly increased in-hospital mortality, independent of other prognostic variables. The adverse impact of delay was most notable in patients with greater iBNP levels (Registry for Acute Decompensated Heart Failure Patients; NCT00366639).

▶ The use of B-type natriuretic peptide (BNP) testing in patients who present to the emergency department (ED) with dyspnea has been shown to be useful in establishing the diagnosis of heart failure (HF) and in aiding appropriate decisions regarding triage to intensive care unit (ICU) care or hospitalization on a medical ward. In this large observational database of patients admitted to the hospital with acute decompensated heart failure (ADHF), Maisel et al found that patients with the longest time to determination of BNP level in the ED had the longest time to initiation of parenteral diuretic therapy, and had longer stays in the ED. This delay in diagnosis highlights the difficulty often encountered in proper diagnosis of HF as the cause of dyspnea, as symptoms and signs on physical examination are very often not specific. Interestingly, those patients with HF who had the longest delay in BNP determination and initiation of parenteral diuretics also had slightly higher hospital mortality.

Other data suggest that the prognosis of patients with dyspnea not because of HF is worsened by intravenous (IV) diuretic administration. Therefore, in cases where the cause of dyspnea is not clear, BNP testing should be performed as early as possible during the ED visit. This can improve diagnostic accuracy, shorten the time to initiation of appropriate therapy, improve use of other diagnostic modalities, shorten ED stay, and improve patients' chances of recovery from their acute illness.

F. Ginsberg, MD

Emergency Cardiac CT for Suspected Acute Coronary Syndrome: Qualitative and Quantitative Assessment of Coronary, Pulmonary, and Aortic Image Quality
Dodd JD, Kalva S, Pena A, et al (Massachusetts Gen Hosp and Harvard Med School, Boston, MA; et al)
AJR Am J Roentgenol 191:870-877, 2008

Objective.—The purpose of this study was to determine whether a dedicated coronary CT protocol provides adequate contrast enhancement and artifact-free depiction of coronary, pulmonary, and aortic circulation.

Materials and Methods.—Dedicated coronary 64-MDCT data sets of 50 patients (27 men; mean age, 54 ± 12.4 years) consecutively admitted from the emergency department with suspected acute coronary syndrome were analyzed. Two independent observers graded overall coronary arterial image quality and qualitative and quantitative contrast opacification, motion, and streak artifacts within the pulmonary arteries and aorta.

Results.—Coronary image quality was excellent in 48 patients (96%) and moderate in two patients (4%). Eleven left main and 22 left upper lobar pulmonary arteries were not visualized. Qualitative evaluation showed pulmonary arterial tree opacification to be excellent except for the right and left lower lateral and posterior segmental branches (52–54% rate of poor opacification). Quantitative evaluation showed four central (8%), six lobar (8%), and 206 segmental (29%) branches had poor contrast opacification (< 200 HU). Nineteen right upper lobar arteries (38%) were slightly and one was severely affected by streak artifact. At the segmental pulmonary artery level, marked differences in contrast enhancement were detected between the upper (292 ± 72 HU) and both the middle (249 ± 85 HU) and the lower lobes (248 ± 76 HU) ($p < 0.01$). Mean aortic opacification was 300 ± 34 HU with excellent contrast homogeneity without severe motion or streak artifacts.

Conclusion.—In the evaluation of patients presenting to the emergency department with suspected acute coronary syndrome, a dedicated coronary CT protocol enables excellent assessment of the coronary arteries and proximal ascending aorta but does not depict the pulmonary vasculature well enough for exclusion of pulmonary embolism.

▶ Differentiating acute coronary syndromes (ACS), pulmonary embolism (PE), and aortic dissection from more benign causes of chest pain is crucial in the emergency department. There has been substantial interest in developing a diagnostic tool for the evaluation of low-to-intermediate risk patients with chest pain because the history and physical examination may be misleading,[1] unnecessary hospitalizations of patients with chest pain result in staggering economic costs to society,[2] and a missed diagnosis may have dire consequences. Coronary CT angiography (CCTA) is a highly effective modality to exclude obstructive epicardial coronary artery disease. The negative predictive value of CCTA for ACS was 100% in a blinded, prospective study of 103 patients with acute chest pain.[3] The study performed by Dodd et al[4] addresses a very important question—Is CCTA a useful test to evaluate the aorta and pulmonary vasculature?

Before proceeding with the answer to this question, it is important to distinguish between the so-called "triple rule out" CT protocol and a dedicated CCTA protocol. A triple rule out CT protocol attempts to visualize the entire pulmonary, coronary, and aortic vasculature simultaneously. Compared with the dedicated CCTA protocol, the triple rule out CT protocol entails greater doses of both ionizing radiation and radiographic contrast, and reduced diagnostic accuracy for significant coronary artery stenosis.[5]

Dodd et al[4] retrospectively analyzed the CCTA of 50 patients with acute chest pain and normal or nondiagnostic electrocardiograms who were judged to be low-to-intermediate risk for ACS. After confirming that the coronary angiographic portions of the studies were excellent, they determined whether the pulmonary vasculature and aorta were adequately opacified with contrast medium, and whether image integrity was maintained. Their results indicate that CCTA achieved excellent coronary artery definition in 96% of patients and excellent opacification of the proximal ascending aorta in 96% of patients, with very minor artifact generation. Unfortunately, a large proportion of left main (22%) and left upper lobe pulmonary arteries (44%) were not visualized with the dedicated coronary CT protocol. Also, there was a significant decrement in the opacification of the pulmonary arteries when looking at the proximal (main) to distal (sub-segmental) flow of contrast medium and differential distribution in the lobar divisions. Based on this study, one may conclude that CCTA is an excellent tool for visualizing the coronary arteries and the proximal ascending aorta, but it cannot reliably exclude PE because the entire pulmonary vasculature is not adequately visualized.

S. B. Heitner, MD
S. W. Werns, MD

References

1. Swap CJ, Nagurney JT. Value and limitations of chest pain history in the evaluation of patients with suspected acute coronary syndromes. *JAMA*. 2005;294:2623-2629.
2. Tosteson AN, Goldman L, Udvarhelyi IS, Lee TH. Cost-effectiveness of a coronary care unit versus an intermediate care unit for emergency department patients with chest pain. *Circulation*. 1996;94:143-150.
3. Hoffmann U, Nagurney JT, Moselewski F, et al. Coronary multidetector computed tomography in the assessment of patients with acute chest pain. *Circulation*. 2006;114:2251-2260.
4. Dodd JD, Kalva S, Pena A, et al. Emergency cardiac CT for suspected acute coronary syndrome: qualitative and quantitative assessment of coronary, pulmonary, and aortic image quality. *AJR Am J Roentgenol*. 2008;191:870-877.
5. Johnson TR, Nikolaou K, Wintersperger BJ, et al. ECG-gated 64-MDCT angiography in the differential diagnosis of acute chest pain. *AJR Am J Roentgenol*. 2007;188:76-82.

Assessing the effectiveness of primary angioplasty compared with thrombolysis and its relationship to time delay: a Bayesian evidence synthesis
Asseburg C, Vergel YB, Palmer S, et al (Univ of York, UK)
Heart 93:1244-1250, 2007

Background.—Meta-analyses of trials have shown greater benefits from angioplasty than thrombolysis after an acute myocardial infarction, but the time delay in initiating angioplasty needs to be considered.

Objective.—To extend earlier meta-analyses by considering 1- and 6-month outcome data for both forms of reperfusion. To use Bayesian statistical methods to quantify the uncertainty associated with the estimated relationships.

Methods.—A systematic review and meta-analysis published in 2003 was updated. Data on key clinical outcomes and the difference between time-to-balloon and time-to-needle were independently extracted by two researchers. Bayesian statistical methods were used to synthesise evidence despite differences between reported follow-up times and outcomes. Outcomes are presented as absolute probabilities of specific events and odds ratios (ORs; with 95% credible intervals (CrI)) as a function of the additional time delay associated with angioplasty.

Results.—22 studies were included in the meta-analysis, with 3760 and 3758 patients randomised to primary angioplasty and thrombolysis, respectively. The mean (SE) angioplasty-related time delay (over and above time to thrombolysis) was 54.3 (2.2) minutes. For this delay, mean event probabilities were lower for primary angioplasty for all outcomes. Mortality within 1 month was 4.5% after angioplasty and 6.4% after thrombolysis (OR = 0.68 (95% CrI 0.46 to 1.01)). For non-fatal reinfarction, OR = 0.32 (95% CrI 0.20 to 0.51); for non-fatal stroke OR = 0.24 (95% CrI 0.11 to 0.50). For all outcomes, the benefit of angioplasty decreased with longer delay from initiation.

Conclusions.—The benefit of primary angioplasty, over thrombolysis, depends on the former's additional time delay. For delays of 30–90 minutes, angioplasty is superior for 1-month fatal and non-fatal outcomes. For delays of around 90 minutes thrombolysis may be the preferred option as assessed by 6-month mortality; there is considerable uncertainty for longer time delays.

▶ Four well-designed, multicenter, randomized trials established that 3 fibrinolytic agents (streptokinase,[1,2] anisolylated plasminogen-streptokinase activator complex,[3] and tissue plasminogen activator[4]) each reduced short-term and long-term mortality in patients with acute myocardial infarction. Nevertheless, the most recent update of the American College of Cardiology/American Heart Association (ACC/AHA) practice guidelines for the management of ST-segment elevation myocardial infarction (STEMI) expressed a preference for primary angioplasty if it can be performed within 90 minutes of first medical contact.[5] Unfortunately, it is well documented that the so-called door-to-balloon time usually exceeds 90 minutes, especially in patients who present during off-hours or who must undergo interhospital transfer to receive percutaneous coronary intervention (PCI).[6] Therefore, it is important to consider the relationship between time to treatment and the relative effectiveness of PCI compared with fibrinolytic therapy.

Asseburg et al[7] performed a meta-analysis of 22 trials that randomized 3760 patients to PCI and 3758 patients to fibrinolytic therapy. This updated meta-analysis confirmed that for the mean angioplasty-related time delay of 54 minutes, that is, the additional time required for angioplasty compared with fibrinolytic therapy, primary angioplasty was associated with lower 1-month and 6-month rates of death, nonfatal reinfarction, and nonfatal stroke. However, as the angioplasty-related time delay increased, the absolute differences between angioplasty and fibrinolytic therapy, and the probability that angioplasty is superior, both diminished. The authors suggest that fibrinolytic therapy may be preferable when the angioplasty-related time delay is 90 minutes. This is consistent with the current practice guideline that recommends fibrinolytic therapy for patients who cannot undergo PCI within 90 minutes of first medical contact.[5]

S. W. Werns, MD

References

1. Gruppo Italiano per lo Studio della Streptochinasi nell'Infarto Miocardico (GISSI). Effectiveness of intravenous thrombolytic treatment in acute myocardial infarction. *Lancet.* 1986;1:397-402.
2. ISIS-2 (Second International Study of Infarct Survival) Collaborative Group. Randomised trial of intravenous streptokinase, oral aspirin, both, or neither among 17,187 cases of suspected acute myocardial infarction. *Lancet.* 1988;2:349-360.
3. AIMS Trial Study Group. Long-term effects of intravenous anistreplase in acute myocardial infarction: final report of the AIMS study. *Lancet.* 1990;335:427-431.
4. Wilcox RG, von der Lippe G, Olsson CG, Jensen G, Skene AM, Hampton JR. Trial of tissue plasminogen activator for mortality reduction in acute myocardial infarction. Anglo-Scandinavian Study of Early Thrombolysis (ASSET). *Lancet.* 1988;2:525-530.
5. Antman EM, Hand M, Armstrong PW, et al. 2007 focused update of the ACC/AHA 2004 guidelines for the management of patients with ST-elevation myocardial infarction: a report of the American College of Cardiology/American Heart Association Task Force on Practice Guidelines. *J Am Coll Cardiol.* 2008; 51:210-247.
6. Nallamothu BK, Bradley EH, Krumholz HM. Time to treatment in primary percutaneous coronary intervention. *N Engl J Med.* 2007;357:1631-1638.
7. Asseburg C, Vergel YB, Palmer S, et al. Assessing the effectiveness of primary angioplasty compared with thrombolysis and its relationship to time delay: a Bayesian evidence synthesis. *Heart.* 2007;93:1244-1250.

Impact of Red Blood Cell Transfusion on Clinical Outcomes in Patients With Acute Myocardial Infarction

Aronson D, Dann EJ, Bonstein L, et al (Rambam Med Ctr and the Bruce Rappaport Faculty of Medicine, Haifa, Israel)
Am J Cardiol 102:115-119, 2008

Divergent views remain regarding the safety of treating anemia with red blood cell (RBC) transfusion in patients with acute coronary syndrome (ACS). We used a prospective database to study effect of RBC transfusion in patients with acute myocardial infarction (MI; n = 2,358). Cox regression models were used to determine the association between RBC transfusion and 6-month outcomes, incorporating transfusion as a time-dependent variable. The models adjusted for baseline variables, propensity for transfusion, and nadir hemoglobin previous to the transfusion. One hundred ninety-two patients (8.1%) received RBC transfusion. Six-month mortality rates were higher in patients receiving transfusion (28.1% vs 11.7%, p <0.0001). The adjusted hazard ratio (HR) for mortality was 1.9 in transfused patients (95% confidence interval [CI] 1.3 to 2.9). Interaction between RBC transfusion and nadir hemoglobin with respect to mortality (p = 0.004) was significant. Stratified analyses showed a protective effect of transfusion in patients with nadir hemoglobin ≤8 g/dL (adjusted HR 0.13, 95% CI 0.03 to 0.65, p = 0.013). By contrast, transfusion was associated with increased mortality in patients with nadir hemoglobin >8 g/dL (adjusted HR 2.2, 95% CI 1.5 to 3.3; p <0.0001). Similar results were obtained for the composite end point of death/MI/heart failure (p for interaction = 0.04). In conclusion, RBC transfusion in patients with acute MI and hemoglobin ≤8 g/dL may be appropriate. The increased mortality observed in transfused patients with nadir hemoglobin above 8 g/dL underscores the clinical difficulty of balancing risks and benefits of RBC transfusion in the setting of ACS.

▶ Anemia is well documented to be a risk factor for poor outcomes in patients with ischemic heart disease. Largely as a result of this fact it has been well established as conventional wisdom that patients with such pathology should have their hemoglobin levels maintained at a level of at least 10 g/dL, especially in the setting of acute ischemia or myocardial infarction (MI). Despite the appearance of a substantial body of literature in the last several years suggesting that transfusion of packed red blood cells (PRBCs) to anemic patients with myocardial ischemia may not be beneficial and may, in fact, be harmful, there remains a high degree of skepticism and, indeed, resistance to this concept. In this study, the investigators used information obtained via a prospectively collected database and analyzed with both traditional methods and propensity analysis to attempt to account for factors that may have influenced the decision to transfuse patients presenting with acute MI. Similar to other studies published in the past few years, these investigators found that in the setting of acute coronary syndrome (ACS), PRBC transfusion, at least when hemoglobin levels are > 8 g/dL, is associated with poor outcomes as defined by a variety of parameters. Transfusion of patients with lower hemoglobin values seemed to confer an outcome benefit. The limitations of stored RBCs to deliver oxygen are well defined, although perhaps not well recognized by clinicians who prescribe their use. Perhaps equally if not more important are the direct adverse effects of stored PRBC including their potential prothrombotic and inflammatory properties, as pointed out by the authors. Despite this additional evidence arguing against the routine transfusion of PRBC in anemic patients with acute MI it remains questionable whether many clinicians are ready to alter their ingrained practice. Although one could certainly take the position, when objectively reviewing the literature to date, that the question of whether or not patients with ischemic heart disease routinely require transfusion has already been answered, as called for by the authors in their concluding statement, randomized controlled trials are likely needed to settle the issue of what the optimal transfusion strategies are in ACS.

D. R. Gerber, DO

Cardiac Arrest

Mild therapeutic hypothermia in patients after out-of-hospital cardiac arrest due to acute ST-segment elevation myocardial infarction undergoing immediate percutaneous coronary intervention
Wolfrum S, Pierau C, Radke PW, et al (Univ of Schleswig-Holstein, Lübeck, Germany)
Crit Care Med 36:1780-1786, 2008

Objective.—Mild therapeutic hypothermia (MTH) has been integrated into international resuscitation guidelines. In the majority of patients, sudden cardiac arrest is caused by myocardial infarction. This study investigated whether a combination of MTH with primary percutaneous coronary intervention (PCI) is feasible, safe, and potentially beneficial in patients after cardiac arrest due to acute myocardial infarction.
Design.—Single-center observational study with a historical control group.
Setting.—University clinic.
Patients.—Thirty-three patients after cardiac arrest with ventricular fibrillation as initial rhythm and restoration of spontaneous circulation who remained unconscious at admission and presented with acute ST elevation myocardial infarction (STEMI).
Interventions.—In 16 consecutive patients (2005–2006), MTH was initiated immediately after admission and continued during primary PCI. Seventeen consecutive patients who were treated in a similar 2-yr observation interval before implementation of MTH (2003–2004) served as a control group. Feasibility, safety, mortality, and neurologic outcome were documented.
Measurements and Main Results.—Initiation of MTH did not result in longer door-to-balloon times compared with the control group (82 vs. 85 mins), indicating that implementation of MTH did not delay the onset of primary PCI. Target temperature (32–34°C) in the MTH group was reached within 4 hrs, consistent with previous trials and suggesting that primary PCI did not affect the velocity of cooling. Despite a tendency to increased bleeding complications and infections, patients treated with MTH tended to have a lower mortality after 6 months (25% vs. 35%, $p = .71$) and an improved neurologic outcome as determined by a Glasgow-Pittsburgh Cerebral Performance Scale score of 1 or 2 (69% vs. 47% in the control group, $p = .30$).
Conclusions.—MTH in combination with primary PCI is feasible and safe in patients resuscitated after cardiac arrest due to acute myocardial infarction. A combination of these therapeutic procedures should be strongly considered as standard therapy in patients after out-of-hospital cardiac arrest due to STEMI.

▶ This is a single-center observational study of a cohort of patients treated with therapeutic hypothermia (TH) during percutaneous coronary intervention (PCI) compared with a cohort of historical controls undergoing coronary intervention without TH. The authors were testing the hypothesis that TH during coronary intervention for acute myocardial infarction (MI) is feasible and does not impair the ability to provide rapid PCI. The authors used external cooling techniques (cold packs and cooling mattresses) and cold intervenous saline infusion to induce hypothermia.

As compared with those patients undergoing PCI in the historical control group, the patients treated with hypothermia just before cardiac catheterization had similar door-to-balloon times. The intervention group achieved the target temperature within 4 hours. The authors concluded that it is feasible to rapidly induce hypothermia in patients undergoing PCI after cardiac arrest because of ST-segment elevation MI, and that the procedures for induction of hypothermia will not slow door-to-balloon times.

This study has important implications. As TH penetrates into clinical practice and becomes a standard of care, it will be important to know how the rapid application of this new innovation affects other time-sensitive goals, such as door-to-balloon time. Just as door-to-balloon time is recognized to be a critical determinant of outcome in patients with acute MI, rapid institution of TH to provide neuroprotection against anoxic brain injury is also a critical action. This study indicates that both of the critical actions can simultaneously (rather than consecutively) be achieved.

S. Trzeciak, MD, MPH

Early predictors of outcome in comatose survivors of ventricular fibrillation and non-ventricular fibrillation cardiac arrest treated with hypothermia: A prospective study

Oddo M, Ribordy V, Feihl F, et al (Lausanne Univ Med Ctr, Switzerland)
Crit Care Med 36:2296-2301, 2008

Objectives.—Current indications for therapeutic hypothermia (TH) are restricted to comatose patients with cardiac arrest (CA) due to ventricular fibrillation (VF) and without circulatory shock. Additional studies are needed to evaluate the benefit of this treatment in more heterogeneous groups of patients, including those with non-VF rhythms and/or shock and to identify early predictors of outcome in this setting.

Design.—Prospective study, from December 2004 to October 2006.

Setting.—32-bed medico-surgical intensive care unit, university hospital.

Patients.—Comatose patients with out-of-hospital CA.

Interventions.—TH to 33 ± 1°C (external cooling, 24 hrs) was administered to patients resuscitated from CA due to VF and non-VF (including asystole or pulseless electrical activity), independently from the presence of shock.

Measurements and Main Results.—We hypothesized that simple clinical criteria available on hospital admission (initial arrest rhythm, duration of CA, and presence of shock) might help to identify patients who eventually survive and might most benefit from TH. For this purpose, outcome was related to these predefined variables. Seventy-four patients (VF 38, non-VF 36) were included; 46% had circulatory shock. Median duration of CA (time from collapse to return of spontaneous circulation [ROSC]) was 25 mins. Overall survival was 39.2%. However, only 3.1% of patients with time to ROSC >25 mins survived, as compared to 65.7% with time to ROSC ≤25 mins. Using a logistic regression analysis, time from collapse to ROSC, but not initial arrest rhythm or presence of shock, independently predicted survival at hospital discharge.

Conclusions.—Time from collapse to ROSC is strongly associated with outcome following VF and non-VF cardiac arrest treated with therapeutic hypothermia and could therefore be helpful to identify patients who benefit most from active induced cooling.

▶ Therapeutic hypothermia (HT) has been shown to improve outcomes in patients with return of spontaneous circulation (ROSC) after cardiac arrest (CA) because of ventricular fibrillation or ventricular tachycardia. However, the landmark randomized controlled trials of HT excluded patients with sustained postresuscitation circulatory shock, and so the best course of action in these patients is unclear.

This was a prospective study conducted between December 2004 and October 2006 in a 32-bed adult medico-surgical ICU of a university hospital. The goal of the study was to compare outcomes in out-of-hospital CA patients who received HT with and without sustained postresuscitation circulatory shock, defined as mean arterial pressure < 60 mm Hg or systolic pressure < 90 mm Hg despite fluid administration leading to the use of norepinephrine (or a cardiac index measured by pulmonary catheter < 2.2 $L/min^{-1}/m^{-2}$ requiring use of dobutamine). The outcome measures were survival and neurological recovery, using Glasgow-Pittsburgh Cerebral Performance categories (CPC), at time of discharge.

The authors found no statistically significant difference in outcome in patients with or without sustained postresuscitation circulatory shock (35.3% vs 42.5% *P*-value 0.52 for survival and 26.5% vs 37.5% *P*-value 0.31 for good neurologic recovery).

This study has several limitations. The first is a relatively small sample size. A second limitation is defining time from collapse to ROSC (ie, unwitnessed collapse may underestimate the duration of CA). Along the same lines, time to cardiopulmonary resuscitation (CPR) and quality of CPR could not be addressed in this study. Importantly, although this study shows no statistical difference in outcomes among patients who receive HT with or without sustained postresuscitation circulatory shock, the study itself does not answer the question as to whether or not HT is beneficial in patients with sustained postresuscitation circulatory shock. Further randomized controlled trials are needed to compare outcomes in patients with sustained postresuscitation circulatory shock who do and do not receive HT.

B. Roberts, MD
S. Trzeciak, MD, MPH

Survival From In-Hospital Cardiac Arrest During Nights and Weekends
Peberdy MA, Ornato JP, Larkin GL, et al (Virginia Commonwealth Univ, Richmond; Yale School of Medicine, New Haven, CN; et al)
JAMA 299:785-792, 2008

Context.—Occurrence of in-hospital cardiac arrest and survival patterns have not been characterized by time of day or day of week. Patient physiology and process of care for in-hospital cardiac arrest may be different at night and on weekends because of hospital factors unrelated to patient, event, or location variables.

Objective.—To determine whether outcomes after in-hospital cardiac arrest differ during nights and weekends compared with days/evenings and weekdays.

Design and Setting.—We examined survival from cardiac arrest in hourly time segments, defining day/evening as 7:00 AM to 10:59 PM, night as 11:00 PM to 6:59 AM, and weekend as 11:00 PM on Friday to 6:59 AM on Monday, in 86 748 adult, consecutive in-hospital cardiac arrest events in the National Registry of Cardiopulmonary Resuscitation obtained from 507 medical/surgical participating hospitals from January 1, 2000, through February 1, 2007.

Main Outcome Measures.—The primary outcome of survival to discharge and secondary outcomes of survival of the event, 24-hour survival, and favorable neurological outcome were compared using odds ratios and multivariable logistic regression analysis. Point estimates of survival outcomes are reported as percentages with 95% confidence intervals (95% CIs).

Results.—A total of 58 593 cases of in-hospital cardiac arrest occurred during day/evening hours (including 43 483 on weekdays and 15 110 on weekends), and 28 155 cases occurred during night hours (including 20 365 on weekdays and 7790 on weekends). Rates of survival to discharge (14.7% [95% CI, 14.3%-15.1%] vs 19.8% [95% CI, 19.5%-20.1%], return of spontaneous circulation for longer than 20 minutes (44.7% [95% CI, 44.1%-45.3%] vs 51.1% [95% CI, 50.7%-51.5%]), survival at 24 hours (28.9% [95% CI, 28.4%-29.4%] vs 35.4% [95% CI, 35.0%-35.8%]), and favorable neurological outcomes (11.0% [95% CI, 10.6%-11.4%] vs 15.2% [95% CI, 14.9%-15.5%]) were substantially lower during the night compared with day/evening (all *P* values <.001). The first documented rhythm at night was more frequently asystole (39.6% [95% CI, 39.0%-40.2%] vs 33.5% [95% CI, 33.2%-33.9%], *P* <.001) and less frequently ventricular fibrillation (19.8% [95% CI, 19.3%-20.2%] vs 22.9% [95% CI, 22.6%-23.2%], *P* <.001). Among in-hospital cardiac arrests occurring during day/evening hours, survival was higher on weekdays (20.6% [95% CI, 20.3%-21%]) than on weekends (17.4% [95% CI, 16.8%-18%]; odds ratio, 1.15 [95% CI, 1.09-1.22]), whereas among in-hospital cardiac arrests occurring during night hours, survival to discharge was similar on weekdays (14.6% [95% CI,

14.1%-15.2%]) and on weekends (14.8% [95% CI, 14.1%-15.2%]; odds ratio, 1.02 [95% CI, 0.94-1.11]).

Conclusion.—Survival rates from in-hospital cardiac arrest are lower during nights and weekends, even when adjusted for potentially confounding patient, event, and hospital characteristics.

▶ It has been reported that nearly 100 000 preventable in-hospital deaths occur in the United States every year. Sudden cardiac arrest (CA) is the most common lethal manifestation of cardiovascular disease. Suboptimal care of CA victims in the hospital could be an important source of increased morbidity and mortality. This study aimed to test the hypothesis that survival from in-hospital CA was lower at night and on weekends. The significance of this research is that it could provide important information that has implications for hospital staffing patterns and resource allocation. This was a registry study using the National Registry of Cardiopulmonary Resuscitation (NRCPR). The authors compared CA occurring after 11:00 PM and on the weekends to CA occurring during day/evening hours on weekdays.

Of the 58 593 CA cases, 28 155 occurred at night and 15 110 occurred on the weekends. The authors found lower survival from in-hospital CA during nights and weekends. This result was held up after multiple adjustments for potential confounders, including patient and hospital characteristics.

The initial rhythm during the off hours was also much more likely to be asystole or pulseless electrical activity, indicating that delays to identification of the CA were likely occurring.

This is an important study that has implications for processes of care and hospital staffing patterns. It can be assumed that delays in identification of the in-hospital CA were occurring, but it is also possible that the quality of CPR during off hours is also suboptimal. Determining whether this is merely an issue of timeliness of identification versus CPR quality would be an important area for future research.

S. Trzeciak, MD, MPH

Delayed Time to Defibrillation after In-Hospital Cardiac Arrest
Chan PS, Krumholz HM, Nichol G, et al (Saint Luke's Mid-America Heart Inst, Kansas City, MO; Yale Univ School of Medicine, New Haven; The Univ of Washington–Harborview Ctr for Prehospital Emergency Care, Seattle; et al)
N Engl J Med 358:9-17, 2008

Background.—Expert guidelines advocate defibrillation within 2 minutes after an in-hospital cardiac arrest caused by ventricular arrhythmia. However, empirical data on the prevalence of delayed defibrillation in the United States and its effect on survival are limited.

Methods.—We identified 6789 patients who had cardiac arrest due to ventricular fibrillation or pulseless ventricular tachycardia at 369 hospitals participating in the National Registry of Cardiopulmonary Resuscitation.

Using multivariable logistic regression, we identified characteristics associated with delayed defibrillation. We then examined the association between delayed defibrillation (more than 2 minutes) and survival to discharge after adjusting for differences in patient and hospital characteristics.

Results.—The overall median time to defibrillation was 1 minute (interquartile range, <1 to 3 minutes); delayed defibrillation occurred in 2045 patients (30.1%). Characteristics associated with delayed defibrillation included black race, noncardiac admitting diagnosis, and occurrence of cardiac arrest at a hospital with fewer than 250 beds, in an unmonitored hospital unit, and during after-hours periods (5 p.m. to 8 a.m. or weekends). Delayed defibrillation was associated with a significantly lower probability of surviving to hospital discharge (22.2%, vs. 39.3% when defibrillation was not delayed; adjusted odds ratio, 0.48; 95% confidence interval, 0.42 to 0.54; P<0.001). In addition, a graded association was seen between increasing time to defibrillation and lower rates of survival to hospital discharge for each minute of delay (P for trend <0.001).

Conclusions.—Delayed defibrillation is common and is associated with lower rates of survival after in-hospital cardiac arrest.

▶ Previous studies have suggested an association between delay in defibrillation attempt and poor survival; however, these studies may have been confounded by the inclusion of cardiac arrests (CAs) with initial rhythms that are unlikely to be shock-responsive or defibrillation-responsive (asystole, or pulseless electrical activity). The authors used the National Registry of Cardiopulmonary Resuscitation (NRCPR) to test the hypothesis that "delays in defibrillation were an important determinant in survival, specifically in patients with pulseless ventricular tachycardia or ventricular fibrillation."

This was a registry study of 6789 patients in 369 hospitals. The authors found that 30.1% of CA was associated with a delay in defibrillation (defined as greater than 2 minutes). The authors performed a multivariate logistic regression analysis to define a number of patient-centered and hospital-centered variables that were independent predictors of having a delay to defibrillation. More importantly, they report that the delay in defibrillation was associated with a sharply lower rate of survival-to-hospital discharge (22.2% vs 39.3% when defibrillation was not delayed; $P > .001$). There was a decline in rate of survival-to-hospital discharge for each minute of delay that was statistically significant for the trend over time.

Although these results are intuitive to a certain degree, they are nonetheless important. As CPR quality is increasingly recognized as a critical determinant of patient outcome, the promptness of defibrillation attempt for appropriate rhythms is also a critical factor. The next important step for this line of clinical research is to investigate why delays in defibrillation attempts actually occur and to apply systematic interventions to decrease the time to defibrillation in experimental studies. Given that ventricular defibrillation and pulseless ventricular tachycardia represent the more salvageable initial rhythms among CA patients, it is conceivable that novel interventions to decrease the time to defibrillation attempt may translate into improved survival.

S. Trzeciak, MD, MPH

Health care costs, long-term survival, and quality of life following intensive care unit admission after cardiac arrest
Graf J, Mühlhoff C, Doig GS, et al (Philipps-Univ Marburg, Baldingerstrasse, Germany; Univ Hosp Aachen, Pauwelsstrasse 30, Germany; Univ of Sydney, Australia; et al)
Crit Care 12:R92, 2008

Introduction.—The purpose of this study was to investigate the costs and health status outcomes of intensive care unit (ICU) admission in patients who present after sudden cardiac arrest with in-hospital or out-of-hospital cardiopulmonary resuscitation.

Methods.—Five-year survival, health-related quality of life (Medical Outcome Survey Short Form-36 questionnaire, SF-36), ICU costs, hospital costs and post-hospital health care costs per survivor, costs per life year gained, and costs per quality-adjusted life year gained of patients admitted to a single ICU were assessed.

Results.—One hundred ten of 354 patients (31%) were alive 5 years after hospital discharge. The mean health status index of 5-year survivors was 0.77 (95% confidence interval 0.70 to 0.85). Women rated their health-related quality of life significantly better than men did (0.87 versus 0.74; $P < 0.05$). Costs per hospital discharge survivor were 49,952 n. Including the costs of post-hospital discharge health care incurred during their remaining life span, the total costs per life year gained were 10,107 n. Considering 5-year survivors only, the costs per life year gained were calculated as 9,816 euro or 14,487 n per quality-adjusted life year gained. Including seven patients with severe neurological sequelae, costs per life year gained in 5-year survivors increased by 18% to 11,566 n.

Conclusion.—Patients who leave the hospital following cardiac arrest without severe neurological disabilities may expect a reasonable quality of life compared with age- and gender-matched controls. Quality-adjusted costs for this patient group appear to be within ranges considered reasonable for other groups of patients.

▶ This study aimed to characterize the 5-year survival and quality of life for patients that were treated in the ICU after cardiac arrest (CA). It was a single-center study that retrospectively identified all patients admitted to the ICU after CA over a 3-year period, and administered a survey to survivors via mail. They assessed 5-year survival, health-related quality of life indices, posthospital health care costs per survivor, cost per life year gained, and cost per quality-adjusted life year. Of the 354 patients, 110 (31%) were alive at 5 years. The authors found reasonable quality of life in these survivors, and costs per life year gained that were not excessive. The authors concluded that the quality-adjusted costs for these CA survivors were comparable with the ranges of quality-adjusted costs for other critically ill population that are routinely cared for in the ICU setting. As the scientific community continues to investigate novel therapies to treat patients with the post-CA syndrome, and in particular the anoxic encephalopathy after CA, it will be important to understand the long-term effects on quality of life for survivors and the associated cost of care. This study represents an important early step in understanding long-term outcomes from CA.

S. Trzeciak, MD, MPH

Pulmonary Embolism/Pulmonary Artery Hypertension

Hospital volume and patient outcomes in pulmonary embolism
Aujesky D, Mor MK, Geng M, et al (Univ of Lausanne, Switzerland; VA Ctr for Health Equity Res and Promotion, Pittsburgh, PA; et al)
CMAJ 178:27-33, 2008

Background.—In numerous high-risk medical and surgical conditions, a greater volume of patients undergoing treatment in a given setting or facility is associated with better survival. For patients with pulmonary embolism, the relation between the number of patients treated in a hospital (volume) and patient outcome is unknown.

Methods.—We studied discharge records from 186 acute care hospitals in Pennsylvania for a total of 15 531 patients for whom the primary diagnosis was pulmonary embolism. The study outcomes were all-cause mortality in hospital and within 30 days after presentation for pulmonary embolism and the length of hospital stay. We used logistic models to study the association between hospital volume and 30-day mortality and discrete survival models to study the association between in-hospital mortality and time to hospital discharge.

Results.—The median annual hospital volume for pulmonary embolism was 20 patients (interquartile range 10–42). Overall in-hospital mortality was 6.0%, whereas 30-day mortality was 9.3%. In multivariable analysis, very-high-volume hospitals ($\geq$ 42 cases per year) had a significantly lower odds of in-hospital death (odds ratio [OR] 0.71, 95% confidence interval [CI] 0.51–0.99) and of 30-day death (OR 0.71, 95% CI 0.54–0.92) than very-low-volume hospitals (< 10 cases per year). Although patients in the very-high-volume hospitals had a slightly longer length of stay than those in the very-low-volume hospitals (mean difference 0.7 days), there was no association between volume and length of stay.

Interpretation.—In hospitals with a high volume of cases, pulmonary embolism was associated with lower short-term mortality. Further research is required to determine the causes of the relation between volume and outcome for patients with pulmonary embolism.

▶ It has previously been demonstrated that hospitals doing high-volume cardiac surgery have better outcomes compared with those doing lower volumes. This is likely true for almost all complex medical interventions. I am not surprised that the same holds true for pulmonary embolism. It would be interesting to see how large-volume institutions' care differs from small institutions'. Is it related to decisions for filter placement? Is it related to decisions that achieve more rapid adequate anticoagulation? Is it related to more appropriate use of thrombolytic therapy?

R. P. Dellinger, MD

Computerised tomography for the detection of pulmonary emboli in intensive care patients—a retrospective cohort study
Licht A, Sibbald WJ, Levin PD (Univ of Toronto, Ontario, Canada)
Anaesth Intensive Care 36:13-19, 2008

Pulmonary emboli are frequently considered as a cause for respiratory deterioration in intensive care unit (ICU) patients, however empirical observation suggests that computerised tomographic (CT) angiography is infrequently positive after the first 24 hours. This study aimed to determine the rate and risk factors for detection of pulmonary emboli by CT angiography in ICU patients.

All patients undergoing CT angiography >24 hours after ICU admission for respiratory deterioration from April 2000 until January 2004 were included. The positivity rate for pulmonary emboli was determined and risk factors analysed.

Seven (6%) out of 113 CT angiograms were positive for pulmonary emboli. All were found in trauma patients. Comparing positive to negative scans, predefined risk factors including head injury (5/7 positive scans, 71% vs. 23/106 negative scans, 22%, $P = 0.005$), spine injury with neurological impairment (4/7, 57% vs. 9/106, 8%, $P = 0.002$) and lower limb injury (3/7, 43% vs. 12/106, 9%, $P = 0.039$) were significantly more frequent in patients with positive scans. Deep vein thrombosis prophylaxis was employed less frequently prior to a positive scan (in 3/7, 43% patients with positive scans vs. 91/106, 86% patients with negative scans $P = 0.015$). Only the predefined risk factors were independently associated with positive CT angiography on limited logistic regression (OR 24.7 per risk factor, 95% CI 2.38 to 255.1, $P = 0.007$).

Pulmonary emboli were infrequently diagnosed using CT angiography in ICU patients admitted for more than 24 hours and found only in patients with recognised risk factors.

▶ Have you ever been on rounds when a resident says, "Could this be pulmonary embolism?" and sort of wish the comment had not been made? Pulmonary embolism appears to be very rare in patients who develop acute respiratory and cardiac symptomatology after ICU admission.

R. P. Dellinger, MD

Investigating suspected acute pulmonary embolism — what are hospital clinicians thinking?
McQueen AS, Worthy S, Keir MJ (Royal Victoria Infirmary, Newcastle upon Tyne, UK)
Clin Radiol 63:642-650, 2008

Aims.—To assess local clinical knowledge of the appropriate investigation of suspected acute pulmonary embolism (PE) and compare this with the 2003 British Thoracic Society (BTS) guidelines as a national reference standard.

Methods.—A clinical questionnaire was produced based on the BTS guidelines. One hundred and eight-six participants completed the questionnaires at educational sessions for clinicians of all grades, within a single NHS Trust. The level of experience amongst participants ranged from final year medical students to consultant physicians.

Results.—The clinicians were divided into four groups based on seniority: Pre-registration, Junior, Middle, and Senior. Forty-six point eight percent of all the clinicians correctly identified three major risk factors for PE and 25.8% recognized the definition of the recommended clinical probability score from two alternatives. Statements regarding the sensitivity of isotope lung imaging and computed tomography pulmonary angiography (CTPA) received correct responses from 41.4 and 43% of participants, respectively, whilst 81.2% recognized that an indeterminate ventilation–perfusion scintigraphy (V/Q) study requires further imaging. The majority of clinicians correctly answered three clinical scenario questions regarding use of D-dimers and imaging (78, 85, and 57.5%). There was no statistically significant difference between the four groups for any of the eight questions.

Conclusions.—The recommended clinical probability score was unfamiliar to all four groups of clinicians in the present study, and the majority of doctors did not agree that a negative CTPA or isotope lung scintigraphy reliably excluded PE. However, questions based on clinical scenarios received considerably higher rates of correct responses. The results indicate that various aspects of the national guidelines on suspected acute pulmonary embolism are unfamiliar to many UK hospital clinicians. Further research is needed to identify methods to improve this situation, as both clinicians and radiologists have a duty to ensure that patients are appropriately investigated.

▶ There is now ample evidence-based medicine support for 2 important clinical conclusions in the approach to management of pulmonary embolism (PE): (1) The importance of pretest clinical probability assessment by the treating physician in patients being evaluated for possible PE; and (2) the use of a standardized prediction score to make this decision.[1-3] One recent study showed that a combination of a nonelevated D-dimer and a low-range prediction score allowed the treating clinician to avoid any diagnostic test for PE.[4] This article again reinforces how slowly and inefficiently evidence-based medicine is integrated into clinical practice. It also points to the value of formalized performance improvement programs, which score physician performance and provide feedback to more quickly integrate evidence-based medicine into clinical practice.

R. P. Dellinger, MD

References

1. The PIOPED Investigators. Value of the ventilation/perfusion scan in acute pulmonary embolism: results of the Prospective Investigation of Pulmonary Embolism Diagnosis (PIOPED). *JAMA*. 1990;263:2753-2759.
2. Stein PD, Fowler SE, Goodman LR, et al. Multidetector computed tomography for acute pulmonary embolism. *N Engl J Med*. 2006;354:2317-2327.
3. Stein PD, Hull RD, Patel KC, et al. D-dimer for the exclusion of acute venous thrombosis and pulmonary embolism. *Ann Intern Med*. 2004;140:589-602.
4. Anderson DR, Kahn SR, Rodger MA, et al. Computed tomographic pulmonary angiography vs ventilation-perfusion lung scanning in patients with suspected pulmonary embolism: a randomized controlled trial. *JAMA*. 2007;298: 2743-2753.

Retrievable Inferior Vena Cava Filters in High-Risk Trauma and Surgical Patients: Factors Influencing Successful Removal
Hermsen JL, Ibele AR, Faucher LD, et al (Univ of Wisconsin-Madison School of Medicine and Public Health, WI; et al)
World J Surg 32:1444-1449, 2008

Background.—An Inferior vena cava filter (IVCF) provides prophylaxis against pulmonary embolism in patients that cannot be anticoagulated. A removable IVCF (R-IVCF) provides prophylaxis during a high-risk period while potentially eliminating long-term complications associated with a permanent IVCF. Factors influencing success of R-IVCF removal are ill-defined.

Methods.—The study was a retrospective review of a prospectively maintained patient registry comprising patients who received an R-IVCF (Bard Recovery™ and G2™) at an academic level 1 trauma center. The influence of time in vivo, filter design, and filter head position on computed abdominal tomographic (CAT) scan (touching caval wall vs. free) on removal success was examined.

Results.—Ninety-two patients each received an R-IVCF. Thirty-nine patients underwent removal attempt and 30 R-IVCFs were removed. Time in vivo did not affect removal success (success: 228 ± 104 days versus unsuccessful: 289 ± 158 days, $p=0.18$). Filter design impacted filter head position (Recovery: 43% touching versus G2: 6% touching,

$p = 0.023$). Position of the filter head influenced removal success (touching: 50% success versus free: 88% success, $p = 0.021$).

Conclusions.—Position of the filter head is the key determinant of removal success. Specific device designs may impact filter head position as was the case with the two designs in this analysis. Time in vivo does not affect removal success.

▶ Bedside placement of vena cava filters and use of retrievable inferior vena cava filters are increasing. For the first time, significant literature is appearing that gives us some idea of performance and safety issues. Four things, however, are clear: (1) Too many of these patients do not get appropriate follow-up for evaluation for removal of the filter; (2) complications do occur although the frequency seems reasonable; (3) length of placement does influence capability to remove (filter becomes imbedded in the inferior vena cava wall); and (4) initial position of the filter also impacts ability to remove.

R. P. Dellinger, MD

Bedside Placement of Removable Vena Cava Filters Guided by Intravascular Ultrasound in the Critically Injured
Spaniolas K, Velmahos GC, Kwolek C, et al (Massachusetts Gen Hosp and Harvard Med School, Boston, MA)
World J Surg 32:1438-1443, 2008

Background.—Bedside placement of removable inferior vena cava filters (RVCF) is increasingly used in critically injured patients. The need for fluoroscopic equipment and specialized intensive care unit beds presents major challenges. Intravascular ultrasound (IVUS) eliminates such problems. The objective of the present study was to analyze the safety and feasibility of IVUS-guided bedside RVCF placement in critically injured patients.

Methods.—Between October 2004 and July 2006 47 IVUS-guided RVCF were placed at the bedside. Medical and trauma registry records were reviewed. Primary outcome was RVCF-related complications.

Results.—The mean patient age was 41 ± 19 years, and the mean Injury Severity Score was 30 ± 12. The right common femoral vein was chosen as the site of access in 40 patients, and the left common femoral vein was the access site in 7 patients. The insertion was performed 3.7 ± 2.5 days after admission. Four patients (8.5%) developed common femoral deep vein thrombosis (DVT) and three (6%) developed a peripheral pulmonary embolism (PE). Complications related to technique were recorded in two patients (4%) and included one misplacement and one access site bleeding with no further associated morbidity. Five patients died during the hospital stay from issues unrelated to RVCF. Forty-one patients were eligible for follow-up. Removal of RVCF was offered only to 8 patients and was performed successfully in 4 (10%) at a mean of 130 days (range: 44-183 days).

Conclusions.—In this study IVUS-guided bedside placement of RVCF was feasible but was also associated with complications. Follow-up was poor, and the rate of removal disappointingly low, underscoring the need for further exploration of the role of RVCF.

▶ Bedside placement of vena cava filters and use of retrievable inferior vena cava filters are increasing. For the first time, significant literature is appearing that gives us some idea of performance and safety issues. Four things, however, are clear: (1) Too many of these patients do not get appropriate follow-up for evaluation for removal of the filter; (2) complications do occur although the frequency seems reasonable; (3) length of placement does influence capability to remove (filter becomes imbedded in the inferior vena cava wall); and (4) initial position of the filter also impacts the ability to remove.

R. P. Dellinger, MD

Computed Tomographic Pulmonary Angiography vs Ventilation-Perfusion Lung Scanning in Patients with Suspected Pulmonary Embolism: A Randomized Controlled Trial
Anderson DR, Kahn SR, Rodger MA, et al (Dalhousie Univ, Halifax, Nova Scotia, Canada; McGill Univ, Montreal, Quebec, Canada; Ottawa Univ, Ontario; et al)
JAMA 298:2743-2753, 2007

Context.—Ventilation-perfusion ($\dot{V}/\dot{Q}$) lung scanning and computed tomographic pulmonary angiography (CTPA) are widely used imaging procedures for the evaluation of patients with suspected pulmonary embolism. Ventilation-perfusion scanning has been largely replaced by CTPA in many centers despite limited comparative formal evaluations and concerns about CTPA's low sensitivity (ie, chance of missing clinically important pulmonary emboli).

Objectives.—To determine whether CTPA may be relied upon as a safe alternative to $\dot{V}/\dot{Q}$ scanning as the initial pulmonary imaging procedure for excluding the diagnosis of pulmonary embolism in acutely symptomatic patients.

Design, Setting, and Participants.—Randomized, single-blinded noninferiority clinical trial performed at 4 Canadian and 1 US tertiary care centers between May 2001 and April 2005 and involving 1417 patients considered likely to have acute pulmonary embolism based on a Wells clinical model score of 4.5 or greater or a positive D-dimer assay result.

Intervention.—Patients were randomized to undergo either $\dot{V}/\dot{Q}$ scanning or CTPA. Patients in whom pulmonary embolism was considered excluded did not receive antithrombotic therapy and were followed up for a 3-month period.

Main Outcome Measure.—The primary outcome was the subsequent development of symptomatic pulmonary embolism or proximal deep vein thrombosis in patients in whom pulmonary embolism had initially been excluded.

Results.—Seven hundred one patients were randomized to CTPA and 716 to V̇/Q̇ scanning. Of these, 133 patients (19.2%) in the CTPA group vs 101 (14.2%) in the V̇/Q̇ scan group were diagnosed as having pulmonary embolism in the initial evaluation period (difference, 5.0%; 95% confidence interval [CI], 1.1% to 8.9%) and were treated with anticoagulant therapy. Of those in whom pulmonary embolism was considered excluded, 2 of 561 patients (0.4%) randomized to CTPA vs 6 of 611 patients (1.0%) undergoing V̇/Q̇ scanning developed venous thromboembolism in follow-up (difference, −0.6%; 95% CI, −1.6% to 0.3%) including one patient with fatal pulmonary embolism in the V̇/Q̇ group.

Conclusions.—In this study, CTPA was not inferior to V̇/Q̇ scanning in ruling out pulmonary embolism. However, significantly more patients were diagnosed with pulmonary embolism using the CTPA approach. Further research is required to determine whether all pulmonary emboli detected by CTPA should be managed with anticoagulant therapy.

Trial Registration.—isrctn.org Identifier: ISRCTN65486961.

▶ Although this study supports the comparable sensitivity of computed tomographic pulmonary angiography (CTPA) with ventilation-perfusion (V/Q) scanning in ruling out pulmonary embolism (PE), it must be remembered that neither test can be used in isolation of important additional variables such as pretest clinical assessment of probability of PE, D-dimer (especially for emergency department patients), and leg ultrasound. More importantly this article supports the use of a "PE unlikely" Wells score and a nonelevated D-dimer as reason to end evaluation for PE.

R. P. Dellinger, MD

Clinical presentation and time-course of postoperative venous thromboembolism: Results from the RIETE Registry
Arcelus JI, Monreal M, Caprini JA, et al (Departamento de Cirugía de la Universidad de Granada y Hosp Virgen de las Nieves, Granada, Spain; Hosp Universitari Germans Trias i Pujol, Badalona, Spain; Evanston Northwestern Healthcare, Evanston, Illinois)
Thromb Haemost 99:546-551, 2008

There is little literature about the clinical presentation and time-course of postoperative venous thromboembolism (VTE) in different surgical procedures. RIETE is an ongoing, prospective registry of consecutive patients with objectively confirmed, symptomatic acute VTE. In this analysis, we analysed the baseline characteristics, thromboprophylaxis and therapeutic patterns, time-course, and three-month outcome of all patients with postoperative VTE. As of January 2006, there were 1,602 patients with postoperative VTE in RIETE: 393 (25%) after major orthopaedic surgery (145 elective hip arthroplasty, 126 knee arthroplasty, 122 hip fracture); 207 (13%) after cancer surgery; 1,002 (63%) after other procedures. The percentage of patients presenting with clinically overt pulmonary embolism (PE) (48%, 48%, and 50% respectively), the average time elapsed from surgery to VTE (22 ± 16, 24 ± 16, and 21 ± 15 days, respectively), and the three-month incidence of fatal PE (1.3%, 1.4%, and 0.8%, respectively), fatal bleeding (0.8%, 1.0%, and 0.2%, respectively), or major bleeding (2.3%, 2.9%, and 2.8%, respectively) were similar in the three groups. However, the percentage of patients who had received thromboprophylaxis (96%, 76% and 52%, respectively), the duration of prophylaxis (17 ± 9.6, 13 ± 8.9, and 12 ± 11 days, respectively) and the mean daily doses of low-molecular-weight heparin (4,252 ± 1,016, 3,260 ± 1,141, and 3,769 ± 1,650 IU, respectively), were significantly lower in those undergoing cancer surgery or other procedures. In conclusion, the clinical presentation, time-course, and three-month outcome of VTE was similar among the different subgroups of patients, but the use of prophylaxis in patients undergoing cancer surgery or other procedures was suboptimal.

▶ This study provides important information on timing of occurrence of postoperative thromboembolism. This diagnosis clearly needs to remain a significant consideration in the differential diagnosis of acute symptomatology during the first month after surgery.

R. P. Dellinger, MD

Cardiopulmonary Resuscitation/Other

Sodium Nitroprusside for Advanced Low-Output Heart Failure
Mullens W, Abrahams Z, Francis GS, et al (Cleveland Clinic, Ohio)
J Am Coll Cardiol 52:200-207, 2008

Objectives.—This study was designed to examine the safety and efficacy of sodium nitroprusside (SNP) for patients with acute decompensated heart failure (ADHF) and low-output states.

Background.—Inotropic therapy has been predominantly used in the management of patients with ADHF presenting with low cardiac output.

Methods.—We reviewed all consecutive patients with ADHF admitted between 2000 and 2005 with a cardiac index ≤2 l/min/m^2 for intensive medical therapy including vasoactive drugs. Administration of SNP was chosen by the attending clinician, nonrandomized, and titrated to a target mean arterial pressure of 65 to 70 mm Hg.

Results.—Compared with control patients (n = 97), cases treated with SNP (n = 78) had significantly higher mean central venous pressure (15 vs. 13 mm Hg; p = 0.001), pulmonary capillary wedge pressure (29 vs. 24 mm Hg; p = 0.001), but similar demographics, medications, and renal function at baseline. Use of SNP was not associated with higher rates of inotropic support or worsening renal function during hospitalization. Patients treated with SNP achieved greater improvement in hemodynamic measurements during hospitalization, had higher rates of oral vasodilator prescription at discharge, and had lower rates of all-cause mortality (29% vs. 44%; odds ratio: 0.48; p = 0.005; 95% confidence interval: 0.29 to 0.80) without increase in rehospitalization rates (58% vs. 56%; p = NS).

Conclusions.—In patients with advanced, low-output heart failure, vasodilator therapy used in conjunction with optimal current medical therapy during hospitalization might be associated with favorable long-term clinical outcomes irrespective of inotropic support or renal dysfunction and remains an excellent therapeutic choice in hospitalized ADHF patients.

▶ Sodium nitroprusside (SNP) has been available as a parenteral agent in cardiovascular medicine for >30 years and is currently recommended as therapy for acute decompensated heart failure (ADHF) by the Heart Failure Society of America (level of evidence: C).[1] The drug exerts its hemodynamic effects by a combination of afterload and preload reduction (through peripheral arterial and pulmonary arterial vasodilatation, as well as venodilatation), resulting in improved cardiac output. The vasodilatation results from liberation of nitric oxide, which may have independent benefits in the treatment of ADHF. Despite the favorable hemodynamic effects, particularly for patients with ADHF and elevated systemic vascular resistance (SVR), 1 study reported that <1% of patients hospitalized for ADHF received SNP.[2] The obstacles to more frequent use of SNP include the risk of thiocyanate toxicity that may occur during high dose or prolonged infusion of SNP. Also, physicians may be reluctant to use SNP in the absence of invasive hemodynamic monitoring, which has not been found to improve outcomes in patients with heart failure.[3] Finally, clinicians may fear that SNP will cause hypotension in patients with ADHF.

The study by Mullens et al[4] is a retrospective analysis of the safety and efficacy of SNP in an extremely morbid population of patients with ADHF who were admitted to a heart failure intensive care unit at the Cleveland Clinic between 2000 and 2005. All of the patients had a cardiac index (CI) [3] 2.0 L/min/m^2 documented by right heart catheterization. The data suggest that treatment with SNP was not associated with an increase in renal failure or the use of inotropic drugs despite a mean baseline CI of 1.6 L/min/m^2 and a mean baseline arterial pressure of 87 mm Hg. The authors postulate that a concomitant increase in cardiac output (the mean CI increased from 1.6 L/min/m^2 to 2.6 L/min/m^2) offsets the reduction in blood pressure during infusion of SNP. Patients treated with SNP achieved greater improvement in hemodynamic measurements during hospitalization, had higher rates of oral vasodilator prescription at discharge, and had lower rates of all-cause mortality during follow-up for a median duration of 25.7 months (29% vs 44%; odds ratio: 0.48; $P = .005$; 95% confidence interval: 0.29 to 0.80).

It is important to note that this was not a randomized or blinded study. The study population was managed at the discretion of the attending cardiologist (with varying degrees of experience using SNP) and followed in a state-of-the-art outpatient setting. Thus, the study design makes it difficult to attribute the remarkable survival benefit solely to treatment with SNP. A potential explanation for the greater survival among the patients who received SNP is the fact that 48% of patients who were treated with SNP were discharged on hydralazine and isosorbide dinitrate (ISDN), compared with only 26% of the patients who were not treated with SNP ($P = .006$). Two randomized, placebo-controlled, double-blind clinical trials demonstrated that the combination of hydralazine and ISDN improves survival in patients with heart failure.[5-7] One can postulate that the hemodyamic improvement that was observed in patients who received SNP resulted in a perception that hydralazine and ISDN would be tolerated. Also, one can speculate that the group of patients who received SNP was more likely to tolerate oral vasodilator therapy. The issue cannot be resolved in the absence of a randomized trial of SNP in patients with ADHF who are discharged from the hospital on comparable medical regimens. Alternative therapies for ADHF, such as milrinone,[8] and nesiritide,[9] have either neutral or possibly adverse effects on survival. Therefore, this study provides welcome evidence that treatment with SNP may have a beneficial effect on the survival of patients who are hospitalized for ADHF.

S. B. Heitner, MD
S. W. Werns, MD

References

1. Heart Failure Society of America. Executive summary: HFSA 2006 Comprehensive Heart Failure Practice Guideline. *J Card Fail.* 2006;12:10-38.
2. Abraham WT, Adams KF, Fonarow GC, et al. In-hospital mortality in patients with acute decompensated heart failure requiring intravenous vasoactive medications: an analysis from the Acute Decompensated Heart Failure National Registry (ADHERE). *J Am Coll Cardiol.* 2005;46:57-64.
3. Binanay C, Califf RM, Hasselblad V, et al. Evaluation study of congestive heart failure and pulmonary artery catheterization effectiveness: the ESCAPE trial. *JAMA.* 2005;294:1625-1633.
4. Mullens W, Abrahams Z, Francis GS, et al. Sodium nitroprusside for advanced low-output heart failure. *J Am Coll Cardiol.* 2008;52:200-207.
5. Cohn JN, Archibald DG, Ziesche S, et al. Effect of vasodilator therapy on mortality in chronic congestive heart failure. Results of a veterans administration cooperative study. *N Engl J Med.* 1986;314:1547-1552.
6. Taylor AL, Ziesche S, Yancy C, et al. Combination of isosorbide dinitrate and hydralazine in blacks with heart failure. *N Engl J Med.* 2004;351:2049-2057.
7. Taylor AL, Ziesche S, Yancy CW, et al. Early and sustained benefit on event-free survival and heart failure hospitalization from fixed-dose combination of isosorbide dinitrate/hydralazine: consistency across subgroups in the African-American Heart Failure Trial. *Circulation.* 2007;115:1747-1753.
8. Cuffe MS, Califf RM, Adams KF Jr, et al. Short-term intravenous milrinone for acute exacerbation of chronic heart failure: a randomized controlled trial. *JAMA.* 2002;287:1541-1547.

9. Sackner-Bernstein JD, Kowalski M, Fox M, Aaronson K. Short-term risk of death after treatment with nesiritide for decompensated heart failure: a pooled analysis of randomized controlled trials. *JAMA.* 2005;293:1900-1905.

Minimally Interrupted Cardiac Resuscitation by Emergency Medical Services for Out-of-Hospital Cardiac Arrest
Bobrow BJ, Clark LL, Ewy GA, et al (Univ of Arizona College of Medicine, Tucson)
JAMA 299:1158-1165, 2008

Context.—Out-of-hospital cardiac arrest is a major public health problem.

Objective.—To investigate whether the survival of patients with out-of-hospital cardiac arrest would improve with minimally interrupted cardiac resuscitation (MICR), an alternate emergency medical services (EMS) protocol.

Design, Setting, and Patients.—A prospective study of survival-to-hospital discharge between January 1, 2005, and November 22, 2007. Patients with out-of-hospital cardiac arrests in 2 metropolitan cities in Arizona before and after MICR training of fire department emergency medical personnel were assessed. In a second analysis of protocol compliance, patients from the 2 metropolitan cities and 60 additional fire departments in Arizona who actually received MICR were compared with patients who did not receive MICR but received standard advanced life support.

Intervention.—Instruction for EMS personnel in MICR, an approach that includes an initial series of 200 uninterrupted chest compressions, rhythm analysis with a single shock, 200 immediate postshock chest compressions before pulse check or rhythm reanalysis, early administration of epinephrine, and delayed endotracheal intubation.

Main Outcome Measure.—Survival-to-hospital discharge.

Results.—Among the 886 patients in the 2 metropolitan cities, survival-to-hospital discharge increased from 1.8% (4/218) before MICR training to 5.4% (36/668) after MICR training (odds ratio [OR], 3.0; 95% confidence interval [CI], 1.1-8.9). In the subgroup of 174 patients with witnessed cardiac arrest and ventricular fibrillation, survival increased from 4.7% (2/43) before MICR training to 17.6% (23/131) after MICR training (OR, 8.6; 95% CI, 1.8-42.0). In the analysis of MICR protocol compliance involving 2460 patients with cardiac arrest, survival was significantly better among patients who received MICR than those who did not (9.1% [60/661] vs 3.8% [69/1799]; OR, 2.7; 95% CI, 1.9-4.1), as well as patients with witnessed ventricular fibrillation (28.4% [40/141] vs 11.9% [46/387]; OR, 3.4; 95% CI, 2.0-5.8).

Conclusions.—Survival-to-hospital discharge of patients with out-of-hospital cardiac arrest increased after implementation of MICR as an alternate EMS protocol. These results need to be confirmed in a randomized trial.

▶ Out-of-hospital cardiac arrest (CA) is a major public health problem and leading cause of death from cardiovascular disease. Despite important advances in cardiopulmonary resuscitation (CPR) and resuscitation science over the past few decades, few patients with out-of-hospital CA survive. A new approach to CPR is minimally interrupted cardiac resuscitation (MICR), also known as cardiocerebral resuscitation. Developed in Tuscon, Arizona in 2003, the approach focuses on minimizing interruption of chest compressions. The MICR protocol is defined by the presence of the following 4 criteria: (1) immediately provided 200 preshock chest compressions; (2) 200 postshock compressions; (3) delayed endotracheal intubation for 3 cycles of rhythm analysis; and (4) early administration of epinephrine (given in the first or second cycle of chest compressions).

The data for this study was collected by the Save Hearts in Arizona Registry and Education (SHARE) program of the Bureau of Emergency Medical Services and Trauma System, a part of the Arizona Department of Health Services. The goal of this study was to investigate whether survival of patients with out-of-hospital CA would improve with MICR. The primary outcome measure was survival-to-hospital discharge and secondary outcome measures were return to spontaneous circulation, favorable neurological outcome, and survival-to-hospital admission. The study was a before-and-after analysis of MICR training of EMS personnel in 2 metropolitan fire departments in Arizona and secondly, they compared patients who received MICR and those who did not receive MICR in 2 metropolitan and 60 additional fire departments throughout the state.

The authors found an increase in survival-to-hospital discharge after MICR training compared with pre-MICR (5.4% vs 1.8%, adjusted odds ratio [OR], 3.0; 95% confidence interval [CI], 1.1-8.9). They also found an increase in survival-to-hospital discharge in those patients receiving MICR versus those who did not receive MICR (9.1% vs 3.8%, adjusted OR, 2.7; 95% CI 1.9-4.1). Neurologic outcomes were also shown to be better in patients receiving MICR based on patient Cerebral Performance Categories (CPC) score after hospital discharge.

This study has several potential confounding variables, most notably the MICR patients were younger. Also, it is unknown if there is any bias by the EMS personnel as to who received MICR, and if there were differences in the quality of chest compressions between the 2 groups. Despite the above limitations, this article demonstrates potential for MICR to increase survival-to-hospital discharge and better neurologic outcomes in patients with out-of-hospital CA. Further research in the form of experimental studies (ie, randomized controlled trials) is warranted.

B. Roberts, MD
S. Trzeciak, MD, MPH

Does the prognosis of cardiac arrest differ in trauma patients?
David J-S, Gueugniaud P-Y, Riou B, et al (Université Lyon 1, Faculté Lyon-Sud, Pierre-Bénite, France; Université Pierre et Marie Curie-Paris-6, France; et al)
Crit Care Med 35:2251-2255, 2007

Objective.—It is proposed to not resuscitate trauma patients who have a cardiac arrest outside the hospital because they are assumed to have a dismal prognosis. Our aim was to compare the outcome of patients with traumatic or nontraumatic ("medical") out-of-hospital cardiac arrest.

Design.—Cohort analysis of patients with out-of-hospital cardiac arrest included in the European Epinephrine Study Group's trial comparing high vs. standard doses of epinephrine.

Setting.—Nine French university hospitals.

Patients.—A total of 2,910 patients.

Interventions.—Patients were successively and randomly assigned to receive repeated high doses (5 mg each) or standard doses (1 mg each) of epinephrine at 3-min intervals.

Measurements and Main Results.—Return of spontaneous circulation, survival to hospital admission and discharge, and secondary outcome measures of 1-yr survival and neurologic outcome were recorded. In the trauma group, patients were younger (42 ± 17 vs. 62 ± 17 yrs, $p < .001$), presented with fewer witnessed out-of-hospital cardiac arrests (62.3% vs. 79.7%), and had fewer instances of ventricular fibrillation as the first documented pulseless rhythm (3.4% [95% confidence interval, 1.2–5.5%] vs. 17.3% [15.8–18.7%]). A return of spontaneous circulation was observed in 91 of 268 trauma patients (34.0% [28.3–39.6%]) compared with 797 of 2,642 medical patients (30.2% [28.4–31.9%]), and more trauma patients survived to be admitted to the hospital (29.9% [24.4–35.3%] vs. 23.5% [22.0–25.2%]). However, there was no significant difference between trauma and medical groups at hospital discharge (2.2% [0.5–4.0%] vs. 2.8% [2.1–3.4%]) and 1-yr survival (1.9% [0.3–3.5%] vs. 2.5% [1.9–3.1%]). Among patients who were discharged, a good neurologic status was observed in two trauma patients (33.3% [4.3–77.7%]) and 37 medical patients (50% [38.1–61.9%]).

Conclusions.—The survival and neurologic outcome of out-of-hospital cardiac arrest were not different between trauma and medical patients. This result suggests that, under the supervision of senior physicians, active resuscitation after out-of-hospital cardiac arrest is as important in trauma as in medical patients.

▶ Many studies have demonstrated a dismal prognosis for patients with trauma-associated cardiac arrest (CA). Although a few recent studies have demonstrated better survival-to-discharge in this population, the literature is still largely pessimistic.

This study by David et al was a secondary analysis of a previous study comparing high versus standard doses of epinephrine in the treatment of out-of-hospital

CA patients. The David et al study compares patients with trauma-associated versus "medical" etiology of arrest with respect to the following outcomes: return of spontaneous circulation, survival-to-hospital admission and hospital discharge, as well as neurologic status and survival at 1 year. The authors found no difference in survival or neurologic outcome in the 2 groups and suggest that active resuscitation is as important in trauma patients as in medical patients.

The generalizability of this French study is somewhat limited because of the high level of physician involvement in the prehospital care of these patients. The fact that these patients received more advance care in the field than they might have in other countries may have elevated the survival rate for the trauma patients. The study is also limited by not discriminating among different mechanisms of trauma in their population that has been shown to affect survival in trauma-associated CA. Nevertheless, this study contributes new data to the literature suggesting that despite the poor prognosis of trauma-associated CA, aggressive resuscitation is as beneficial to trauma as nontrauma CA patients.

D. Lundy, MD
S. Trzeciak, MD, MPH

Improving In-Hospital Cardiac Arrest Process and Outcomes With Performance Debriefing

Edelson DP, Litzinger B, Arora V, et al (Univ of Chicago, Chicago, IL; et al)
Arch Intern Med 168:1063-1069, 2008

Background.—Recent investigations have documented poor cardiopulmonary resuscitation (CPR) performance in clinical practice. We hypothesized that a debriefing intervention using CPR quality data from actual in-hospital cardiac arrests (resuscitation with actual performance integrated debriefing [RAPID]) would improve CPR performance and initial patient survival.

Methods.—Internal medicine residents at a university hospital attended weekly debriefing sessions of the prior week's resuscitations, between March 2006 and February 2007, reviewing CPR performance transcripts obtained from a CPR-sensing and feedback-enabled defibrillator. Objective metrics of CPR performance and initial return of spontaneous circulation were compared with a historical cohort in which a similar feedback-delivering defibrillator was used but without RAPID.

Results.—Cardiopulmonary resuscitation quality and outcome data from 123 patients resuscitated during the intervention period were compared with 101 patients in the baseline cohort. Compared with the control period, the mean (SD) ventilation rate decreased (13 [7]/min vs 18 [8]/min; $P < .001$) and compression depth increased (50 [10] vs 44 [10] mm; $P = .001$), among other CPR improvements. These changes correlated with an increase in the rate of return of spontaneous circulation in the RAPID group (59.4% vs 44.6%; $P=.03$) but no change in survival to discharge (7.4% vs 8.9%; $P=.69$).

Conclusions.—The combination of RAPID and real-time audiovisual feedback improved CPR quality compared with the use of feedback alone and was associated with an increased rate of return of spontaneous circulation. Cardiopulmonary resuscitation sensing and recording devices allow for methods of debriefing that were previously available only for simulation-based education; such methods have the potential to fundamentally alter resuscitation training and improve patient outcomes.

Trial Registration.—Clinicaltrials.gov Identifier: NCT00228293.

▶ The quality of CPR is now recognized to be a critical determinant of survival for patients who suffer cardiac arrest (CA). In particular, the rate and depth of chest compressions and avoidance of hyperventilation are recognized to be important factors. Therefore, measuring the quality of CPR and finding new ways to provide feedback to providers about their performance are very important to improving CPR quality.

This was a prospective observational study performed in a university medical center. The hospital uses defibrillators and monitors that have CPR-sensing capabilities. Via an impedance technique, the defibrillators can measure and record the rate of compression, depth of compression, and frequency of ventilations in addition to pauses in chest compressions, defibrillation attempts, and so forth. The control group for this study was a previously published cohort of CA victims. The intervention group was a cohort of patients enrolled over a 1-year period in which the house staff responsible for responding to CA and providing CPR received weekly debriefing sessions of the previous week's resuscitations, in which the trainees reviewed the details of the quality measures of recent CAs. The authors called the intervention period and its training sessions "resuscitation with actual performance integrated debriefing (RAPID)." They tested the hypothesis that the RAPID debriefing intervention would enhance CPR quality and also improve initial patient survival, defined as the rate of return of spontaneous circulation.

There were 123 patients in the RAPID cohort and 101 patients in the control cohort. They found that the RAPID cohort was associated with a decrease in the rate of ventilation, and an increase in the depth of chest compressions. These CPR improvements were also associated with an increase in the rate of return of spontaneous circulation (59.4% for the RAPID group vs 44.6% in controls; $P=.03$). There was no difference among the groups in survival to hospital discharge.

The investigators report a new and viable alternative to conventional training in CPR and CA management. The performance-integrated debriefing improves CPR quality. As quality of CPR is an important determinant of survival, it is conceivable that these new innovations for training may translate to improved clinical outcomes.

S. Trzeciak, MD, MPH

Vasopressin and Epinephrine vs. Epinephrine Alone in Cardiopulmonary Resuscitation

Gueugniaud P-Y, David J-S, Chanzy E, et al (Univ of Lyon 1, France; SAMU 93, Bobigny, France; et al)
N Engl J Med 359:21-30, 2008

Background.—During the administration of advanced cardiac life support for resuscitation from cardiac arrest, a combination of vasopressin and epinephrine may be more effective than epinephrine or vasopressin alone, but evidence is insufficient to make clinical recommendations.

Methods.—In a multicenter study, we randomly assigned adults with out-of-hospital cardiac arrest to receive successive injections of either 1 mg of epinephrine and 40 IU of vasopressin or 1 mg of epinephrine and saline placebo, followed by administration of the same combination of study drugs if spontaneous circulation was not restored and subsequently by additional epinephrine if needed. The primary end point was survival to hospital admission; the secondary end points were return of spontaneous circulation, survival to hospital discharge, good neurologic recovery, and 1-year survival.

Results.—A total of 1442 patients were assigned to receive a combination of epinephrine and vasopressin, and 1452 to receive epinephrine alone. The treatment groups had similar baseline characteristics except that there were more men in the group receiving combination therapy than in the group receiving epinephrine alone (P=0.03). There were no significant differences between the combination-therapy and the epinephrine-only groups in survival to hospital admission (20.7% vs. 21.3%; relative risk of death, 1.01; 95% confidence interval [CI], 0.97 to 1.05), return of spontaneous circulation (28.6% vs. 29.5%; relative risk, 1.01; 95% CI, 0.97 to 1.06), survival to hospital discharge (1.7% vs. 2.3%; relative risk, 1.01; 95% CI, 1.00 to 1.02), 1-year survival (1.3% vs. 2.1%; relative risk, 1.01; 95% CI, 1.00 to 1.02), or good neurologic recovery at hospital discharge (37.5% vs. 51.5%; relative risk, 1.29; 95% CI, 0.81 to 2.06).

Conclusions.—As compared with epinephrine alone, the combination of vasopressin and epinephrine during advanced cardiac life support for out-of-hospital cardiac arrest does not improve outcome. (ClinicalTrials.gov number, NCT00127907.)

▶ Epinephrine has been the cornerstone of vasoactive drug therapy in the treatment of cardiac arrest (CA). Some experimental data have suggested that there may be an added benefit of vasopressor administration instead of catecholamines alone. Conceptually, it makes sense that stimulation of vasopressin receptors in addition to stimulation of catecholamine receptors may augment blood flow to vital organs during CA resuscitation. However, there was no high-level clinical data to be able to advocate the routine use of vasopressin in addition to epinephrine.

The authors aimed to test the hypothesis that the addition of vasopressin to epinephrine would improve clinical outcome for CA victims. They tested this hypothesis with a randomized double-blind placebo controlled trial in a large multicenter network in France.

There were nearly 3000 patients enrolled in this trial. There was no significant difference in survival-to-hospital admission, survival-to-discharge, or 1-year survival in the combination (epinephrine plus vasopressin) versus epinephrine alone groups.

This large multicenter clinical trial identifies that vasopressin in combination with epinephrine does not improve outcomes compared with epinephrine alone in the treatment of CA. This trial has important implications with respect to future consensus treatment recommendations for CA.

S. Trzeciak, MD, MPH

Transfusion of Packed Red Blood Cells in Patients with Ischemic Heart Disease

Gerber DR (Univ of Medicine and Dentistry of New Jersey-Robert Wood Johnson Med School at Camden, Cooper Univ Hosp, Camden, NJ)
Crit Care Med 36:1068-1074, 2008

Objective.—To review the current literature concerning the utility of and complications associated with transfusion of packed red blood cells (PRBC) in medical and surgical patients with ischemic heart disease.

Data Sources, Study Selection, and Data Extraction.—The PubMed database of the National Library of Medicine was searched for all studies investigating the use of PRBC in medical and surgical patients with cardiac disease published since 1999. Relevant background literature from before that date was reviewed for inclusion as well.

Data Synthesis.—An extensive body of literature has accumulated evaluating the safety and efficacy of transfusion as a therapeutic modality in a wide variety of critically ill patients, including patients with cardiac disease. Most, but not all, of these studies have been retrospective in nature, and methodologies have varied from study to study. Some have involved retrospective reviews of patient records, some have been retrospective analyses of detailed databases prospectively collected for other purposes, and some have been prospective randomized or observational studies. Despite the variability in data sources and study design, with a handful of exceptions, the preponderance of data indicates that transfusion of PRBC in the population of patients with ischemic heart disease is of limited clinical utility and may carry the potential for serious adverse consequences.

Conclusions.—Based on the current literature, there appears to be no indication for routine transfusion in patients with non-ST-elevation acute coronary syndrome, although anemic patients with ST-elevation myocardial infarction may benefit from this intervention. However, the specific indications for transfusion in this population remain ill-defined.

▶ This important article continues to support more judicious use of packed red blood cell transfusion in critically ill patients. First was the Transfusion Requirements in Critical Care (TRIC) study, which demonstrated that the general ICU patient did not benefit from maintaining transfusion thresholds higher than 7 g/dL.[1] In fact, there was a trend toward better outcome when the more conservative transfusion approach was used. Next came literature support for no benefit of higher hemoglobin levels to facilitate weaning from mechanical ventilation, along with mounting evidence of negative effects of transfused blood in postoperative patients. This article supports conservative transfusion policy as well for non-ST elevation coronary syndrome. ST segment myocardial infarction patients may benefit from transfusion. Current thinking is that patients with acute hemorrhage also should have a more liberal threshold for transfusion. With the risk of infection secondary to transfused blood products, it is important that we avoid transfusion for the sake of transfusion in ICU patients because it increases complications of ICU stay, especially infection.

R. P. Dellinger, MD

Reference

1. Hébert PC, Wells G, Blajchman MA, et al. A multicenter, randomized, controlled clinical trial of transfusion in critical care. *N Engl J Med.* 1999;340:409-417.

3 Hemodynamics and Monitoring

Noninvasive Cardiac Output Determination Using Applanation Tonometry-Derived Radial Artery Pulse Contour Analysis in Critically Ill Patients
Compton F, Wittrock M, Schaefer J-H, et al (Univ Med Berlin, Campus Benjamin Franklin, Germany)
Anesth Analg 106:171-174, 2008

Conventional thermodilution cardiac output (CO) monitoring is limited mainly to intensive care units and operating rooms because it requires the use of invasive techniques. To reduce the potential for complications and to broaden the applicability of hemodynamic monitoring, noninvasive methods for CO determination are being sought. Applanation tonometry allows noninvasive CO estimation through pulse contour analysis, but the method has not been evaluated in critically ill patients. We therefore performed noninvasive radial artery applanation tonometry in 49 critically ill medical intensive care unit patients and compared CO estimates to invasive CO measurements obtained using a pulmonary artery catheter or the PiCCO® transpulmonary thermodilution system. One-hundred-sixteen measurements were performed, and patients were receiving vasopressor support during 78 measurements. When the data were analyzed with bias and precision statistics, a large bias of 2.03 $L \cdot min^{-1} \cdot m^{-2}$ and a high percentage error of 85% were found between the invasive measurements and applanation tonometry-derived CO estimates, with the noninvasive CO results being significantly lower than the invasive ones ($P < 0.001$). There was no significant difference in bias between the patients who were receiving vasopressor support and those who were not ($P = 0.874$) or between patients with good and poor applanation tonometry pressure waveform signal quality ($P = 0.071$). Whereas a significant increase in the invasively determined CO was observed when a fluid bolus was administered ($n = 7$, $P = 0.016$), these changes were not reflected by the noninvasive method. We conclude that radial artery applanation tonometry is not suitable to determine CO in critically ill hemodynamically unstable patients.

▶ Noninvasive or less invasive strategies for monitoring critically ill patients are almost always preferable if they are valid, reliable, and cost-effective. Many critically ill patients are already having their blood pressure monitored via an arterial catheter commonly placed in the radial artery. At present, the waveform generated is typically only used for its systolic, mean, and diastolic readings. This is unfortunate as there are a lot of data encoded in the waveform itself and ignoring this data would be similar to only recording the maximum and minimum voltage of electrocardiogram (ECG) leads. This study of applanation pulse contour analysis for the determination of cardiac output (CO) takes the concept 1 step further by recording radial arterial pulse through a noninvasive tonometer placed on the skin of the distal forearm over the radial artery. Unfortunately, it underestimated CO at baseline and further underestimated the effect of a volume challenge. These limitations effectively render this approach as not valid or reliable under the conditions studied. An important limitation of this study that favors this approach receiving further study although is that the CO calculated from this device was compared with a variable standard and in some cases to a methodology not considered the gold standard.

T. Dorman, MD

Ultrasound evaluation of central veins in the intensive care unit: effects of dynamic manoeuvres

Samy Modeliar S, Sevestre M-A, de Cagny B, et al (Service de Néphrologie, Unité de Réanimation, Amiens, France; Service de Chirurgie Vasculaire et Thoracique, Amiens, France; et al)
Intensive Care Med 34:333-338, 2008

Objective.—To determine: (1) the proportion of small (< 5 mm) or thrombosed internal jugular veins (IJV) and femoral veins (FV) in which catheter placement would be difficult without ultrasound guidance; (2) which position increases central vein sizes and may facilitate cannulation of these vessels.

Design.—Prospective study.

Setting.—Twelve-bed adult medical intensive care unit.

Patients and Participants.—Sixty patients (62 ± 19 years, SAPS II score 36 ± 17).

Interventions.—Ultrasound examinations of the IJV and FV in supine, Trendelenburg (T) and reverse Trendelenburg (Ti) positions.

Measurements and Results.—Maximum diameter and cross-sectional area (CSA) were measured. Venous catheter placement would have been difficult (diameter < 5 mm) or even impossible (thrombosis) for 22% of right IJV, 13% of left IJV, 2% of left and 2% of right FV. In the T position, the CSA of the IJV increased (right IJV: 1.7 ± 1.4 to 2.01 ± 1.34 cm^2, left IJV: 1.18 ± 0.81 to 1.34 ± 0.85 cm^2; $p < 0.05$) and theCSA of the FV decreased (right FV: 1.42 ± 0.61 to 1.22 ± 0.58 cm^2, left FV: 1.51 ± 0.62 to 1.26 ± 0.58 cm^2; $p < 0.05$). In the Ti position, the CSA of the IJV decreased (right IJV: 1.7 ± 1.4 to 1.35 ± 1.35 cm^2, left IJV: 1.18 ± 0.81 to 0.87 ± 0.62 cm^2; $p < 0.05$) and the CSA of the FV increased (right FV: 1.42 ± 0.61 to 1.66 ± 0.65 cm^2, left FV: 1.51 ± 0.62 to 1.65 ± 0.68 cm^2; $p < 0.05$). In two-thirds of patients, the right IJV was significantly larger than the left IJV.

Conclusions.—Ultrasonography should be performed before at least central venous catheter placement to detect the presence of deep vein thrombosis or vessels less than 5 mm in diameter. Some positions increase veins' diameter at least internally, T position increasing IJV size and Ti position increasing FV size.

▶ The use of ultrasound (US) by intensive care physicians is increasing rapidly across many different application areas in the ICU. The US has likely had the greatest growth as to use during central line insertion. Not only does US identify the location of a vein, but perhaps more importantly can identify small central veins (asymmetry in size of veins is now identified to be common) and veins which are clotted. The authors show significant value with use of US. They show the increase in size of the internal jugular vein with Trendelenburg (T) position and the increase in size of femoral vein with reverse Trendelenburg position (Ti). The former is not of great clinical import because standard technique is to use T position when inserting a neck or chest central line; the use of Ti for femoral line insertion is typically not done, but perhaps should be according to the results of this article.

R. P. Dellinger, MD

Continuous and intermittent cardiac output measurement in hyperdynamic conditions: pulmonary artery catheter vs. lithium dilution technique
Costa MG, Della Rocca G, Chiarandini P, et al (Azienda Ospedaliero Universitaria di Udine, Italy; et al)
Intensive Care Med 34:257-263, 2008

Objective.—This study aimed to assess the level of agreement of both intermittent cardiac output monitoring by the lithium dilution technique (CO_{Li}) and continuous cardiac output monitoring (PulseCO$_{Li}$) using the arterial pressure waveform with intermittent thermodilution using a pulmonary artery catheter (CO_{PAC}).
Design.—Prospective, single-center evaluation.
Setting.—University Hospital Intensive Care Unit.
Patients.—Patients ($n = 23$) receiving liver transplantation.
Intervention.—Pulmonary artery catheters were placed in all patients and CO_{PAC} was determined using thermodilution. CO_{Li} and PulseCO$_{Li}$ measurements were made using the LiDCO system.
Measurements and Main Results.—Data were collected after intensive care unit admission and every 8 h until the 48th hour. A total of 151 CO_{PAC}, CO_{Li} and PulseCO$_{Li}$ measurements were analysed. Bias and 95% limit of agreement were 0.11 lmin^{-1} and -1.84 to $+2.05$ lmin^{-1} for CO_{PAC} vs. CO_{Li} ($r = 0.88$) resulting in an overall percentage error of 15.6%. Bias and 95% limit of agreement for CO_{PAC} vs. PulseCO$_{Li}$ were 0.29 lmin^{-1} and -1.87 to $+2.46$ lmin^{-1} ($r = 0.85$) with a percentage error of 16.8%. Subgroup analysis revealed a percentage error of 15.7%

for CO_{PAC} vs. CO_{Li} and 15.1% for CO_{PAC} vs. $PulseCO_{Li}$ for data pairs less than 8 lmin^{-1}, and percentage errors of 15.5% and 18.5% respectively for data pairs higher than 8 lmin^{-1}.

Conclusion.—In patients with hyperdynamic circulation, intermittent and continuous CO values determined using the LiDCO system showed good agreement with those obtained by intermittent pulmonary artery thermodilution.

▶ This article demonstrates the correlations between standard thermodilution methodologies used with a pulmonary artery catheter (PAC) and similar variables obtained from a lithium dilution approach. If one is using the lithium approach, then this article offers some reassurance that the variables obtained do indeed correlate with those obtained from a standard PAC. The inclusion and exclusion criteria are critical in such a study. This small study was performed in 23 patients undergoing an orthotopic liver transplant, but excluded any patient with pre-existing cardiac or pulmonary disease, fulminant hepatic failure, hepatopulmonary syndrome, or pulmonary hypertension. This obviously limits the use of the correlated findings to those liver transplant patients who are totally healthy. Furthermore, no patients received inotropic agents during the study, a further significant limitation. Finally, a correlation between PAC and less invasive approaches is intriguing but what I hope for in the future are tools that include well-studied clinical approaches, for example, protocols, to help standardize and improve care and outcomes.

T. Dorman, MD

Heparinized solution vs. saline solution in the maintenance of arterial catheters: a double blind randomized clinical trial
Del Cotillo M, Grané N, Llavoré M, et al (Hosp Mútua de Terrassa, Spain)
Intensive Care Med 34:339-343, 2008

Objectives.—The objectives were to analyze the effectiveness of heparinized solution vs. saline solution for the maintenance of arterial catheters and to detect changes in the activated partial thromboplastin time (aPTT) and platelet count in the samples extracted from both groups of arterial catheters.

Design.—Randomized, double blind, placebo-controlled clinical trial.

Setting.—Intensive Care Unit of a third-level hospital in Terrassa, Barcelona, Spain.

Patients.—One hundred and thirty-three patients were included in the trial. The selection criteria were: adults, informed consent, not receiving either full-dose anticoagulant or fibrinolytic treatment, and no thrombocytopenia.

Interventions.—Sixty-five patients received heparinized solution (1 IU/ml) and 68 received saline solution.

Measurements.—Arterial catheter functionality was compared in the groups every 8 h and at catheter removal. Patency, reliability of arterial pressure, and curve quality were used to evaluate the functionality of the catheters. Blood was drawn, discarding 7.5 ml, from the arterial catheter and from the venous catheter simultaneously for coagulation tests.

Results.—The median duration of catheters being in place was 5.1 days (IQR = 8.1) in the heparin group, and 5.4 (IQR = 7.3) in the saline group ($p = 0.7$). Kaplan–Meier curves showed no differences between groups ($p = 0.6$). The number of manipulations required to maintain the patency of the arterial catheters was 35% vs. 40% ($p = 0.5$). The heparin group had a significantly longer aPTT (2.1 ± 1.3 vs. 1.25 ± 0.3, $p = 0.001$).

Conclusions.—The use of heparinized solution for arterial catheter maintenance does not appear to be justified. It did not increase the duration of the catheters, nor did it improve their functionality significantly. On the other hand, heparin Na altered aPTT significantly.

▶ These authors looked at an area where there is conflicting opinion, that is, the value of low-concentration heparin as part of a saline solution for maintenance of continuous flow in arterial catheters. Some studies have supported use in that it prolongs average duration of use of the line, whereas others have shown no significant differences. This very well-designed study supports no value of heparinized solution over saline solution. When one considers the growing concern of heparin-induced thrombocytopenia and its potentially catastrophic results, saline without heparin should be used.

R. P. Dellinger, MD

Lack of an Effect of Body Mass on the Hemodynamic Response to Arginine Vasopressin During Septic Shock
Lam SW, Bauer SR, Cha SS, et al (Columbia Univ Med Ctr, New York; Cleveland Clinic, OH; Mayo Clinic, Rochester, MN)
Pharmacotherapy 28:591-599, 2008

Study Objective.—To determine whether body mass alters the effectiveness of a fixed-dose infusion of arginine vasopressin.

Design.—Retrospective medical record review.

Setting.—All intensive care units of a tertiary medical center.

Patients.—Sixty-six mechanically ventilated patients who received a fixed-dose intravenous infusion of arginine vasopressin at 0.04 U/minute as the sole agent for hemodynamic support during septic shock.

Measurements and Main Results.—Patients were divided into four groups on the basis of body mass index. Effectiveness was measured as hemodynamic stability, which was defined as the proportion of patients achieving a mean arterial pressure (MAP) of 65 mm Hg or higher, the magnitude of the change in MAP at 1 hour, and the need for additional rescue vasopressors. Secondary outcomes included mortality and length of stay. Baseline characteristics of all four groups were comparable for age, sex, and severity of illness determined by using Acute Physiology and Chronic Health Evaluation II (APACHE II), Simplified Acute Physiology II (SAPS II), and Sequential Organ Failure Assessment (SOFA) scores. The only significant differences in baseline characteristics among the groups were in their central venous pressures. The four groups similarly achieved hemodynamic stability at 1 hour after the administration of arginine vasopressin (p=0.41). We observed no significant differences among groups in the magnitude of MAP change (p=0.62), need for rescue catecholamine vasopressors (p=0.17), 28-day mortality rates (p=0.31), or length of stay in the intensive care unit (p=0.43).

Conclusion.—Body mass index did not alter the effects of arginine vasopressin on hemodynamic stability or changes in MAP when the drug was administered as a fixed-dose infusion of 0.04 U/minute. Our results do not support weight-based dosing of vasopressin, unlike the dosing for catecholamine vasopressors (Table 2).

▶ Critically ill patients commonly require vasoactive substance infusions to control hemodynamics and avoid morbidity and mortality. Most infusions are administered according to weight-based protocols. Arginine vasopressin, a fad at present for treating hypotension related to septic shock and in a few other vasodilated hypotensive states, is typically not administered based upon weight-based protocols. This retrospective study, in an attempt to evaluate the effect of weight on vasopressin dosing, used body mass index (BMI) as a surrogate for weight and found no association, seemingly justifying a non-weight-based approach to administration (Table 2). It should be noted, however, that BMI is not solely determined by weight and thus may have obscured any relationship. More importantly, though, is that the dose

TABLE 2.—Multivariate Analysis of Variables Potentially Affecting the Response to Arginine Vasopressin

Variable	OR	95%CI[a]	p Value
SOFA score	0.80	0.58–1.11	0.177
AACHE II score	0.95	0.821–1.10	0.500
Age	0.97	0.92–1.02	0.291
Use of β-blocker on day of AVP infusion	1.04	0.25–4.37	0.956
Body mass index	1.05	0.95–1.16	0.376
Male sex	1.32	0.31–5.72	0.709
Corticosteroid use during arginine vasopressin infusion	1.40	0.05–36.0	0.841

OR–odds radio: CI = confidence interval: SOFA = Sequential Organ Failure Assessment: APACHE II = Acute Physiology and Chronic Health Evaluation II.

[a]All 95% CIs crossed 1, signifying that none of the variables were independent predictors of the hemodynamic response to AVP.

(Reprinted from Lam SW, Bauer SR, Cha SS, et al. Lack of an effect of body mass on the hemodynamic response to arginine vasopressin during septic shock. *Pharmacotherapy.* 2008;28:591-599, with permission of the American College of Clinical Pharmacology.)

administered in these patients may be supramaximal and thus a relationship to weight may have been missed. Interestingly, a subset of patients with serial creatinines experienced an improvement in creatinine during vasopressin infusion. Despite the fact that volume status and administration are not presented, thus making the interpretation difficult, this interesting finding should be evaluated in future prospective trials.

T. Dorman, MD

Effect of the implementation of NICE guidelines for ultrasound guidance on the complication rates associated with central venous catheter placement in patients presenting for routine surgery in a tertiary referral centre
Wigmore TJ, Smythe JF, Hacking MB (Royal Marsden NHS Foundation Trust, London, UK; Imperial College London, UK)
Br J Anaesth 99:662-665, 2007

Background.—The National Institute for Clinical Excellence (NICE) guidelines of 2002 recommended the use of ultrasound (US) for central venous catheterization in order to minimize complications associated with central line placement. An ongoing audit of line placement by anaesthetists in the theatre complex of a tertiary referral centre looked at the associated complication rates. The objective of the study was to compare complication rates pre- and post-implementation of NICE guidelines.

Methods.—This prospective, single centre audit looked at all patients in whom a central venous catheter was placed for surgery. Complication rates were assessed for procedures that were performed pre- and post-implementation of NICE guidelines. In total, 438 patients were identified for the study, and the procedures were performed either by trainee or by consultant anaesthetists.

Results.—The pre- and post-implementation complication rates were 10.5% (16/152) and 4.6% (13/284), respectively, representing an absolute risk reduction of 5.9% (95% CI 0.5–11.3%). Comparison of those procedures in which US was used when compared with the landmark technique after implementation found a reduction of 6.9% in complications (95% CI 1.4–12.4%). The reduction in complication rates was larger for specialist registrars than for consultants (11.2% vs 1.6%).

Conclusions.—The implementation of NICE guidelines has been associated with a significant reduction in complication rates in our tertiary referral centre. In the light of the cross-speciality evidence of US superiority and our results, it is imperative that routine use of US guidance becomes more widespread (Table 1).

▶ This article examines the National Institute for Clinical Excellence (NICE) guidelines recommending the use of ultrasound (US) guidance as the preferred method of insertion for both elective and emergency central line insertion. US guidance has been shown to decrease complications including arterial

TABLE 1.—Main Outcome Measures Pre- And Post-Implementation of NICE Guidelines.
*In Eight Cases, Both SpR and Consultant Attempted Insertion on the Same Patient

	Before implementation of NICE guidelines ($n=152$)	After implementation of NICE guidelines ($n=284$)
Operator		
Consultant	64 (42.1%)	126 (44.4%)
SpR	88 (57.9%)	158 (55.6%)
Ultrasound uptake	19 (12.5%)	169 (59.5%)
Complications		
Overall	16 (10.5%)	13 (4.6%)

(Reprinted from Wigmore TJ, Smythe JF, Hacking MB, et al. Effect of the implementation of NICE guidelines for ultrasound guidance on the complication rates associated with central venous catheter placement in patients presenting for routine surgery in a tertiary referral centre. Br J Anaesth. 2007;99:662-665, with permission from The Board of Management and Trustees of the British Journal of Anaesthesia, Oxford University Press.)

puncture, pneumothorax, hematoma, and hemothorax as well as decreasing the time to cannulation and number of attempts. The greatest effect on complication rate is seen in the less experienced operator. Table 1 summarizes the results showing an absolute risk reduction in favor of ultrasound of 6.9%.

Despite this evidence, a recent survey of pediatric anesthetics by Tovey and colleagues[1] showed only 39% routinely used ultrasound and in North America a study of cardiovascular anesthesiologists found only 15% used ultrasound routinely.[2]

Having been trained without US, we use landmarks to insert lines and on occasion tell the fellows to "get the probe out of the way" so we can just put in the line. This study showed that even with an experienced operator, complications are decreased with the use of ultrasound. The training for this procedure was a 1-day course. We should all get on board and learn to do lines with the benefit of US. Patient safety demands it and those coming out of fellowship will likely all have the training to use it, pushing the standard-of-care in the direction of US.

A. Spevetz, MD
C. Bekes, MD

References

1. Tovey G, Stokes M. A survey of the use of 2D ultrasound guidance for insertion of central venous catheters by UK consultant paediatric anaesthetists. *Eur J Anaesthesiol.* 2007;24:71-75.
2. Bailey PL, Glance LG, Eaton MP, Parshall B, McIntosh S. A survey of the use of ultrasound during cental venous catheterization. *Anesth Analg.* 2007;104:491-497.

Use of bladder pressure to correct for the effect of expiratory muscle activity on central venous pressure

Qureshi AS, Shapiro RS, Leatherman JW (Univ of Minnesota, Minneapolis, MN)
Intensive Care Med 33:1907-1912, 2007

Objective.—To assess whether subtracting the expiratory change in intra-abdominal (bladder) pressure (ΔIAP) from central venous pressure (CVP) provides a reliable estimate of transmural CVP in spontaneously breathing patients with expiratory muscle activity.

Design and setting.—Prospective observational study in a medical ICU.

Patients.—Twenty-four spontaneously breathing patients with central venous and bladder catheters: 18 with no clinical evidence of active expiration (group 1) and 6 with active expiration (group 2).

Interventions.—Patients in group 1 were coached to change their breathing pattern to one of active expiration for several breaths; those in group 2 were asked to sip water through a straw to briefly interrupt active expiration.

Measurements and results.—During active expiration end-expiratory CVP (uncorrected CVP) and ΔIAP were measured; ΔIAP was subtracted from uncorrected CVP to obtain corrected CVP. End-expiratory CVP during relaxed breathing (best CVP) was assumed to represent the best estimate of transmural CVP. The absolute difference between corrected CVP and best CVP was much less than the difference between uncorrected CVP and best CVP (2.3 ± 2.0 vs. 12.5 ± 4.7 mmHg).

Conclusions.—In patients with active expiration, subtracting ΔIAP from end-expiratory CVP yields a more reliable (and lower) estimate of transmural CVP than does the uncorrected CVP value.

▶ Although there are drawbacks in using a pressure measurement as an indicator for response to fluid challenge, it is the variable that is quickest to ascertain in the patient presenting with hypotension and/or tissue hypoperfusion. Because the values of central venous pressure (CVP) >12 mm Hg to14 mm Hg usually make response to fluid challenge very unlikely, any patient condition that would overestimate CVP as a true reflection of right atrial transmural filling would be important to control for. The use of expiratory change in intra-abdominal (bladder) pressure subtracted from the CVP in the actively expired patient appears to be an appropriate correction factor that should be performed in patients being fluid resuscitated to a CVP target who are spontaneously breathing with active expiration.

R. P. Dellinger, MD

The Effects of Vasodilation on Cardiac Output Measured by PiCCO
Yamashita K, Nishiyama T, Yokoyama T, et al (Kochi Med School, Nankoku, Japan; The Univ of Tokyo, Japan)
J Cardiothorac Vasc Anesth 22:688-692, 2008

Objectives.—The purpose of this study was to investigate the effects of vasodilation on cardiac output (CO) measured by pulse contour method using PiCCO (Pulsion Medical Systems AG, Munich, Germany) in comparison with CO by the thermodilution method.

Design.—A prospective observational study.

Settings.—An operating room in a university hospital.

Participants.—Twenty patients scheduled for off-pump coronary artery bypass grafting.

Interventions.—After anesthesia induction with midazolam, fentanyl, and vecuronium, the PiCCO catheter and pulmonary artery catheter were inserted. Before the initiation of surgery, progressively higher infusions of prostaglandin E1 (PGE1) were administered for vasodilation.

Measurements and Main Results.—CO was measured before PGE1 (control); at PGE1 0.01, 0.02, and 0.04 μg/kg/min; and 15 minutes after stopping PGE1 infusion. Systemic vascular resistances (SVRs) at PGE1 0.02 and 0.04 μg/kg/min were significantly lower than the control value. The correlation coefficient (R^2) at each point, percentage error, and limits of agreement (bias ± 2 standard deviation of bias) were 0.89, 17, −0.21 ± 0.53 before PGE1; 0.72, 27, −0.31 ± 0.93 at 0.01 μg/kg/min; 0.53, 40, −0.62 ± 1.41 at 0.02 μg/kg/min; 0.57, 34, −0.61 ± 1.26 at 0.04 μg/kg/min; and 0.97, 21, −0.14 ± 0.69 L/min 15 minutes after the end of infusion, respectively.

Conclusions.—PiCCO may not be an alternative to thermodilution measurement without recalibration when SVR decreases by infusion of PGE1 ≥0.02 μg/kg/min (Table 1).

▶ Patients always prefer less invasive approaches to care. Physicians also prefer less invasive approaches when the data support their reliability and validity. Cardiac output (CO) monitoring using arterial pulse waveform analysis is a highly attractive solution to the concerns regarding the use of pulmonary artery catheters (PAC). Their acceptance into clinical practice has been slowed by several factors of which the most concerning is their reliability in a variety of clinical situations. Furthermore, the seemingly constant change in hemodynamic status of a patient who is critically ill requires a device that remains stable throughout the changing conditions of vascular volume, vasoreactive status, inotropic state, and compliance of the system. These authors, having evaluated PiCCO in comparison with a standard PAC, have demonstrated that PiCCO-derived values are not stable under vasodilatory conditions, in this case induced by prostaglandin E1 (PGE1). In fact, as can be seen in Table 1, errors in calculation as high as 40% may exist. These errors in calculated CO should not lead clinicians into not using these less invasive devices

TABLE 1.—Changes of CO and Hemodynamic Variables, Mean Difference (Bias) Between CO by PiCCO and CO by the Bolus Thermodilution Method, Lower Limits of Agreement (Bias – 2 SD), Upper Limits of Agreement (Bias + 2 SD), and Percentage Error (Mean CO·2 SD^{-1})

	Control (After Calibration)	PGE1 0.01 µg/kg/min	PGE1 0.02 mg/kg/min	PGE1 0.04 mg/kg/min	Post PGE1
CO by PiCCO (L/min)	3.0 ± 0.8	3.3 ± 0.8	3.2 ± 0.8†	3.4 ± 0.8*†	3.1 ± 0.7
CO by bolus thermodilution method (L/min)	3.2 ± 0.7	3.6 ± 0.9*	3.8 ± 1.0*	3.9 ± 0.9*	3.2 ± 0.6
Systemic vascular resistance (dynes·sec·cm^{-5})	2,099 ± 518	1,900 ± 528	1,743 ± 505*	1,604 ± 355*	2,073 ± 426
Heart rate (beat/min)	53 ± 10	56 ± 10	58 ± 11	58 ± 11	53 ± 10
Mean arterial pressure (mmHg)	75 ± 12	74 ± 15	73 ± 12	72 ± 12	74 ± 12
Mean pulmonary artery pressure (mmHg)	16 ± 5	15 ± 4	14 ± 4	14 ± 3	17 ± 4
Central venous pressure (mmHg)	7 ± 4	8 ± 4	6 ± 4	7 ± 4	7 ± 3
Bias (L/min)	–0.21 (–0.35 ~ –0.08)	–0.31 (–0.55 ~ –0.07)	–0.62 (–0.98 ~ –0.26)	–0.61 (–0.92 ~ –0.29)	–0.14 (–0.31 ~ –0.04)
Lower limits of agreement (L/min)	–0.75 (–0.98 ~ –0.51)	–1.24 (–1.65 ~ –0.83)	–2.02 (–2.64 ~ –1.41)	–1.86 (–2.41 ~ –1.31)	–0.82 (–1.13 ~ –0.52)
Upper limits of agreement (L/min)	0.32 (0.08 ~ 0.55)	0.62 (0.21 ~ 1.03)	0.79 (0.17 ~ 1.40)	0.64 (0.10 ~ 1.20)	0.55 (0.26 ~ 0.86)
Percentage error (%)	17	27	40	34	21

NOTE. Data are expressed as mean ± standard deviation (SD); 95% confidence interval in parentheses.
* $p < 0.05$ versus control (calibration).
† $p < 0.05$ versus cardiac output by bolus thermodilution method.
(Reprinted from Yamashita K, Nishiyama T, Yokoyama T, et al. The effects of vasodilation on cardiac output measured by PiCCO. J Cardiothorac Vasc Anesth. 2008;22:688-692, with permission from Elsevier.)

because they can be mitigated by recalibration of the device. Thus, clinicians should strongly consider frequent recalibration of these devices despite manufacturers recommendation for less frequent calibration until more definitive evidence exists.

T. Dorman, MD

4 Burns

Emergence of the USA300 Strain of Methicillin-Resistant *Staphylococcus aureus* in a Burn-Trauma Unit
Wibbenmeyer LA, Kealey GP, Latenser BA, et al (The Univ of Iowa Carver College of Medicine, Iowa City, IA)
J Burn Care Res 29:790-797, 2008

Community-associated methicillin-resistant *Staphylococcus aureus* (MRSA), particularly USA300, is a major pathogen in the outpatient setting. We suspected that USA300 had been introduced into our burn-trauma unit (BTU) when three burn patients presented with numerous simultaneous abscesses. We did molecular typing on 206 MRSA isolates from all patients on the BTU who had MRSA isolated from either nares cultures or clinical specimens obtained between April 11, 2002 and October 24, 2006. We reviewed medical records for all patients who had USA300 and for 75 control patients. Twenty-five of 206 (12.1%) patients who were colonized (n = 3) or infected (n = 22) with MRSA had USA300. Thirteen patients had abscesses drained surgically and eight had necrotizing fasciitis excised. Seven patients had burns (mean burn size 11.8 ± 3.4%), of whom four (66.7%) acquired numerous simultaneous (3-33) abscesses. Fourteen patients acquired USA300 outside of the BTU, and three acquired this strain on the BTU. Cases were more likely to have been hospitalized or to have had an operation in the 6 months before they were hospitalized than were controls ($P = .001$ for both). To our knowledge, this is the first study to describe numerous simultaneous MRSA abscesses in burn patients. The MRSA strain USA300 may be introduced onto burn units from the community by patients admitted with skin and soft tissue infections, especially abscesses and necrotizing fasciitis. Burn patients may be at risk for numerous abscesses with USA300, because they have open wounds and their immune systems may be compromised.

▶ Most health care-associated methicillin-resistant *Staphylococcus aureus* (MRSA) infections are because of the USA100 strain; however, the USA300 strain is growing in prevalence and is more difficult to control. A policy of placing all patients with complex wounds or necrotizing fasciitis in contact isolation until nasal swab and wound culture results are known helps prevent the spread of MRSA USA300 in a unit. Although it may be expensive and time-consuming to don and doff gowns every time you enter and exit a patient room, the savings may be more than just dollars if you choose to adopt this practice. The other practice that should be part of every entry and exit into a patient's room should be hand washing, a habit that will also help to prevent the spread of MRSA USA300, vancomycin-resistant enterococci (VRE), and other pathogens.

In our unit, we had hoped that by identifying patients who were at high risk for bringing MRSA into the unit, we could use selective isolation practices, thereby bringing about what we anticipated would be a significant time and cost savings. Unfortunately, MRSA USA300 strain has become ubiquitous in our health care system. To prevent MRSA outbreaks, we continue to place all patients in contact precautions on admission and continuing weekly surveillance cultures. In my experience, patients who had partial thickness burns or areas of donor sites within the past 1-6 months and now complain of "bug bites" or "severe acne" in these areas have multiple abscesses that require intravenous (IV) antibiotics and often, surgical incision and drainage of what I now call "miliary MRSA."

B. A. Latenser, MD

Base deficit and lactate: Early predictors of morbidity and mortality in patients with burns
Andel D, Kamolz LP, Roka J, et al (Med Univ Vienna, Austria)
Burns 33:973-978, 2007

Severe burn results in severe and unique physiological changes called burn shock. Historically, resuscitation has been guided by a combination of basic laboratory values, invasive monitoring and clinical findings, but the optimal guide to the endpoint of resuscitation still remains controversial. Two hundred and eighty patients, who were admitted to our Burn Unit, were enrolled in this prospective study. Resuscitation of these patients was undertaken according to the current standard of care. Parkland formula was used as a first approximation of acquired fluid administration rates; final fluid administration was adapted in order to meet clinical needs. The aim of this study was to evaluate if plasma lactate (PL) and base deficit (BD) are useful early parameters to estimate the severity of a burn. One of the main objectives was to evaluate if BD and its changes due to fluid resuscitation adds additional information in comparison to the evaluation of PL alone. The results of this study indicate that initial PL and BD level (Day 0) are useful parameters to separate survivors from non-survivors.

Moreover, an outcome predictor of shock and effective resuscitation could be defined by evaluating the changes of BD on Day 1. Normalization of the BD within 24 h is associated with a better chance of survival.

One explanation for this phenomenon might be the fact that many burn patients are still sub-optimally resuscitated; in summary, measuring PL and BD may help to identify critically injured patients either for enhancement of treatment, or selection of therapeutic options.

▶ The debate rages about base deficit and lactate levels during the burn resuscitation period and their predictive powers for outcomes. Although there are guidelines for fluid resuscitation, each burn unit, and often each burn surgeon, modifies one of the more commonly used resuscitation protocols. Some of the more commonly used parameters to judge the effectiveness of a resuscitation include urine output, heart rate, mental status, temperature, and blood pressure trends. For those patients requiring more monitoring, a central venous catheter, or less commonly a pulmonary artery catheter, may be used, but there are drawbacks to the more invasive monitoring lines. Clinical investigations are underway in burn centers around the country to evaluate the usefulness of other real-time monitoring technologies. Gastric tonometry has been evaluated to assess resuscitation but has not proven to be effective. Technologies such as the lithium dilution cardiac output (LiDCO), and less invasive cardiac output monitoring using the esophagus or trachea, may provide very useful as monitoring tools. Until there is good evidence that either laboratory or technological data are effective, we will continue to use indirect, and very gross, evidence of perfusion and resuscitation such as urine output.

B. A. Latenser, MD

A Systematic Review of Heparin to Treat Burn Injury
Oremus M, Hanson MD, Whitlock R, et al (McMaster Univ, Hamilton, ON, Canada)
J Burn Care Res 28:794-804, 2007

This systematic review was conducted to assess the evidence for using heparin to treat burn injury. The following databases were searched for relevant studies: MEDLINE, EMBASE, CINAHL, The Cochrane Central Database of Controlled Trials, Web of Science, and BIOSIS. Additional searches involved the reference lists of included studies, the "grey " literature (eg, government reports), and consultations with experts to obtain unpublished manuscripts. Included studies were summarized descriptively and in tabular form, and assessed for methodological quality. A metaanalysis was conducted to obtain a summary estimate for the association between heparin use and postburn mortality. Nine studies were abstracted and included in the review. Five studies contained adult and pediatric patients, one contained adults only, and three contained pediatric patients only. Burn etiologies included flame, scald, thermal, or smoke inhalation. Heparin administration was done topically, subcutaneously, intravenously, or via aerosol. Heparin was reported to have a beneficial impact on mortality, graft and wound healing, and pain control. For mortality, the overall estimate (relative risk) of heparin's effect was 0.32 (95% confidence interval = 0.18–0.57). Heparin's reported benefits may be severely biased because the abstracted studies were beset by poor methodological quality (eg, inadequate definitions of treatment and outcome, no control of confounding). Given poor study quality, there is no strong evidence to indicate that heparin can improve clinical outcomes in the treatment of burn injury. Further research is needed to assess the clinical utility of using heparin in the treatment of burn injury.

▶ Although heparin is best known for its anticoagulant effects, it has antiinflammatory and antiangiogenic properties and a capacity for wound healing. These additional properties may be explained by the action of heparin on secretory products released from neutrophils. Heparin binds, stabilizes, and activates locally produced growth factors that may enhance wound healing. Finally, not all heparins are anticoagulants. Heparin may be modified to produce a nonanticoagulant derivative with minimal hemostatic activity. A variety of investigators have advocated the use of heparin as a topical adjunct in burn healing and as an inhaled therapy with pulmonary injury. Although these studies have increased our knowledge of burn care, the quality of available data and inconsistencies in contemporary investigation do not support the routine use of heparin in management specific to burn injury.[1] Heparins clearly have a role in prophylaxis and thromboembolic complication management for burn-injured patients. Remarkably, in this review, a computer literature search yielded over 450 citations. When screening for quality and consistency in methodology was complete only 9 studies were available for rigorous evaluation.

D. J. Dries, MSE, MD

Reference

1. McCall JE, Cahill TJ. Respiratory care of the burn patient. *J Burn Care Res*. 2005; 26:200-206.

Positive Fungal Cultures in Burn Patients: A Multicenter Review
Ballard J, Edelman L, Saffle J, et al (Univ of Utah, Salt Lake City)
J Burn Care Res 29:213-221, 2008

Fungal infections are increasingly common in burn patients. We performed this study to determine the incidence and outcomes of fungal cultures in acutely burned patients. Members of the American Burn Association's Multicenter Trials Group were asked to review patients admitted during 2002–2003 who developed one or more cultures positive for fungal organisms. Data on demographics, site(s), species and number of cultures, and presence of risk factors for fungal infections were collected. Patients were categorized as untreated (including prophylactic topical antifungal therapy), nonsystemic treatment (nonprophylactic topical antifungal therapy, surgery, removal of foreign bodies), or systemic treatment (enteral or parenteral therapy). Fifteen institutions reviewed 6918 patients, of whom 435 (6.3%) had positive fungal cultures. These patients had mean age of 33.2 ± 23.6 years, burn size of 34.8 ± 22.7%TBSA, and 38% had inhalation injuries. Organisms included *Candida species* (371 patients; 85%), yeast non-*Candida* (93 patients, 21%), *Aspergillus* (60 patients, 14%), other mold (39 patients, 9.0%), and others (6 patients, 1.4%). Systemically treated patients were older, had larger burns, more inhalation injuries, more risk factors, a higher incidence of multiple positive cultures, and significantly increased mortality (21.2%), compared with nonsystemic (mortality 5.0%) or untreated patients (mortality 7.8%). In multivariate analysis, increasing age and burn size, number of culture sites, and cultures positive for *Aspergillus* or other mold correlated with mortality. Positive fungal cultures occur frequently in patients with large burns. The low mortality for untreated patients suggests that appropriate clinical judgment was used in most treatment decisions. Nonetheless, indications for treatment of fungal isolates in burn patients remain unclear, and should be developed.

▶ Burn patients with significant injuries are at risk for fungal infections for a variety of reasons: nonintact skin, impaired immune system, systemic antibiotics, central venous catheters, Foley catheters, endotracheal tubes, total parenteral nutrition (TPN), and topical antimicrobials. The difficulty comes when you try to quantify the risk(s) for each factor. Not surprisingly, the risk of fungal infection increases with burn size. Several items complicate categorization of this issue: burn center practices vary widely regarding description, diagnosis, and treatment of fungal infections. Additionally, infections with *Aspergillus* or other mold are notoriously difficult to diagnose until well advanced and carry an especially grim prognosis. Future collaborations between burn centers through the American Burn Association's MultiCenter Trials Group should help to define a fungal infection and outline optimal treatment protocols. Because fungal infections are more common than one might think, practitioners must be aware of patients at high risk.

B. A. Latenser, MD

Acute Renal Failure in Intensive Care Burn Patients (ARF in Burn Patients)
Mustonen K-M, Vuola J (Helsinki Univ Hosp, Finland)
J Burn Care Res 29:227-237, 2008

The purpose of this study was to establish the incidence and mortality of burn patients with acute renal failure (ARF) at the Helsinki Burn Centre and to analyze the associated factors. The files of 238 intensive care (ICU) patients of a total of 1380 burn patients admitted to our institution between November 1988 and December 2001 were studied retrospectively. Of all admitted burn patients, 17.2% needed ICU. According to our criteria (S-Cr >120 μmol/l = 1.4 mg/dl), 39.1% of the ICU patients suffered from ARF and one in three of these required renal replacement therapy. The proportion of all admitted burn patients requiring renal replacement therapy was 2.3%. The mortality of ICU patients with ARF was 44.1% whereas that of patients without ARF was only 6.9%. Renal function recovered in all survivors. The nonsurvivors had a larger burned total body surface area, were older, and had more inhalation injuries and a higher abbreviated burn severity index score. The prognosis for patients with early ARF was worse than that for patients with late ARF. Rhabdomyolysis caused by flame injury was associated with high mortality. In this study we observed that ARF is associated with higher mortality even in minor burns when compared with patients without ARF. Flame burn with rhabdomyolysis and subsequent ARF predicts very poor survival. If a patient with severe ARF survives, the renal failure recovers over time.

▶ Traditional mortality rates for burn patients have been grossly calculated by adding the patient's age to the total body surface area burned, known as the Baux score. A newer, more accurate mortality predictor has distinguished between partial and full thickness burns, with the formula involving the patients' age plus the total body surface area of full thickness burns plus 0.6 the body surface area partial thickness burns. Older data showed dismal outcomes for patients with burns and subsequent renal failure. This study found differences between early and late acute renal failure (ARF) based on etiologies. The early etiologies are preventable and showed higher mortality rates compared with the late development of renal failure. Not surprisingly, the nonsurvivors were significantly older and had larger burns than survivors. Delay in resuscitation leads to worse outcomes in patient with or without renal failure. One important concept is that even in minor burns, mortality rates are higher in patients with ARF. Additionally, mortality rates are higher in patients with renal failure. Despite these facts, renal failure requiring dialysis should not preclude the aggressive resuscitation and intervention for burn patients, as the outcomes for survival and ultimate recovery of renal function are continuously improving.

B. A. Latenser, MD

Effects of treatments on the mortality of Stevens-Johnson syndrome and toxic epidermal necrolysis: A retrospective study on patients included in the prospective EuroSCAR Study

Schneck J, Fagot J-P, Sekula P, et al (Univ Med Ctr Freiburg; Inserm Hôpital Saint-Antoine, Paris)
J Am Acad Dermatol 58:33-40, 2008

Background.—No treatment modality has been established as standard for patients with Stevens-Johnson syndrome and toxic epidermal necrolysis.

Objective.—We sought to evaluate the effect of treatment on mortality in a large cohort of patients with Stevens-Johnson syndrome or toxic epidermal necrolysis.

Methods.—Data on therapy were retrospectively collected from patients in France and Germany enrolled in EuroSCAR, a case-control study of risk factors.

Results.—Neither intravenous immunoglobulins nor corticosteroids showed any significant effect on mortality in comparison with supportive care only. Compared with supportive care, odds ratios for death were 1.4 (95% confidence interval: 0.6-4.3) for intravenous immunoglobulins in France and 1.5 (0.5-4.4) in Germany, and 0.4 (0.1-1.7) for corticosteroids in France and 0.3 (0.1-1.1) in Germany.

Limitations.—Such an observational study with retrospective data collection has obvious limitations, including heterogeneity between the countries, supportive care, treatment doses, and durations.

Conclusions.—We found no sufficient evidence of a benefit for any specific treatment. The trend for a beneficial effect of corticosteroids deserves further exploration.

▶ Surgical trauma is associated with a prothrombotic state in which the coagulation cascade is activated, resulting in thrombin generation and formation of fibrin clots. Normally, this state obtains for a matter of days postoperatively, but in some cases, it may persist and lead to vascular thrombotic complications like deep vein thrombosis (DVT), pulmonary embolism (PE), acute myocardial infarction (AMI), transient ischemic attacks (TIAs), or stroke. In the case of a total hip arthroplasty procedure, for example, recent practice has included some weeks of coverage with low molecular weight heparin (LMWH) postoperatively as a preventive measure. Many surgeons are reluctant to undertake this as the approach is beset by concerns for balancing risks of hemorrhage versus benefits of prevention. There has therefore been a need for a reliable method of surveillance. The authors here present a study of the use of measured levels of urine prothrombin fragments 1 and 2 (uF1 + 2) for such an application.

B. A. Latenser, MD

The Relationship of Body Mass Index and Functional Outcomes in Patients With Acute Burns

Farrell RT, Gamelli RL, Aleem RF, et al (Univ Med Ctr, Maywood, IL)
J Burn Care Res 29:102-108, 2008

Obesity may contribute to the functional decline in elderly adults. It can also increase the risk of mortality in burn patients. However, little data exist regarding the relationship between obesity and functional outcomes in patients with burns. Data were collected regarding admission body mass index (BMI), length of stay, TBSA burn, inhalation injury, age, sex, discharge disposition, and discharge functional independence measure (FIM) scores for 221 patients. We used the classification and regression trees (CART) method to determine the strongest predictors of discharge disposition and FIM scores. Patients older than 59, with 0 to 30.75%

TBSA burn, and a BMI of less than 27 were more likely to return home when compared with matched patients with a greater BMI. Regardless of age and BMI, patients with greater than 30.75% TBSA burn were less likely to return home (27.6%) posthospitalization when compared with patients with less than 30.75% TBSA burn (82.8%). Patients aged 54 to 72 years with less than 22.50% TBSA burn and a higher BMI (>25.15) demonstrated lower FIM locomotion scores than corresponding patients with a lower BMI (<25.15). Older patients (>72.5 years) with burns less than 22.50% TBSA and a larger BMI (>31.25) had lower transfer FIM scores when compared with matched patients with a smaller BMI (≤31.25). Among patients with greater than 22.50 TBSA burn, women demonstrated lower FIM transfer and locomotion scores when compared with men. BMI may contribute to lower functional scores and the likelihood of discharge to an inpatient setting in elderly patients with less severe burns.

▶ Unfortunately, obesity has become an everyday reality for all health care clinicians. Although a number of factors influence outcomes and discharge disposition for burn patients, this is the first study that nicely demonstrates how obese middle-aged patients and elderly patients suffering from even small burns are less likely to return home at the time of discharge. As discharge from the hospital needs to be planned well in advance of the actual event, and patients with obesity may present severe challenges to the burn care team, being able to predict those patients who will require placement on discharge can decrease length of stay and prevent costly unnecessary hospital days. Factors weighing into the decision-making process of discharge disposition need to be familiar to the team. For those for whom the functional independence measure (FIM) is a new concept, this article contains a nice description of the variables and the scale, a tool that could be used for a variety of situations.

B. A. Latenser, MD

Comparison of premortem clinical diagnosis and autopsy findings in patients with burns
Kallinen O, Partanen TA, Maisniemi K, et al (Helsinki Univ Hosp, Finland)
Burns 34:595-602, 2008

Introduction.—Despite the diagnostic advancements, some clinically important diagnoses remain undetected during intensive care in burn patients. The aim of this study was to compare the premortem clinical diagnoses and autopsy findings.

Patients and methods.—A retrospective review of all burn deaths during 1995-2005 was conducted. The clinical diagnoses and autopsy reports were reviewed, and diagnostic discrepancies were classified into four categories, according to the impact on the treatment.

Results.—Overall mortality during the study period was 5.4%. Altogether 74 deaths were recorded, of which 71 were included in the study. Typical patient was a 58-year-old male with flame burn of %TBSA 49, ABSI 10. Clinical diagnostic discrepancies were found in 14.1% of the patients; one diagnostic discrepancy was recorded in each of the patients. Of these diagnostic discrepancies, 8.5% were considered major, and 5.6% would have altered the clinical outcome or therapy, if known at the time. Diagnostic discrepancies consisted of one cardiovascular, seven respiratory and two gastrointestinal missed diagnoses. The most common missed diagnosis was pneumonia.

Conclusion.—This study emphasizes the usefulness of autopsies to provide valuable clinical data for the treatment of burn patients. It also highlights the few missed diagnoses which may occur in burn patients.

▶ Information gained from autopsies may provide clinical data, uncover missed diagnoses, reveal congenital defects/abnormalities, and provide a powerful educational tool for all clinicians. In the United States, many burn deaths are covered under state laws that mandate autopsy for any traumatic death or death in a hospital within 24 hours of admission. Because of laws in Finland mandating autopsy, the authors were able to obtain a 100% autopsy rate over the 10-year study period. With only 86% complete concordance with premortem diagnoses, the autopsy findings of pneumonia, pulmonary embolus, myocardial infarction, and kidney, liver, and spleen necrosis provide an opportunity for improvement. Some of the findings would have altered the patient care strategy, as the findings of probable nonsurvivable diagnoses would have moved those patients to a comfort care category. Clinicians working in nonburn or trauma settings where the state may mandate autopsy should consider approaching the family for autopsy consent in those cases not mandated by law.

B. A. Latenser, MD

American Burn Association Practice Guidelines Burn Shock Resuscitation
Pham TN, Cancio LC, Gibran NS (Univ of Washington Burn Ctr, Seattle; U.S. Army Inst of Surgical Research, Fort Sam Houston, TX)
J Burn Care Res 29:257-266, 2008

Background.—The triage and initial treatment of burn patients have been guided by estimates of the total burned surface area (TBSA). The goal of fluid resuscitation is to support organ perfusion with the least of amount of fluid possible and the least cost to the patient physiologically. Fluid therapy must be tailored to the specific patient, and hemodynamic endpoints indicative of adequate tissue perfusion require close monitoring. Resuscitation issues include type and rate of fluid given as well as adjunct measures.

Guidelines.—Patients, whether adults or children, with over 20% TBSA require formal fluid resuscitation based on estimates of body size and surface area burned. The crystalloid need is met by 2 to 4 ml/kg body weight/%TBSA over the initial 24 hours. The fluid given should be titrated to obtain a urinary output of 0.5 ml/kg/hr in adults and 1 ml/kg/hr for young children. The most popular resuscitation formulas include lactated Ringer's (LR) solution, which is effective against hypovolemia and extracellular sodium deficits resulting from thermal injury. If hypertonic saline fluid is used, smaller fluid volumes are appropriate. Large volumes of hypertonic saline fluid can raise the risk of hypernatremia and should only be used by experienced burn physicians with close monitoring of plasma sodium levels. The addition of colloids to resuscitation can lower the total volume requirements, especially after the first 12 to 24 hours, but further study is required to document any other benefits.

For pediatric patients, both vigilance and precision are required in conducting resuscitation measures. Weight-based formulas to determine the amount of fluid are probably insufficient. Body surface area plus estimated needs based on burn size are more accurate, but glucose homeostasis must also be considered in children. Maintenance fluids should be given to pediatric patients in addition to the fluid needed to ameliorate the burn injury.

Patients with full-thickness injuries, inhalation injury, and delayed resuscitation often require increased fluid volumes. Patients who are awake and alert and have moderately sized burns may benefit from oral resuscitation.

Adjunct Measures.—Antioxidant therapy, specifically using high-dose ascorbic acid, presents an option that may reduce the formation of edema and the fluid requirements of burn patients. This adjunct measure requires validation before it reaches the level of a treatment standard. Plasma exchange is designed to restore the patient's preinjury leukocyte state by removing part of the patient's plasma volume and adding fresh frozen plasma and albumin. The evidence supporting this measure is scant.

Conclusions.—Although the data are insufficient to support a standard treatment for burn shock resuscitation, measures are available to meet the challenges posed in these patients' initial treatment. Further research is required to support most of the approaches and the adjunct measures.

▶ Although there is insufficient class I data to support a specific resuscitation protocol, certain guidelines may optimize patient outcomes. Another mass casualty event such as the World Trade Center bombings in 2001 could result in a multitude of burn victims that exceed regional burn center capabilities. In such an event, burn patients would be kept in local and/or regional critical care units until transportation to burn centers around the country could be arranged. In that instance, practitioners with critical care skills should have the knowledge to provide emergency burn care for up to 72 hours for critically burned patients. This rational template for burn patient resuscitation, based on current practices in United States burn centers, should be used as a reference for those clinicians who seldom care for burns.

B. A. Latenser, MD

Lightning injury: A review
Ritenour AE, Morton MJ, McManus JG, et al (U.S. Army Institute of Surgical Research, Fort Sam Houston, TX)
Burns 34:585-594, 2008

Lightning is an uncommon but potentially devastating cause of injury in patients presenting to burn centers. These injuries feature unusual symptoms, high mortality, and significant long-term morbidity. This paper will review the epidemiology, physics, clinical presentation, management principles, and prevention of lightning injuries.

▶ Although injury due to lightning is a rare event, much of what we think we know about how lightning-induced injury may be more based on myth than fact. There are entire textbooks written on lightning injury, delving into the physics of the injury and the myriad symptoms, as well as later sequelae that may affect patients. Unless one has a special interest in the subject, reading an entire textbook on the subject of lightning injuries is unnecessary. This thorough review not only provides educated guidance for those caring for patients who have sustained injuries due to lightning, but also reminds us of some (not so) commonsense practices to avoid being struck by lightning.

B. A. Latenser, MD

Safety and Efficacy of an Intensive Insulin Protocol in a Burn-Trauma Intensive Care Unit
Cochran A, Davis L, Morris SE, et al (Burn Ctr, Univ of Utah, Salt Lake City, UT)
J Burn Care Res 29:187-191, 2008

Aggressive glycemic management in critically ill patients with acute burn injury or life-threatening soft-tissue infections has not been thoroughly evaluated. An intensive insulin protocol with target glucose values of less than 120 mg/dl was implemented in October 2005 in our regional Burn-Trauma intensive care unit. We reviewed our initial experience with this protocol to evaluate the safety and efficacy of aggressive glycemic control in these patient groups. Patients were placed on the intensive insulin protocol based upon the need for glycemic management during their hospitalization for burn or soft-tissue disease. Patient information prospectively collected while on protocol included all measured blood glucose values, total daily insulin use, and incidence of hypoglycemic episodes, defined as serum glucose <60 mg/dl. Thirty patients (17 burns, 13 soft-tissue infections) were placed on the intensive insulin protocol during the first 16 months of use. The mean daily blood glucose level for burn patients was 115.9 mg/dl and for soft-tissue disease patients was 119.5 mg/dl. There was a 5% incidence of hypoglycemic episodes per protocol day. All hypoglycemic episodes were treated by holding the insulin infusion, and no episode had known adverse effects. Hyperglycemia in critically ill patients with burns and extensive soft-tissue disease can be effectively managed with an insulin protocol that targets blood glucose values of less than 120 mg/dl with minimal incidence of hypoglycemia. A multicenter prospective randomized trial would provide the ideal forum for evaluating clinical outcome benefits of using an intensive insulin protocol.

▶ Ever since the landmark article by Van den Berghe in 2001, glycemic control for critically ill patients in a variety of settings has remained a hot topic. There is great debate about which patient populations will benefit, what the target glucose values should be, how monitoring should be conducted, the effect of hypoglycemic events, and the cost/benefit ratio. What is agreed on is that burn patients benefit from aggressive glycemic management. Hemmila et al[1] recently published their findings using a blood glucose target of 100 to 140 mg/dL (hospital-wide policy) and concluded that an elevated blood glucose was a nonspecific marker for infection. Their historical controls seemed to be a sicker patient population, leading me to conclude that the findings of improved outcomes using the 100 to 140 mg/dL range blood glucose are not generalizable. Mann et al[2] performed a survey of American Burn Association-verified burn centers and found that 73% of all centers used an intensive insulin protocol with the upper limit of 120 mg/dL. Although the focus of this article is to evaluate protocol safety, the protocol outlined by the authors is easy for nursing staff and more inexperienced housestaff to understand and follow. If anyone is interested in a simpler method of strict glycemic control (in our medical intensive care unit (MICU), there are no less than 7 separate insulin protocols), I would recommend this protocol. This is an instance where simplicity leads to decreasing errors and enhanced patient safety and outcomes.

B. A. Latenser, MD

References

1. Hemmila MR, Taddonio MA, Arbabi S, Maggio PM, Wahl WL. Intensive insulin therapy is associated with reduced infectious complications in burn patients. *Surgery.* 2008;144:629-637.
2. Mann EA, Pidcoke HF, Salinas J, Holcomb JB, Wolf SE, Wade CE. The impact of intensive insulin protocols and restrictive blood transfusion strategies on glucose measurement in American Burn Association (ABA) verified burn centers. *J Burn Care Res.* 2008;29:718-723.

Use of Inhaled Heparin/N-acetylcystine in Inhalation Injury: Does it help?
Holt J, Saffle JR, Morris SE, et al (Univ of Utah Health Sciences Ctr, Salt Lake City, UT)
J Burn Care Res 29:192-195, 2008

Inhaled heparin/N-acetylcystine (AHA) has been reported to decrease mortality in children with inhalation injury. The use of AHA therapy in adult burn patients with inhalation injury has not been evaluated. We hypothesized that patients who received AHA therapy in the management of inhalation injury would have better pulmonary mechanics and better clinical outcomes than patients who did not. This study is a retrospective chart review of pulmonary mechanics and clinical outcomes in all inpatients identified in the institutional ABA/TRACS database as having sustained inhalation injury from 1999 to 2005. Patients were not assigned to a treatment group. One hundred and fifty patients with inhalation injury were identified. Sixty-two patients were treated with AHA during the first 72 hours of admission. Treatment occurred mostly in patients admitted after 2002, with only 18 patients receiving AHA from 1999 through 2002. Treated and untreated patients did not differ in age or TBSA burn injury, nor did any studied clinical outcome differ between treated and untreated groups. In addition, there was no difference in pulmonary findings at 1 week after injury between treated and untreated patients. Although best Pao_2 was higher in treated patients during the first 72 hours, this was not a durable finding, and the best Pao_2/Fio_2 ratio was unaffected by treatment. Importantly, the use of AHA in adults with inhalation injury did not affect clinical outcomes. A prospective, randomized trial would be of benefit to delineate the clinical benefits of AHA treatment for inhalation injury.

▶ Once the Galveston group published their findings in 1998 that the use of inhaled heparin/N-acetylcystine in pediatric burn patients with inhalation injury decreased mortality rates by up to 40%, the practice slowly made its way into current burn care treatment for both adult and pediatric patients. Many recent publications and protocols have come to include the Galveston model, including dosing and duration of administration regimens. However, the fantastic results obtained by Galveston have not been reproducible up to this point. Although this particular study did not randomize patients, leading to potential selection bias, the patients do seem similar in both groups. Holt and colleagues have provided another example of a treatment regimen becoming part of the "standard of care" without thorough testing or evidence of efficacy in adult burn patients with inhalation injury. Although appealing, until there is a prospective randomized study, the treatment regimen cannot be recommended as mainstream therapy.

B. A. Latenser, MD

5 Infectious Disease

Nosocomial/Ventilator-Acquired Pneumonia

Effectiveness of Chlorhexidine Bathing to Reduce Catheter-Associated Bloodstream Infections in Medical Intensive Care Unit Patients
Bleasdale SC, Trick WE, Gonzalez IM, et al (Rush Univ Med Ctr; Cook County Bureau of Health Services; et al)
Arch Intern Med 167:2073-2079, 2007

Objective.—To determine whether patients bathed daily with chlorhexidine gluconate (CHG) have a lower incidence of primary bloodstream infections (BSIs) compared with patients bathed with soap and water.

Methods.—The study design was a 52-week, 2-arm, crossover (ie, concurrent control group) clinical trial with intention-to-treat analysis. The study setting was the 22-bed medical intensive care unit (MICU), which comprises 2 geographically separate, similar 11-bed units, of the John H. Stroger Jr (Cook County) Hospital, a 464-bed public teaching hospital in Chicago, Illinois. The study population comprised 836 MICU patients. During the first of 2 study periods (28 weeks), 1 hospital unit was randomly selected to serve as the intervention unit in which patients were bathed daily with 2% CHG-impregnated washcloths (Sage 2% CHG cloths; Sage Products Inc, Cary, Illinois); patients in the concurrent control unit were bathed daily with soap and water. After a 2-week wash-out period at the end of the first period, cleansing methods were crossed over for 24 more weeks. Main outcome measures included incidences of primary BSIs and clinical (culture-negative) sepsis (primary outcomes) and incidences of other infections (secondary outcomes).

Results.—Patients in the CHG intervention arm were significantly less likely to acquire a primary BSI (4.1 vs 10.4 infections per 1000 patient days; incidence difference, 6.3 [95% confidence interval, 1.2-11.0). The incidences of other infections, including clinical sepsis, were similar between the units. Protection against primary BSI by CHG cleansing was apparent after 5 or more days in the MICU.

Conclusion.—Daily cleansing of MICU patients with CHG-impregnated cloths is a simple, effective strategy to decrease the rate of primary BSIs.

Trial Registration.—clinicaltrials.gov Identifier: NCT00130221.

▶ Catheter-related sepsis is one of the major noscomial infections found in the hospital. A variety of technological approaches to prevention of catheter infection have been studied including antimicrobial/antiseptic-bonded catheter material, use of subcutaneous cuffs, and use of chlorhexidine-impregnated patches at the insertion site.[1] However, simpler approaches may be equally effective. Chlorhexidine skin preparation[2] and chlorhexidine-soaked patches at the catheter insertion site[3] have also been shown to be efficacious. This prospective crossover study similarly demonstrates that a simple daily bath with a 2% chlorhexidine-soaked washcloth decreases catheter-related bloodstream infection (bacteremia or candidemia) by approximately 60% compared with daily washing with soap and water. Given that technological solutions like antimicrobial/antiseptic-bonded catheters have an incremental cost of several hundred dollars, it seems advisable to first consider adopting low-tech solutions such as chlorhexidine washcloth baths.

A. Kumar, MD

References

1. Raad I, Hanna H, Maki D. Intravascular catheter-related infections: advances in diagnosis, prevention, and management. *Lancet Infect Dis.* 2007;7:645-657.
2. Kumar A, Ostromecki A, Direnfeld J, et al. Prospective randomized trial of 10% povidone-iodine versus 0.5% tincture of chlorhexidine as cutaneous antisepsis for prevention of central venous catheter infection. *Clin Infect Dis.* 2000;31: 1001-1007.
3. Maki, DG, Mermel, LA, Kluger, D, et al. The efficacy of a chlorhexidine-impregnated sponge (BiopatchTM) for the prevention of intravascular catheter-related infection: a prospective, randomized controlled multicenter study. 40th Interscience Conference on Antimicrobial Agents and Chemotherapy, #1430, 2000.

Utility of bilateral bronchoalveolar lavage for the diagnosis of ventilator-associated pneumonia in critically ill surgical patients
Jackson S-R, Ernst NE, Mueller EW, et al (Univ of Cincinnati, OH; et al)
Am J Surg 195:159-163, 2008

Background.—Bronchoalveolar lavage (BAL) is recommended to facilitate the diagnosis of ventilator-associated pneumonia (VAP). It is unclear if bilateral sampling improves the accuracy of BAL.

Methods.—Consecutive patients with clinical suspicion for VAP were analyzed. All patients underwent bilateral BAL. A threshold of >10^4 colony-forming units (cfu)/mL was diagnostic for VAP (VAP positive). Samples were concordant if the organism(s) and thresholds from both lungs were diagnostically consistent. Organisms ≤10^4 cfu/mL with growth on the contralateral sample >10^4 cfu/mL were considered false-negative samples.

Results.—Between November 2005 and April 2006, 73 patients were considered clinically suspicious for VAP. Forty-four (60%) patients were

VAP positive. Twenty-eight (64%) VAP patients had concordant samples. Overall, there were 15 false-negative samples. Sole use of the unilateral samples to guide treatment would have inappropriately directed antibiotic avoidance and/or discontinuation in 25% of VAP patients. Influence of the chest radiograph was equivocal because of the presence of bilateral infiltrates in 80% of discordant samples.

Conclusions.—Bilateral BAL improves the accuracy of bronchoscopy in diagnosing VAP. Unilateral BAL may be insensitive in patients with clinically significant contralateral infection.

▶ Whether or not to treat patients with suspected ventilator-associated pneumonia (VAP) with empiric antibiotics as directed by consensus guidelines or treat based on finding significant organisms on invasive sampling, bronchoalveolar lavage (BAL), or protected specimen brushes remains an area of controversy despite decades of opinion and scores of studies.[1,2] This study muddies the water a bit by suggesting that performing a unilateral procedure in the region of the radiographic infiltrate in contrast to a bilateral procedure may not be sufficient for making a diagnosis of VAP or defining the offending organism. In this trial, 15% of the BAL procedures performed on the side of the infiltrate yielded a false-negative result. In addition, the results of a unilateral BAL alone would have led to an incorrect diagnosis in one-quarter of the patients. Of course, all of these results need to be balanced by the observation that we all recognize it is important to start the correct antibiotic as soon as feasible.[3] We have seen that in septic shock there is an increase in mortality associated with each hour of delay in the administration of effective antibiotics after the onset of hypotension.[4] Although this has not been proven in the setting of VAP, it does make sense that the initial therapy will be based on consensus guideline recommendations, and the results of the BAL will likely serve to either confirm effective treatment choice or assist in the antibiotic change when the empiric treatment is ineffective.[1] We are still waiting for a study to show that the correct diagnostic and therapeutic approach improves long-term outcome in the setting of VAP. This is partly related to the influence of the underlying comorbid condition that necessitated the need for mechanical ventilatory support in the first place.

R. P. Dellinger, MD

References

1. American Thoracic Society and The Infectious Disease Society of America. Guidelines for the management of adults with hospital-acquired, ventilator-associated, and healthcare-associated pneumonia. *Am J Respir Crit Care Med.* 2005;171: 388-416.
2. Fagon JY, Chastre J, Wolff M, et al. Invasive and noninvasive strategies for management of suspected ventilator-associated pneumonia. a randomized trial. *Ann Int Med.* 2000;132:621-630.
3. Kollef MH. Appropriate antibiotic therapy for ventilator-associated pneumonia and sepsis: a necessity, not an issue for debate. *Intens Care Med.* 2003;29:147-149.
4. Kumar A, Roberts D, Wood KE, et al. Duration of hypotension before initiation of effective antimicrobial therapy is the critical determinant of survival in human septic shock. *Crit Care Med.* 2006;34:1589-1596.

Candidemia and candiduria in critically ill patients admitted to intensive care units in France: incidence, molecular diversity, management and outcome

Bougnoux M-E, Kac G, Aegerter P, et al (Université René Descartes, Paris; Hôpital Européen Georges Pompidou, Paris; Hôpital Ambroise-Paré, Boulogne Billancount, France)
Intensive Care Med 34:292-299, 2008

Objective.—To determine the concomitant incidence, molecular diversity, management and outcome of nosocomial candidemia and candiduria in intensive care unit (ICU) patients in France.

Design.—A 1-year prospective observational study in 24 adult ICUs.

Patients.—Two hundred and sixty-two patients with nosocomial candidemia and/or candiduria.

Measurements and results.—Blood and urine samples were collected when signs of sepsis were present. Antifungal susceptibility of *Candida* strains was determined; in addition, all blood and 72% of urine *C. albicans* isolates were analyzed by using multi-locus sequence type (MLST). The mean incidences of candidemia and candiduria were 6.7 and 27.4/1000 admissions, respectively. Eight percent of candiduric patients developed candidemia with the same species. The mean interval between ICU admission and candidemia was 19.0 ± 2.9 days, and 17.2 ± 1.1 days for candiduria. *C. albicans* and *C. glabrata* were isolated in 54.2% and 17% of blood and 66.5% and 21.6% of urine *Candida*-positive cultures, respectively. Fluconazole was the most frequently prescribed agent. In all candidemic patients, the prescribed curative antifungal agent was active in vitro against the responsible identified strain. Crude ICU mortality was 61.8% for candidemic and 31.3% for candiduric patients. Seventy-five percent of the patients were infected with a unique *C. albicans* strain; cross-transmission between seven patients was suggested in one hospital.

Conclusions.—Candidemia is late-onset ICU-acquired infection associated with high mortality. No difference in susceptibility and genetic background were found between blood and urine strains of *Candida* species.

▶ Choosing ideal antibiotics in the setting of shock is of paramount importance. "Typical infections" in critically ill patients are changing. The use of broad-spectrum antibacterials, parenteral nutrition, increased use and numerous varieties of invasive devices, and extended life expectancy of chronically ill patients present a greater challenge for clinicians to choose the "correct or ideal" antibiotic regime. The new paradigm may need to include antifungals, in addition to antibacterials coupled with more aggressive prevention as part of the standard arsenal. This article suggests that, in prolonged ICU admissions, both candiduria and candidemia are becoming more commonly encountered infectious causes of shock with alarmingly high mortality. Although the spectrum of antifungals has increased since the study was conducted, fluconazole and amphotericin derivatives were mostly used. The minimum inhibitory concentrations (MICs) for fluconazole against *Candida albicans* remained acceptable in this study. More importantly, the argument of using empiric or broad-spectrum antifungals may not be the answer for combating the associated high mortality rate. Fluconazole can be a good first choice as *C albicans* is most often encountered. Rather, the more rapid implementation of antimicrobials, prompt identification of infectious causes of shock, and considering fungal infections higher on the differential diagnosis are important. It should be almost dogmatic that patients with indwelling catheters, females with urinary devices, immunosuppressed patients, and burn patients should be considered candidates at risk of fungal infections in the setting of new-onset shock and after a prolonged ICU stay that undoubtedly included a course of board-spectrum antibacterial medications. An important point for ICU patients is the time course in which fungal infections should be considered, approximately 17 days for the onset of candiduria and approximately 19 days for candidemia. Additionally, there was an average delay of 4 days between blood sampling and positive blood cultures, a diagnostic challenge that plagues early institution of antimicrobials and choosing the "appropriate regime." Regular implementation of antifungals in certain critically ill populations requires a broad study to consider such a question. Such an addition would likely recycle the problem of new resistance patterns and pressures. The balance of improving mortality or simply worsening resistance patterns is the clinical question that needs to be answered. However, a low threshold to implement antifungals should be considered in ICU populations with prolonged hospitalizations, particularly when patients fail to respond to standardized aggressive shock management. This article advocates developing expedient methods for diagnosing aggressive fungal infections. Likewise, clinicians need to consider instituting antifungals earlier with greater suspicion in the appropriate critically ill population. Ultimately, clinicians should become the masters of the obvious, prevention. Shortening antibiotic duration of treatments, avoiding invasive devices, finding ways to shorten ICU stays, and earlier mobilization of patients may be the most effective and efficient help offered for patients on all fronts.

R. Nanda, DO
C. Bekes, MD, MPH

A Comparative Study of Community-Acquired Pneumonia Patients Admitted to the Ward and the ICU
Restrepo MI, Mortensen EM, Velez JA, et al (Univ Texas Health Science Ctr, San Antonio, TX; VERDICT, South Texas Veterans Health Care System Audie L. Murphy Division, San Antonio, TX)
Chest 133:610-617, 2008

Background.—Limited information is available on the health-care utilization of hospitalized patients with community-acquired pneumonia (CAP) depending on the location of care. Our aim was to compare the clinical characteristics, etiologies, and outcomes of patients with CAP who were admitted to the ICU with those admitted who were to the ward service.

Methods.—A retrospective cohort study, at two tertiary teaching hospitals, one of which was a Veterans Affairs hospital, and the other a county hospital. Eligible subjects had been admitted to the hospital with a diagnosis of CAP between January 1, 1999, and December 31, 2001, had a confirmatory chest radiograph, and a hospital discharge *International Classification of Diseases*, ninth revision, diagnosis of pneumonia. Subjects were excluded from the study if they had designated "comfort measures only" or had been transferred from another acute care hospital or were nursing home patients. Bivariate and multivariable analysis evaluated 30-day and 90-day mortality as the dependent measures.

Results.—Data were abstracted on 730 patients (ICU, 145 patients; wards, 585 patients). Compared to ward patients, ICU patients were more likely to be male ($p = 0.001$), and to have congestive heart failure ($p = 0.01$) and COPD ($p = 0.01$). ICU patients also had higher mean pneumonia severity index scores (112 [SD, 35] vs 83 [SD, 30], respectively; $p = 0.02$). Patients admitted to the ICU had a longer mean length of hospital stay (12 days [SD, 10 days] vs 7 days [SD, 17 days], respectively; $p = 0.07$), and a higher 30-day mortality rate (23% vs 4%, respectively; $p < 0.001$) and 90-day mortality rate (28% vs 8%, respectively; $p < 0.001$) compared to ward patients.

Conclusions.—ICU patients present with more severe disease and more comorbidities. ICU patients stay longer in the hospital and have a much higher mortality rate when compared to ward patients. Management strategies should be designed to improve clinical outcomes in ICU patients.

▶ This study confirms that severe community-acquired pneumonia (CAP) has a higher pneumonia severity index (PSI) score, longer length of stay, and higher 30- and 90-day mortality rate than less severe forms of CAP. It was interesting to note that the etiologic organisms, when found on culture, were similar between the ICU and ward patients. This observation might lead the clinician to question the recommended antibiotic regimens from the 2007 Infectious Diseases Society of America/American Thoracic Society (IDSA/ATS) consensus guidelines for adult patients with CAP.[1]

Unfortunately, this was a retrospective study and we are not given any information that allows us to understand how the decision was made to admit a patient to the ward or the ICU. There are a number of recommendations to help the clinician determine who has severe CAP versus a less severe form, but we are clueless as to the rationale that was followed by these 2 institutions. Nonetheless, the conclusion does support the notion that severe CAP, at least as defined by admission to the ICU, has a higher mortality rate and longer length of stay.

R. A. Balk, MD

Reference

1. Marshall RP, Webb PD, Bellingan CJ, et al. Angiotensin converting enzyme insertion/deletion polymorphism is associated with susceptibility and outcome in acute respiratory distress syndrome. *Am J Respir Crit Care Med.* 2002;166:646-650.

Angiotensin-Converting Enzyme Insertion/Deletion Polymorphism and Risk and Outcome of Pneumonia

van de Garde EMW, Endeman H, Deneer VHM, et al (St. Antonius Hosp, Nieuwegein, The Netherlands)
Chest 133:220-225, 2008

Background.—Recent studies have suggested involvement of the angiotensin-converting enzyme (ACE) insertion/deletion (I/D) polymorphism in the susceptibility to and severity of community-acquired pneumonia (CAP) in Asian populations. We have explored the hypothesis that the ACE I/D polymorphism affects the risk and outcome of CAP in a Dutch white population.

Methods.—This is a hospital-based prospective observational study including patients with CAP admitted between October 2004 and August 2006. All patients were genotyped, and pneumonia severity and clinical outcome were compared between patients with II, ID, and DD genotypes of the ACE gene. Pneumonia severity was assessed on day of hospital admission and consecutively on days 2, 3, 5, and 10 of hospital stay using the acute physiology score (APS). Outcomes evaluated were duration of hospital stay, ICU admittance, and in-hospital and 28-day mortality rates. To study the association between ACE genotype and risk of pneumonia, the distribution of the ACE I/D polymorphism was compared with healthy control subjects from the same geographic region.

Results.—In total, 200 patients with pneumonia and 200 control subjects were included in the study. Mean age of the patients was 63 years. APS scores were not different between the genotype groups on any of the days, and all clinical outcomes (duration of hospital stay, ICU admittance, in-hospital and 28-day mortality rates) were comparable between the three genotype groups. The ACE I/D genotype distribution was identical for patients and control subjects ($p = 0.973$).

Conclusions.—The ACE I/D polymorphism is not associated with risk and outcome of CAP in the Dutch white population.

▶ The role of angiotensin-converting enzyme (ACE) in the pathogenesis and development of pneumonia and/or acute respiratory distress syndrome (ARDS) has been suggested by recent studies. The observation of specific deletion polymorphisms on intron 16 of the ACE gene and an increase in pneumonia development in elderly Japanese patients led these authors to test this hypothesis in a group of Dutch patients with pneumonia. Whether this relationship with pneumonia is specific to the Japanese population or was not evident in the specific group of Dutch patients enrolled in this study remains to be seen with further study. The attractive part of defining a role for ACE in the pathogenesis of pneumonia is the potential to easily block this effect by the use of ACE inhibitors. We will await additional studies to help answer this important question.

R. A. Balk, MD

SMART-COP: A Tool for Predicting the Need for Intensive Respiratory or Vasopressor Support in Community-Acquired Pneumonia

Charles PGP, Wolfe R, Whitby M, et al (Austin Health, Heidelberg; Monash Univ; Princess Alexandra Hosp, Woolloongabba; et al)
Clin Infect Dis 47:375-384, 2008

Background.—Existing severity assessment tools, such as the pneumonia severity index (PSI) and CURB-65 (tool based on confusion, urea level, respiratory rate, blood pressure, and age ≥65 years), predict 30-day mortality in community-acquired pneumonia (CAP) and have limited ability to predict which patients will require intensive respiratory or vasopressor support (IRVS).

Methods.—The Australian CAP Study (ACAPS) was a prospective study of 882 episodes in which each patient had a detailed assessment of severity features, etiology, and treatment outcomes. Multivariate logistic regression was performed to identify features at initial assessment that were associated with receipt of IRVS. These results were converted into a simple points-based severity tool that was validated in 5 external databases, totaling 7464 patients.

Results.—In ACAPS, 10.3% of patients received IRVS, and the 30-day mortality rate was 5.7%. The features statistically significantly associated with receipt of IRVS were low systolic blood pressure (2 points), multilobar chest radiography involvement (1 point), low albumin level (1 point), high respiratory rate (1 point), tachycardia (1 point), confusion (1 point), poor oxygenation (2 points), and low arterial pH (2 points): SMART-COP. A SMART-COP score of ≥3 points identified 92% of patients who received IRVS, including 84% of patients who did not need immediate admission to the intensive care unit. Accuracy was also high in the 5 validation databases. Sensitivities of PSI and CURB-65 for identifying the need for IRVS were 74% and 39%, respectively.

Conclusions.—SMART-COP is a simple, practical clinical tool for accurately predicting the need for IRVS that is likely to assist clinicians in determining CAP severity.

▶ There have been a number of attempts to define patients with severe community-acquired pneumonia (CAP) using clinical indices.[1-3] The pneumonia severity index (PSI) and a tool based on confusion, urea level, respiratory rate, blood pressure (BP), and age [3]65 years (CURB-65) have been 2 of the most popular systems, but require laboratory values in addition to clinical parameters.[2,3] This article discusses the value of systolic BP, multilobar chest radiography involvement, albumin level, respiratory rate, tachycardia, confusion, oxygenation, and arterial pH (SMART-COP) to predict the need for intensive respiratory or vasopressor support (IRVS). Although not the same as severe CAP, the use of IRVS therapy typically signifies a need for management in the intensive care unit. The authors have compared the SMART-COP tool with other scoring tools. As seen by the receiver operating characteristic (ROC) curve in Fig 2 in the original article, SMART-COP performed better at defining a group of patients with severe CAP who require the use of IRVS. In addition to correlating with the use of IRVS, the SMART-COP score also correlated with mortality rate. The SMART-COP score seems to be a good predictor of severe CAP and will likely be used based on its ease of use and performance ability.

R. A. Balk, MD

References

1. Mandell LA, Anzueto RG, Hollander A, et al. Infectious Disease Society of America/American Thoracic Society Consensus Guidelines on the management of community-acquired pneumonia in adults. *Clin Infect Dis.* 2007;44:S27-S72.
2. Fine MJ, Auble TE, Yealy DM, et al. A prediction rule to identify low risk patients with community acquired pneumonia. *N Engl J Med.* 1997;336:243-250.
3. Lim WS, van der Eerden MM, Laing R, et al. Defining community acquired pneumonia severity on presentation to hospital: an international derivation and validation study. *Thorax.* 2003;58:377-382.

Silver-Coated Endotracheal Tubes and Incidence of Ventilator-Associated Pneumonia: The Nascent Randomized Trial

Kollef MH, Afessa B, Anzueto A, et al (Washington Univ School of Medicine, St Louis; Mayo Clinic College of Medicine, Rochester, MN; South Texas Veterans Health Care System Audie L. Murphy Division, San Antonio, Texas)
JAMA 300:805-813, 2008

Context.—Ventilator-associated pneumonia (VAP) causes substantial morbidity. A silver-coated endotracheal tube has been designed to reduce VAP incidence by preventing bacterial colonization and biofilm formation.

Objective.—To determine whether a silver-coated endotracheal tube would reduce the incidence of microbiologically confirmed VAP.

Design, Setting, and Participants.—Prospective, randomized, single-blind, controlled study conducted in 54 centers in North America. A total of 9417 adult patients (≥18 years) were screened between 2002 and 2006. A total of 2003 patients expected to require mechanical ventilation for 24 hours or longer were randomized.

Intervention.—Patients were assigned to undergo intubation with 1 of 2 high-volume, low-pressure endotracheal tubes, similar except for a silver coating on the experimental tube.

Main Outcome Measures.—Primary outcome was VAP incidence based on quantitative bronchoalveolar lavage fluid culture with 10^4 colony-forming units/mL or greater in patients intubated for 24 hours or longer. Other outcomes were VAP incidence in all intubated patients, time to VAP onset, length of intubation and duration of intensive care unit and hospital stay, mortality, and adverse events.

Results.—Among patients intubated for 24 hours or longer, rates of microbiologically confirmed VAP were 4.8% (37/766 patients; 95% confidence interval [CI], 3.4%-6.6%) in the group receiving the silver-coated tube and 7.5% (56/743; 95% CI, 5.7%-9.7%) ($P = .03$) in the group receiving the uncoated tube (all intubated patients, 3.8% [37/968; 95% CI, 2.7%-5.2%] and 5.8% [56/964; 95% CI, 4.4%-7.5%] [$P=.04$]), with a relative risk reduction of 35.9% (95% CI, 3.6%-69.0%; all intubated patients, 34.2% [95% CI, 1.2%-67.9%]). The silver-coated endotracheal tube was associated with delayed occurrence of VAP ($P=.005$). No statistically significant between-group differences were observed in durations of intubation, intensive care unit stay, and hospital stay; mortality; and frequency and severity of adverse events.

Conclusion.—Patients receiving a silver-coated endotracheal tube had a statistically significant reduction in the incidence of VAP and delayed time to VAP occurrence compared with those receiving a similar, uncoated tube.

Trial Registration.—clinicaltrials.gov Identifier: NCT00148642.

▶ Ventilator-associated pneumonia (VAP) is one of the major preventable causes of morbidity and mortality in the ICU. The pathogenesis is thought to be related to colonization of the oropharynx with bacterial pathogens followed by migration of these pathogens into the lung through microaspiration of pooled secretions around the endotracheal cuff. Biofilm formation on the surface of the endotracheal tube may contribute to VAP by shielding pathogens from direct contact with antimicrobials and effectively providing a protected reservoir for the pathogen. The use of antimicrobial/antiseptic-impregnated central venous catheters has shown a high degree of efficacy in reducing the risk of infusion-related sepsis.[1] Similarly, silver-coated urinary catheters substantially reduce the risk of nosocomial urinary tract infections.[2]

This study demonstrates that a similar approach can reduce the risk of VAP by as much as a third. As such, it is an important demonstration of how technological innovation can be harnessed to optimize patient care. Although no formal recommendations recommend use of antiseptic/antimicrobial-impregnated catheters yet, it seems likely that use of these devices will become the standard of practice in the near future, at least for select patients likely to be intubated for more than short periods of time.

A. Kumar, MD

References

1. Hockenhull JC, Dwan KM, Smith GW, et al. The clinical effectiveness of central venous catheters treated with anti-infective agents in preventing catheter-related bloodstream infections: a systematic review. *J Crit Care Med.* 2009;37:702-712.
2. Karchmer TB, Giannetta ET, Muto CA, et al. A randomized crossover study of silver-coated urinary catheters in hospitalized patients. *Arch Intern Med.* 2000; 160:3294-3298.

Polyurethane cuffed endotracheal tubes to prevent early postoperative pneumonia after cardiac surgery: A pilot study
Poelaert J, Depuydt P, De Wolf A, et al (Ghent Univ, Belgium; Ghent Univ Hosp, Belgium; et al)
J Thorac Cardiovasc Surg 135:771-776, 2008

Objective.—Patients receiving mechanical ventilation through an endotracheal tube are at increased risk for pneumonia. Because microaspiration of contaminated supraglottic secretions past the endotracheal tube cuff is considered to be central in the pathogenesis of ventilator-associated and postoperative pneumonia, better sealing of the upper trachea by the endotracheal tube cuff could possibly reduce this risk. We therefore postulated that use of a polyurethane cuffed tube would prevent early postoperative pneumonia through this mechanism in a population of cardiac surgical patients.

Methods.—In a prospective, single-blind, randomized study, patients scheduled for cardiac surgery were allocated to intubation with a polyurethane cuffed endotracheal tube or the routinely used polyvinyl chloride cuffed endotracheal tube. Patients were scheduled for routine or emergency cardiac surgery and admitted to an 8-bed cardiac surgical intensive care unit of a tertiary care hospital.

Results.—A total of 134 patients were available for analysis (67 in each group). Whereas mortality was not different between the groups, the incidence of early postoperative pneumonia and empirical prescription of antibiotic therapy were significantly lower in the polyurethane group than in the polyvinyl chloride group (23% vs 42%, $P < .03$). Intensive care unit and hospital stays were not significantly different between the two study subsets (3 ± 5 days vs 3 ± 4 days and 16 ± 9 vs 17 ± 11 days, respectively). In a multivariate regression analysis, preoperative serum creatinine levels (odds ratio 1.85, confidence interval 1.02–3.37, $P = .04$) and perioperative transfusion (odds ratio 1.50, confidence interval 1.08–3.37, $P = .015$) were independently associated with increased risk of early postoperative pneumonia, whereas use of a polyurethane endotracheal tube was protective (odds ratio 0.31, confidence interval 0.13–0.77, $P = .01$).

Conclusion.—Polyurethane cuffed endotracheal tubes can reduce the frequency of early postoperative pneumonia in cardiac surgical patients.

▶ Nosocomial pneumonia, and specifically ventilator-associated pneumonia (VAP), continues to be a significant complication in patients who are in an ICU. It is associated with increased morbidity and mortality and is being considered by Centers for Medicare and Medicaid Services as one of the nonpayment diagnoses for 2009. One of the contributors to VAP is microaspiration of upper airway and oral flora. Approaches to reduce this risk include the following: decreased leakage of flora around an endotracheal tube (ETT), improved suctioning of secretions, and neutralization of pathogens.[1] Additional measures that have been shown to decrease the development of VAP include peptic ulcer disease prophylaxis, deep vein thrombosis prophylaxis, elevation of the head of bed, and holding sedation daily. A recent update on the guidelines and recommended practices to reduce VAP has been published.[2]

One of the contributors to VAP, leakage of flora, is felt to be facilitated through channels that form in the cuff of a standard ETT cuff.[3] Polyurethane cuffs are ultrathin and were designed to prevent formation of folds in the cuff and thus theoretically reduce the likelihood leakage of secretions around the cuff. This pilot study by Poelaert sought to evaluate the impact of using polyurethane-cuffed ETTs on the prevention of early postoperative pneumonia. They performed a single-blind, randomized trial to evaluate this in cardiac surgical patients. Through a multivariable analysis they found that the polyurethane cuff was protective and resulted in a 70% decreased risk of developing pneumonia (OR 0.31, CI 0.13-0.77). Although the study may show a promising method to decrease patients' risks, some of the limitations of the study should be highlighted. Although they required all of the Johanson criteria plus 2 additional criteria to diagnose VAP, they did not require microbiologic confirmation of the diagnosis. Although there may not be a gold standard for diagnosing pneumonia, this is a significant problem for this trial, especially in a patient population that is notable for postoperative atelectasis and pulmonary edema, which makes it extremely difficult to confidently and accurately diagnose a "new or evolving infiltrate," which was one of the criteria used in this for diagnosis. Even though this potential misclassification of patients should be equally distributed between the groups, it seriously limits the ability of researchers to confidently state that they decreased the incidence of early postoperative pneumonia among cardiac surgical patients. Interestingly, there was an association with blood units transfused and the incidence of pneumonia. This finding raises further questioning of their outcome variable and diagnosis of pneumonia. Were there patients who had transfusion-related lung injury with a protracted inflammatory response and had patchy findings on chest X-ray misclassified as having pneumonia?

One very interesting finding, not reported in the results but noted in the discussion, was that early postoperative antibiotic use was decreased by half in the intervention population. One could hypothesize that with decreased secretions and need for suctioning, the clinical provider's suspicion of pneumonia was decreased, suggesting that in general we may be overtreating noninfectious airway secretions with antibiotics. This could be the most important result of this intervention and a very interesting outcome variable to track in follow-up to this pilot study.

Despite the limitations described above, the authors report findings from a very interesting and potentially important pilot study. It is well known that there are many challenges with studies that seek to evaluate the impact of an intervention on the development of pneumonia. These challenges include the definition used for VAP, separating the risk of mortality in the baseline ICU population from those who develop a VAP, and determining the exact role of the prevention.[4] Given the significant morbidity and mortality associated with VAP, we need to continue to explore interventions to decrease the risk of VAP development.

E. A. Martinez, MD, MHS

References

1. Kollef MH, Afessa B, Anzueto A, et al. Silver-coated endotracheal tubes and incidence of ventilator-associated pneumonia: the NASCENT randomized trail. *JAMA.* 2008;300:805-813.
2. Muscedere J, Dodek P, Keenan S, Fowler R, Cook D, Heyland D. Comprehensive evidence-based clinical practice guidelines for ventilator-associated pneumonia: prevention. *J Crit Care.* 2008;23:126-137.
3. Lorente L, Lecuona M, Jimenez A, Mora ML, Sierra A. Influence of an endotracheal tube with polyurethane cuff and subglottic secretion drainage on pneumonia. *Am J Respir Crit Care Med.* 2007;176:1079-1083.
4. Chastre J. Preventing ventilator-associated pneumonia: could silver-coated endotracheal tubes be the answer? *JAMA.* 2008;300:842-844.

Miscellaneous

Duration of Red-cell Storage and Complications after Cardiac Surgery
Koch CG, Li L, Sessler DI, et al (Cleveland Clinic Foundation, OH)
N Engl J Med 358:1229-1239, 2008

Background.—Stored red cells undergo progressive structural and functional changes over time. We tested the hypothesis that serious complications and mortality after cardiac surgery are increased when transfused red cells are stored for more than 2 weeks.

Methods.—We examined data from patients given red-cell transfusions during coronary-artery bypass grafting, heart-valve surgery, or both between June 30, 1998, and January 30, 2006. A total of 2872 patients received 8802 units of blood that had been stored for 14 days or less ("newer blood"), and 3130 patients received 10,782 units of blood that had been stored for more than 14 days ("older blood"). Multivariable logistic regression with propensity-score methods was used to examine the effect of the duration of storage on outcomes. Survival was estimated by the Kaplan–Meier method and Blackstone's decomposition method.

Results.—The median duration of storage was 11 days for newer blood and 20 days for older blood. Patients who were given older units had higher rates of in-hospital mortality (2.8% vs. 1.7%, P=0.004), intubation beyond 72 hours (9.7% vs. 5.6%, P<0.001), renal failure (2.7% vs. 1.6%, P=0.003), and sepsis or septicemia (4.0% vs. 2.8%, P=0.01). A composite of complications was more common in patients given older blood (25.9% vs. 22.4%, P=0.001). Similarly, older blood was associated with an increase in the risk-adjusted rate of the composite outcome (P=0.03). At 1 year, mortality was significantly less in patients given newer blood (7.4% vs. 11.0%, P<0.001).

Conclusions.—In patients undergoing cardiac surgery, transfusion of red cells that had been stored for more than 2 weeks was associated with a significantly increased risk of postoperative complications as well as reduced short-term and long-term survival.

▶ Many studies have now demonstrated that blood transfusion is associated with increased risk of infection and, possibly, mortality even after correction for comorbidities and severity of illness.[1,2] This is thought to be a consequence of red blood cell transfusion-associated immunosuppression. Many questions regarding this phenomenon remain open. For example, it is unclear whether survival can truly be adversely affected by transfusion and whether the effect is specific to particular characteristics of the blood being transfused.

This retrospective study helps to address these questions by analyzing a large cohort of patients who received blood transfusion while undergoing coronary artery bypass grafting or heart valve repair/replacement. They demonstrate that patients receiving older blood had a significantly higher risk of sepsis/septicemia and in-hospital mortality even after correction for other factors. Although such a retrospective study cannot demonstrate direct causality, it does suggest that a randomized study to address this question is urgently required. If these results hold up, the factors associated with older blood that lead to increased risk of infection should be studied; it is possible that modification of blood may lead to elimination of the risk with older blood. In the meantime, it is reasonable to suggest that critically ill and high-risk operative patients should have priority for use of relatively fresh blood.

A. Kumar, MD

References

1. Shorr AF, Jackson WL, Shorr AF, Jackson WL. Transfusion practice and nosocomial infection: assessing the evidence. *Curr Opin Crit Care.* 2005;11:468-472.
2. Shorr AF, CRIT Study Group. Red blood cell transfusion and ventilator-associated pneumonia: a potential link? *Crit Care Med.* 2004;32:666-674.

Transfusion of fresh frozen plasma in critically ill surgical patients is associated with an increased risk of infection
Sarani B, Dunkman WJ, Dean L, et al (Univ of Pennsylvania, Philadelphia, PA)
Crit Care Med 36:1114-1118, 2008

Objective.—To determine whether there is an association between transfusion of fresh frozen plasma and infection in critically ill surgical patients.

Design.—Retrospective study.

Setting.—A 24-bed surgical intensive care unit in a university hospital.

Patients.—A total of 380 non-trauma patients who received fresh frozen plasma from 2004 to 2005 were compared with 2,058 nontrauma patients who did not receive fresh frozen plasma.

Interventions.—None.

Measurements and Main Results.—We calculated the relative risk of infectious complication for patients receiving and not receiving fresh frozen plasma. *T*-test allowed comparison of average units of fresh frozen plasma transfused to patients with and without infectious complications to describe a dose-response relationship. We used multivariate logistic regression analysis to evaluate the association between fresh frozen plasma and infectious complication, controlling for the effect of red blood cell transfusion, Acute Physiology and Chronic Health Evaluation II, and patient age. A significant association was found between transfusion of fresh frozen plasma and ventilator-associated pneumonia with shock (relative risk 5.42, 2.73–10.74), ventilator-associated pneumonia without shock (relative risk 1.97, 1.03–3.78), bloodstream infection with shock (relative risk 3.35, 1.69–6.64), and undifferentiated septic shock (relative risk 3.22, 1.84–5.61). The relative risk for transfusion of fresh frozen plasma and all infections was 2.99 (2.28–3.93). The *t*-test revealed a significant dose-response relationship between fresh frozen plasma and infectious complications ($p = .02$). Chi-square analysis showed a significant association between infection and transfusion of fresh frozen plasma in patients who did not receive concomitant red blood cell transfusion ($p < .01$), but this association was not significant in those who did receive red blood cells in addition to fresh frozen plasma. The association between fresh frozen plasma and infectious complications remained significant in the multivariate model, with an odds ratio of infection per unit of fresh frozen plasma transfused equal to 1.039 (1.013–1.067). This odds ratio resembled that noted for each unit of packed red blood cells, 1.074 (1.043–1.106).

Conclusions.—Transfusion of fresh frozen plasma is associated with an increased risk of infection in critically ill patients.

▶ Fresh frozen plasma (FFP) is used in various ways in surgical intensive care units. Some programs use this blood product as a colloid resuscitation fluid. In other settings, it is aggressively used even when the international normalized ratio (INR) is minimally elevated. The increase in risk of infection associated with each unit of FFP infused was similar in magnitude to the risk associated with administration of each unit of packed red blood cells (RBCs), approximately 4%. Immunomodulation associated with transfusion has been reported for several years and observed clinically for decades.[1-3] Specific mechanisms for immunomodulation and increased infection risk with FFP administration, however, are less clear. A number of possibilities exist. For example, antigens and fibrin degradation products having immunomodulatory properties are noted in FFP. White cell products are also present, even after leukoreduction.[4,5] The implications of this work warrant further study. Routine use of FFP in the nonbleeding coagulopathic patient should be reconsidered and these individuals given other forms of fluid therapy.[6] We may also need to reconsider the risk-benefit ratio associated with the prophylactic use of FFP. Given this new view of risk associated with use of FFP, the role of vitamin K and newer synthetic products for reversal of coagulopathy must be reexamined. It will be important in subsequent trials to identify the incremental risk associated with the use of FFP in conjunction with packed RBC infusion. This data does not allow discrimination of an immunomodulatory effect in patients receiving FFP and packed RBCs. Prospective trials with larger

and packed RBCs
ber of patients

es, MSE, MD

ion. *Am J Ther.* 2002;9:

TRIM: what does it mean

n-induced immunosuppres-

4. Gajic O, Rana R, Mendez JL, et al. Acute lung injury after blood transfusion in mechanically ventilated patients. *Transfusion.* 2004;44:1468-1474.
5. Gajic O, Dzik W, Toy P. Fresh frozen plasma and platelet transfusion for non-bleeding patients in the intensive care unit: benefit or harm? *Crit Care Med.* 2006;34:S170-S173.
6. Abdel-Wahab OI, Healy B, Dzik WH. Effect of fresh-frozen plasma transfusion on prothrombin time and bleeding in patients with mild coagulation abnormalities. *Transfusion.* 2006;46:1279-1285.
7. Brand A. Immunological aspects of blood transfusions. *Transpl Immunol.* 2002; 10:183-190.

Detection of Bloodstream Infections in Adults: How Many Blood Cultures Are Needed?
Lee A, Mirrett S, Reller LB, et al (Department of Medicine, Robert Wood Johnson Med School, New Brunswick, New Jersey; Duke Univ Med Ctr, Durham, North Carolina)
J Clin Microbiology 45:3546-3548, 2007

Although several reports have shown that two to three 20-ml blood cultures are adequate for the detection of bacteremia and fungemia in adults, a recent study (F. R. Cockerill et al., *Clin. Infect. Dis.* 38:1724–1730, 2004) found that two blood cultures detected only 80% of bloodstream infections and that three blood cultures detected 96% of episodes. We reviewed data at two university hospitals to determine whether the recent observations by Cockerill et al. are applicable more widely. We assessed all blood cultures obtained from adult inpatients from 1 January 2004 through 31 December 2005 at Robert Wood Johnson University Hospital and Duke University Medical Center. All instances in which ≥3 blood cultures per patient were obtained during a 24-h period were included. The medical records of patients who met the inclusion criteria were reviewed retrospectively to determine the clinical significance of the positive blood culture (true infection versus contamination). Data were analyzed to determine the cumulative sensitivity of blood cultures obtained sequentially during the 24-h time period. Of 629 unimicrobial episodes with ≥3 blood cultures obtained during the 24-h period, 460 (73.1%) were detected with the first blood culture, 564 (89.7%) were detected with the first two blood cultures, 618 (98.2%) were detected with the first three blood cultures, and 628 (99.8%) were detected with the first four blood cultures. Of 351 unimicrobial episodes with ≥4 blood cultures obtained during the 24-h period, 257 (73.2%) were detected with the first blood culture, 308 (93.9%) were detected with the first two blood cultures, 340 (96.9%) were detected with the first three blood cultures, and 350 (99.7%) were detected with the first four blood cultures. Among unimicrobial episodes, *Staphylococcus aureus* was more likely to be detected with the first blood culture (approximately 90% detected with the first blood culture). There were 58 polymicrobial episodes in which ≥3 blood cultures were obtained. Forty-seven (81.0%) were detected with the first blood culture, 54 (93.1%) were detected with the first two blood cultures, and 58 (100%) were detected with the first three blood cultures. The results of this study indicate that two blood cultures in a 24-h period will detect approximately 90% of bloodstream infections in adults. To achieve a detection rate of >99%, as many as four blood cultures may be needed. The previously held axiom that virtually all bloodstream infections can be detected with two to three blood cultures may no longer be valid but may also depend on the definition of the 'first' blood culture obtained (see Materials and Methods and Discussion in the text).

▶ One of the most common diagnostic procedures in the ICU or anywhere in the hospital is the blood culture. Despite its low yield, it continues to be used on a routine basis in all patients with even the most modest indication of possible infection. The reason for this is the high risk of adverse events when bacteremia/fungemia is missed. If we are going to use this test with the frequency with which it continues to be used, it is incumbent on physicians to make most effective use of the test. Unfortunately, we often fail to do so. For example, in many cases, suboptimal volumes of blood are frequently drawn and incubated with a substantial decrease in sensitivity for true bacteremia/fungemia. In this study, it is shown that the standard 2 blood cultures detect only 90% of bacteremias that are detected by a total of 4 or more cultures. To achieve 99% sensitivity of bacteremia/fungemia, 3 or more cultures appear to be required. Prudent physicians may want to consider additional blood cultures in high-risk patients.

A. Kumar, MD

Quantitative Detection of *Staphylococcus aureus* and *Enterococcus faecalis* DNA in Blood To Diagnose Bacteremia in Patients in the Intensive Care Unit
Peters RPH, Van Agtmael MA, Gierveld S, et al (VU University Med Ctr, Amsterdam, The Netherlands)
J Clin Microbiol 45:3641-3646, 2007

Direct detection of bacterial DNA in blood offers a fast alternative to blood culture and is presumably unaffected by the prior use of antibiotics. We evaluated the performance of two real-time PCR assays for the quantitative detection of *Staphylococcus aureus* bacteremia and for *Enterococcus faecalis* bacteremia directly in blood samples, without prior cultivation. Whole-blood samples for PCR were obtained simultaneously with blood cultures from patients admitted to the intensive care unit of our hospital. After the extraction of DNA from 200 µl of blood, real-time PCR was performed for the specific detection and quantification of *S. aureus* and *E. faecalis* DNA. The sensitivity for bacteremia of the *S. aureus* PCR was 75% and that of the *E. faecalis* PCR was 73%, and both tests had high specificity values (93 and 96%, respectively). PCR amplification reactions were positive for *S. aureus* for 10 (7%) blood samples with negative blood cultures, and 7 (4%) PCR reactions were positive for *E. faecalis*. The majority of these PCR results were likely (50%) or possibly (42%) related to infection with the specific microorganism, based on clinical data and radiological and microbiological investigations. PCR results were concordant for 95% of paired whole-blood samples, and blood culture results were concordant for 97% of the paired samples. We conclude that the detection of *S. aureus* and *E. faecalis* DNA in blood by real-time PCR enables a rapid diagnosis of bacteremia and that a positive DNAemia is related to proven or possible infection with the specific microorganism in the majority of patients with negative blood cultures.

▶ One of the most common diagnostic procedures in the ICU or anywhere in the hospital is the blood culture. Despite its low yield, it continues to be used on a routine basis in all patients with even the most modest indication of possible infection. The reason for this is the high risk of adverse events when bacteremia/fungemia is missed. If we are going to use this test with the frequency with which it continues to be used, it is incumbent on physicians to make most effective use of the test. Unfortunately, we often fail to do so. For example, in many cases, suboptimal volumes of blood are frequently drawn and incubated with a substantial decrease in sensitivity for true bacteremia/fungemia. In this study, it is shown that the standard 2 blood cultures detect only 90% of bacteremias that are detected by a total of 4 or more cultures. To achieve 99% sensitivity of bacteremia/fungemia, 3 or more cultures appear to be required. Prudent physicians may want to consider additional blood cultures in high-risk patients.

For further reading on this subject, I suggest an article by Louie et al.[1]

A. Kumar, MD

Reference

1. Louie RF, Tang Z, Albertson TE, et al. Multiplex polymerase chain reaction detection enhancement of bacteremia and fungemia. *Crit Care Med.* 2008;36: 1487-1492.

Timing of Specimen Collection for Blood Cultures from Febrile Patients with Bacteremia
Riedel S, Bourbeau P, Swartz B, et al (Univ of Iowa College of Medicine; Geisinger Med Ctr, Danville, Pennsylvania)
J Clin Microbiol 46:1381-1385, 2008

Bloodstream infections are an important cause of morbidity and mortality. Physician orders for blood cultures often specify that blood specimens be collected at or around the time of a temperature elevation, presumably as a means of enhancing the likelihood of detecting significant bacteremia. In a multicenter study, which utilized retrospective patient chart reviews as a means of collecting data, we evaluated the timing of blood culture collection in relation to temperature elevations in 1,436 patients with bacteremia and fungemia. The likelihood of documenting bloodstream infections was not significantly enhanced by collecting blood specimens for culture at the time that patients experienced temperature spikes. A subset analysis based on patient age, gender, white blood cell count and specific cause of bacteremia generally also failed to reveal any associations.

▶ Blood cultures, as noted, are one of the most commonly used diagnostic tests in the hospital setting. However, physicians and nurses frequently have significant misconceptions about their optimal use. For example, all too frequently, insufficient numbers of cultures or blood volume is used to achieve maximal sensitivity for detection of true bacteremia/fungemia. Another common error is to draw cultures only when there is fever. This study points out that the presence of fever does not significantly increase the probability of a positive culture. Waiting for a fever spike before blood culture wastes time (and potentially) can delay therapy. A better understanding of the best use of our most common tools would seem to be indicated for all health care workers.

A. Kumar, MD

Mortality Associated with Bloodstream Infection after Coronary Artery Bypass Surgery
Olsen MA, Krauss M, Agniel D (Washington Univ School of Medicine, St. Louis, MO)
Clin Infect Dis 46:1537-1546, 2008

Background.—Mortality attributable to bloodstream infection (BSI) is still controversial. We studied the impact of BSI on mortality after coronary artery bypass surgery, including the specific impact of different etiologic organisms.

Methods.—Our cohort consisted of 4515 patients who underwent coronary artery bypass procedures at a university hospital from 1996 through

2004. We used Society of Thoracic Surgery data supplemented with laboratory and infection control data. Mortality dates were identified using Society of Thoracic Surgery data and the Social Security Death Index. BSI within 90 days after surgery was defined by a positive blood culture result. Cox proportional hazards and propensity score models were used to analyze the association between BSI and mortality.

Results.—Patients with BSI had a 4.2-fold increased risk of death (95% confidence interval [CI], 3.0–5.9) 2–90 days after coronary artery bypass surgery, compared with uninfected patients. The risk of death was higher among patients with BSI due to gram-negative bacteria (hazard ratio [HR], 6.8; 95% CI, 3.9–12.0) and BSI due to *Staphylococcus aureus* (HR, 7.2; 95% CI, 3.3–15.7) and lowest among patients with BSI caused by gram-positive bacteria other than *S. aureus* (HR, 2.2; 95% CI, 1.1–4.6). The risk of death was highest among patients who developed BSI but had the lowest likelihood of infection (HR, 10.0; 95% CI, 3.5–28.8) and was lowest among patients who developed BSI but had the highest likelihood of infection (HR, 2.3; 95% CI, 1.2–4.6).

Conclusions.—BSIs due to gram-negative bacteria and BSIs due to *S. aureus* contributed significantly to mortality. Mortality attributable to BSI was highest among patients predicted to be least likely to develop infection and was lowest among severely ill patients who were most likely to develop infection. BSI appears to be an important contributor to death after coronary artery bypass surgery, particularly among the healthiest patients.

▶ According to the Centers for Disease Control and Prevention the rate of catheter-related bloodstream infections (BSIs) in ICUs ranges from 1.8 to 5.2 per 1000 catheter-days. Essentially, every cardiac surgical patient has central access for their surgical procedure and many patients will require these during the perioperative period to infuse vasoactive agents and monitor hemodynamic parameters. Although central lines remain an important adjunct for our management of complex patients, the risks of central catheters are real and up to a third of patients who develop a catheter-related BSI will die. Patients can also develop a BSI for other reasons, including hematogenous spread of infection from a distant site (pneumonia, surgical site infection, urinary infection).

Olsen and colleagues report their analysis of the attributable mortality of the development of a BSI in patients following coronary artery bypass (CAB) surgery. They reviewed data on over 4000 patients in a single center and defined a BSI as *any* positive blood culture ≤ 90 days after the primary surgical procedure. If the organism was a potential skin contaminant (coagulase-negative staphylococci or *Streptococcus viridans* group), then ≥2 positive cultures were required, unless only 1 set of blood cultures were drawn, plus a temperature > 38.6°C or < 36°C, chills, hypotension, and treatment with antibiotics. Although this is not the "standard" definition used for surveillance of bloodstream infections, it nonetheless is a clinically important outcome measure. One hundred fifty-one patients (3.3%) were diagnosed with at least 1 BSI. Of these, 51 (38%) died within 90 days after surgery. The rate of developing a BSI was not significantly different by year over the length of the study and 40% of the BSIs were defined as central catheter-related BSIs. Using a time-dependent variable for BSI, the Cox hazard ratio (adjusted risk) for mortality was higher among patients who developed a BSI (4.19, 95% CI, 2.97-5.92) at any given time. When they looked at the risk based on the organism identified, they showed that this varied and that there was a 7-fold increase risk of mortality associated with gram-negative and *Staphylococcus aureus* bacteremia compared with patients who did not develop a BSI.

The authors further went on to assess the attributable risk of developing a BSI using propensity scoring. The predicted probability of developing a BSI ≤ 90 days postoperatively was broken down into quintiles with equal numbers of patients in each. Those patients who did not develop an infection were grouped similarly based on the relevant covariates (predictors). The groups were then compared to identify the relative risk of mortality based on the risk of developing a BSI. The authors report that those patients who had the lowest risk of developing a BSI (described as an overall lower risk population or "healthiest patients") had the highest risk of mortality, should they develop a BSI. Only 2% of the lowest risk patients in the no-BSI group died, compared with 13% in the BSI group. This translates into a high attributable risk of the BSI on mortality. The attributable risk of the BSI on mortality in the highest risk group ("least healthy") is lower. The highest BSI-risk group had a lower attributable risk most likely secondary to the likelihood of dying regardless of whether they developed a BSI. The authors address some important confounders to these findings. They report in their discussion that most of these lowest risk patients had a BSI with *S. aureus* and more than 85% of these had an associated surgical site infection, which was the source of their positive blood cultures.

Although this study has important limitations inherent to its observational and retrospective nature, it also has some very important strengths. They reviewed over 4000 patients, utilized the Society of Thoracic Surgeons (STS) database (cardiac surgical specific risk factors) for risk stratification, and used rigorous statistical methods. Furthermore they identify important opportunities for improving outcomes among cardiac surgical patients.

Recent studies have shown that the implementation of evidence-based practices reduces the incidence of catheter-related BSI (CR-BSI) by over 60%,[1] and 40% of the BSIs in this study were CR-BSI. However, in the lowest risk patients who developed BSIs, CR-BSIs would most likely not be the targeted intervention, but strategies to reduce the risk of surgical site infections such as those defined in the Surgical Care Improvement Project (SCIP) would be.

E. A. Martinez, MD, MHS

Reference

1. Pronovost P, Needham D, Berenholtz S, et al. An intervention to decrease catheter-related bloodstream infections in the ICU. *N Engl J Med.* 2006;355:2725-2732.

Femoral vs Jugular Venous Catheterization and Risk of Nosocomial Events in Adults Requiring Acute Renal Replacement Therapy: A Randomized Controlled Trial

Parienti J-J, Thirion M, Mégarbane B, et al (Côte de Nacre Univ Hosp Ctr, Caen; Cochin Univ Hosp Ctr, Paris; Univ of Paris)
JAMA 299:2413-2422, 2008

Context.—Based on concerns about the risk of infection, the jugular site is often preferred over the femoral site for short-term dialysis vascular access.

Objective.—To determine whether jugular catheterization decreases the risk of nosocomial complications compared with femoral catheterization.

Design, Setting, and Patients.—A concealed, randomized, multicenter, evaluator-blinded, parallel-group trial (the Cathedia Study) of 750 patients from a network of 9 tertiary care university medical centers and 3 general hospitals in France conducted between May 2004 and May 2007. The severely ill, bed-bound adults had a body mass index (BMI) of less than 45 and required a first catheter insertion for renal replacement therapy.

Intervention.—Patients were randomized to receive jugular or femoral vein catheterization by operators experienced in placement at both sites.

Main Outcome Measures.—Rates of infectious complications, defined as catheter colonization on removal (primary end point), and catheter-related bloodstream infection.

Results.—Patient and catheter characteristics, including duration of catheterization, were similar in both groups. More hematomas occurred in the jugular group than in the femoral group (13/366 patients [3.6%] vs 4/370 patients [1.1%], respectively; $P=.03$). The risk of catheter colonization at removal did not differ significantly between the femoral and jugular groups (incidence of 40.8 vs 35.7 per 1000 catheter-days; hazard ratio [HR], 0.85; 95% confidence interval [CI], 0.62-1.16; $P=.31$). A prespecified subgroup analysis demonstrated significant qualitative heterogeneity by BMI (P for the interaction term <.001). Jugular catheterization significantly increased incidence of catheter colonization vs femoral catheterization (45.4 vs 23.7 per 1000 catheter-days; HR, 2.10; 95% CI, 1.13-3.91; $P=.017$) in the lowest tercile (BMI <24.2), whereas jugular catheterization significantly decreased this incidence (24.5 vs 50.9 per 1000 catheter-days; HR, 0.40; 95% CI, 0.23-0.69; $P<.001$) in the highest tercile (BMI >28.4). The rate of catheter-related bloodstream infection was similar in both groups (2.3 vs 1.5 per 1000 catheter-days, respectively; $P=.42$).

Conclusion.—Jugular venous catheterization access does not appear to reduce the risk of infection compared with femoral access, except among adults with a high BMI, and may have a higher risk of hematoma.

Trial Registration.—clinicaltrials.gov Identifier: NCT00277888.

▶ Central venous catheterization is an almost universal element of ICU care. The femoral insertion site is often used in emergency situations but has a reputation as being prone to increased risk of infection relative to the internal jugular site, the other commonly used access point. A series of retrospective studies over the last 30 years have attempted to ascertain the optimum site of central venous catheter insertion for purposes of minimizing risk of catheter infection. The results of those studies have been inconsistent and contradictory with some indicating higher infection risk at each site.[1,2]

This study represents the first randomized trial to address this question and suggests the question should not be "Which site is preferred?" but rather "When is one site preferred over the other?" The answer to that seems to be dependent on body mass index with the femoral site having a higher incidence of catheter colonization (though not catheter-related bloodstream infection) in heavier patients and the internal jugular site being higher risk in thinner. These results should be considered when placing central venous catheters on a nonemergency basis.

A. Kumar, MD

References

1. Richet H, Hubert B, Netemberg G. Prospective multicenter study of vascular catheter-related complications and risk factors for positive central-catheter cultures in intensive care unit patients. *J Clin Microbiol.* 1990;28:2520-2525.
2. Harden JL, Kemp L, Mirtallo J. Femoral catheters increase risk of infection in total parenteral nutrition patients. *Nutr Clin Pract.* 1995;10:60-66.

Empirical Fluconazole versus Placebo for Intensive Care Unit Patients: A Randomized Trial

Schuster MG, Edwards Jr. JE, Sobel JD, et al (Univ of Pennsylvania, Philadelphia; UCLA Med Ctr, Torrance, CA; Wayne State Univ Detroit, MI)
Ann Intern Med 149:83-90, 2008

Background.—Invasive infection with *Candida* species is an important cause of morbidity and mortality in intensive care unit (ICU) patients. Optimal preventive strategies have not been clearly defined.

Objective.—To see whether empirical fluconazole improves clinical outcomes more than placebo in adult ICU patients at high risk for invasive candidiasis.

Design.—Double-blind, placebo-controlled, randomized trial conducted from 1995 to 2000.

Setting.—26 ICUs in the United States.

Patients.—270 adult ICU patients with fever despite administration of broad-spectrum antibiotics. All had central venous catheters and an Acute Physiology and Chronic Health Evaluation II score greater than 16.

Intervention.—Patients were randomly assigned to either intravenous fluconazole, 800 mg daily, or placebo for 2 weeks and were followed for 4 weeks thereafter. Two hundred forty-nine participants were available for outcome assessment.

Measurements.—A composite primary outcome that defined success as all 4 of the following: resolution of fever; absence of invasive fungal infection; no discontinuation because of toxicity; and no need for a nonstudy, systemic antifungal medication (as assessed by a blinded oversight committee).

Results.—Only 44 of 122 (36%) fluconazole recipients and 48 of 127 (38%) placebo recipients had a successful outcome (relative risk, 0.95 [95% CI, 0.69 to 1.32; $P = 0.78$]). The main reason for failure was lack of resolution of fever (51% for fluconazole and 57% for placebo). Documented invasive candidiasis occurred in 5% of fluconazole recipients and 9% of placebo recipients (relative risk, 0.57 [CI, 0.22 to 1.49]). Seven (5%) fluconazole recipients and 10 (7%) placebo recipients had adverse events resulting in discontinuation of the study drug. Discontinuation because of abnormal liver test results occurred in 3 (2%) fluconazole recipients and 5 (4%) placebo recipients.

Limitations.—Twenty-one randomly assigned patients were not included in the analysis because they either did not meet entry criteria or did not have postbaseline assessments. Fewer fungal infections than anticipated occurred in the control group. Confidence bounds were wide and did not exclude potentially important differences in outcomes between groups.

Conclusion.—In critically ill adults with risk factors for invasive candidiasis, empirical fluconazole did not clearly improve a composite outcome more than placebo.

▶ ICU presence of invasive *Candida* infection in critically ill ICU patients is associated with a marked increase in morbidity and mortality. Although only 1% to 2% of all ICU patients ever develop invasive candidiasis,[1,2] *Candida* infections can account for as many as 5% to 10% of all blood isolates[3] or cases of septic shock[4] in the ICU. *Candida* infections may be substantially underdiagnosed given the difficulty in determining the presence of invasive infection with this organism. *Candida* are often thought to be present as colonizers at a variety of sites in critically ill infected patients. However, it is possible that these isolates may represent true but unrecognized invasive infection.

In this randomized study, Schuster and colleagues test the possibility that empirical fluconazole administration in high-risk patients with fever unresponsive to broad-spectrum antibiotics leads to improved fever resolution and decreased subsequent documentation of invasive *Candida*. Unfortunately, the small improvement in fever resolution and decreased occurrence of invasive *Candida* infection failed to even approach statistical significance. However, this question may not be fully resolved. Closer examination of the study suggests an unusually low rate of *Candida* infection in the control group, suggesting that a larger study may have been required to adequately examine this question. For the present, though, there is no documented benefit of empirical antifungal therapy in high-risk antibiotic-treated ICU patients with unresolving fever.

A. Kumar, MD

References

1. Eggimann P, Garbino J, Pittet D. Epidemiology of Candida species infections in critically ill non-immunosuppressed patients. *Lancet Infect Dis.* 2003;3:685-702.
2. Blumberg HM, Jarvis WR, Soucie JM, et al. Risk factors for candidal bloodstream infections in surgical intensive care unit patients: the NEMIS prospective multicenter study. The National Epidemiology of Mycosis Survey. *Clin Infect Dis.* 2001;33:177-186.
3. National Nosocomial Infections Surveillance System. National nosocomial infections surveillance (NNIS) system report, data summary from January 1992 to June 2002 (issued August 2002). *Am J Infect Control.* 2002;30:458-475.
4. Kumar A, Roberts D, Wood KE, et al. Duration of hypotension before initiation of effective antimicrobial therapy is the critical determinant of survival in human septic shock. *Crit Care Med.* 2006;34:1589-1596.

Cytomegalovirus Reactivation in Critically Ill Immunocompetent Patients

Limaye AP, Kirby KA, Rubenfeld GD, et al (Univ of Washington Med)
JAMA 300:413-422, 2008

Context.—Cytomegalovirus (CMV) infection is associated with adverse clinical outcomes in immunosuppressed persons, but the incidence and association of CMV reactivation with adverse outcomes in critically ill persons lacking evidence of immunosuppression have not been well defined.

Objective.—To determine the association of CMV reactivation with intensive care unit (ICU) and hospital length of stay in critically ill immunocompetent persons.

Design, Setting, and Participants.—We prospectively assessed CMV plasma DNAemia by thrice-weekly real-time polymerase chain reaction (PCR) and clinical outcomes in a cohort of 120 CMV-seropositive, immunocompetent adults admitted to 1 of 6 ICUs at 2 separate hospitals at a large US tertiary care academic medical center between 2004 and 2006. Clinical measurements were assessed by personnel blinded to CMV PCR results. Risk factors for CMV reactivation and association with hospital and ICU length of stay were assessed by multivariable logistic regression and proportional odds models.

Main Outcome Measures.—Association of CMV reactivation with prolonged hospital length of stay or death.

Results.—The primary composite end point of continued hospitalization (n = 35) or death (n = 10) by 30 days occurred in 45 (35%) of the 120 patients. Cytomegalovirus viremia at any level occurred in 33% (39/120; 95% confidence interval [CI], 24%-41%) at a median of 12 days (range, 3-57 days) and CMV viremia greater than 1000 copies/ mL occurred in 20% (24/120; 95% CI, 13%-28%) at a median of 26 days (range, 9-56 days). By logistic regression, CMV infection at any level (adjusted odds ratio [OR], 4.3; 95% CI, 1.6-11.9; $P = .005$) and at greater than 1000 copies/mL (adjusted OR, 13.9; 95% CI, 3.2-60; $P = .001$) and the average CMV area under the curve (AUC) in $\log_{10}$ copies per milliliter (adjusted OR, 2.1; 95% CI, 1.3-3.2; $P < .001$) were independently associated with hospitalization or death by 30 days. In multivariable partial proportional odds models, both CMV 7-day moving average (OR, 5.1; 95% CI, 2.9-9.1; $P < .001$) and CMV AUC (OR, 3.2; 95% CI, 2.1-4.7; $P < .001$) were independently associated with a hospital length of stay of at least 14 days.

Conclusions.—These preliminary findings suggest that reactivation of CMV occurs frequently in critically ill immunocompetent patients and is associated with prolonged hospitalization or death. A controlled trial of CMV prophylaxis in this setting is warranted.

▶ Cytomegalovirus (CMV) infection/reactivation is a major infectious complication in immunosuppressed patients, particularly those who have undergone organ transplantation. Antiviral prophylaxis of this infection is the standard of care in high-risk organ transplant patients where it clearly improves outcome including survival. Intensive care unit (ICU) patients, though not specifically immunosuppressed, are almost invariably immunocompromised in the broad sense due to nutritional deficiency, organ failure, altered barrier function, and altered immune responsiveness. Many of these patients are at risk for reactivation of latent CMV infection.

In this prospective observational study, Limaye and colleagues examine the frequency and impact of CMV reactivation in nonimmunosuppressed CMV-seropositive ICU patients. The study clearly demonstrates reactivation in a large subset (about a third) of CMV-seropositive patients admitted to ICU. They further demonstrate that such reactivation (and the degree of viremia) is associated with increased mortality and ICU length of stay. Given the fact that prophylactic antiviral therapy improves outcome in transplant patients, this study strongly suggests that similar therapy must be studied in this patient cohort. Although insufficient data exists to support such prophylactic therapy at this time, we may come to a different conclusion after additional investigations into this question are performed.

A. Kumar, MD

Clinical Significance and Predictors of Community-Onset *Pseudomonas aeruginosa* Bacteremia
Cheong HS, Kang C-I, Wi YM, et al (Sungkyunkwan Univ School of Medicine, Seoul, Republic of Korea; et al)
Am J Med 121:709-714, 2008

Background.—*Pseudomonas aeruginosa* bacteremia is a serious and possibly fatal condition. It is important to determine the likelihood of *P. aeruginosa* bacteremia when Gram-negative sepsis is suspected in community-onset infection.

Methods.—We performed a retrospective cohort study to identify the risk factors for *P. aeruginosa* infection in community-onset Gram-negative bacteremia.

Results.—A total of 106 patients with *P. aeruginosa* bacteremia and a total 508 patients with *E. coli* bacteremia were included in this study. Factors associated with *P. aeruginosa* bacteremia in the multivariate analysis included presentation with neutropenia, presentation with septic shock, indwelling central venous catheter, and health-care-associated infection (all P <.05). The 30-day mortality rate was 26.4% in patients with *P. aeruginosa* and 13.6% in those with *E. coli* bacteremia (P <.001). Multivariate analysis demonstrated that risk factors for mortality included a *P. aeruginosa* bacteremia, inappropriate initial antimicrobial therapy, a higher Charlson's weighted index of comorbidity, and a higher Pitt bacteremia score (all P <.05). In addition, urinary tract infection and benign pancreatobiliary disease were found to be protective factors for mortality based on multivariate analysis (all *P* <.05).

Conclusions.—Our data suggest that initial empirical antimicrobial coverage of *P. aeruginosa* should be seriously considered in patients with neutropenia, presentation with septic shock, indwelling central venous catheter, or health-care-associated infection, when Gram-negative sepsis is suspected in community-onset infection.

▶ Many studies have demonstrated the adverse impact of inappropriate initial empiric antimicrobial therapy on outcome of life-threatening infections including those due to *Pseudomonas* and other resistant organism infection. One of the reasons for administration of inappropriate therapy is the failure to recognize the risk of resistant organisms in particular clinical scenarios. One such scenario is the "community-acquired" infection. In the past, chronically ill patients with a variety of comorbidities (renal failure, organ transplant, cancer, inflammatory bowel disease, etc) spent prolonged periods of time in the hospital. The term "community-acquired" infection accurately denoted patients infected with community pathogens with a low degree of antibiotic resistance. However, recent decades have seen the growth of a large group of aged and chronically ill patients who live in the community or chronic health care environment who possess many of the risk factors formerly associated with the nosocomial setting.

This study examines the risk factors for isolation of *Pseudomonas aeruginosa*, a pathogen resistant to standard regimens used for "community-acquired" infections from patients presenting to the hospital from the community. Factors that were associated with *Pseudomonas* (in contrast to *Escherichia coli*) bacteremia included neutropenia, a central venous catheter, chronic nursing/medical facility residence, and, most notably, presentation with septic shock. This study gives strong credence to the concept that septic shock is intrinsically a risk factor for resistant organisms in community-acquired infection and that its presence mandates empiric broad-spectrum therapy akin to that used in immunosuppressed patients.

A. Kumar, MD

Bacteremia in Previously Hospitalized Patients: Prolonged Effect From Previous Hospitalization and Risk Factors for Antimicrobial-Resistant Bacterial Infections
Chen S-Y, Wu GH-M, Chang S-C, et al (Natl Taiwan Univ Hosp, Taipei)
Ann Emerg Med 51:639-646, 2008

Study objective.—Patients who came from the community but were recently discharged from the hospital have a higher risk of contracting antimicrobial-resistant bacterial infections. Our objectives are to determine the time from previous hospital discharge that affects subsequent antimicrobial susceptibility pattern and risk factors for antimicrobial-resistant infection in bacteremia in recently discharged patients.

Methods.—Excluding patients of hospital-acquired, patients with regular health care-associated exposure, and patients whose previous hospitalization was not at our hospital, a total of 789 nonduplicated bacteremia episodes from community adult patients were enrolled in a 1-year study period. Antimicrobial-resistant bacteria, including multidrug-resistant Gram-negative bacilli, methicillin-resistant *Staphylococcus aureus*, and vancomycin-resistant enterococci causing bacteremia, were logistically analyzed according to different posthospitalization periods (3 to 90 days, 91 to 180 days, 181 to 360 days, and no hospitalization in the past 360 days) to identify the independent effect from previous hospitalization on subsequent antimicrobial-resistant bacteremia.

Results.—Of the 789 bacteremia patients, the proportion of antimicrobial-resistant bacteremia is 14.6% (95% confidence interval [CI] 9.8% to 19.4%) for 3 to 90 days, 9.6% (95% CI 1.6% to 17.6%) for 91 to 180 days, and 6.4% (95% CI 0% to 13.4%) for 181 to 360 days since last hospitalization and 1.0% (95% CI 0.1% to 1.9%) for no hospitalization within the last 360 days. Risk of antimicrobial-resistant bacteremia decreased monthly after discharge by an odds ratio of 0.83 (95% CI 0.76 to 0.90) ($P<.01$). Previous carriage of antimicrobial-resistant bacteria in the past 360 days and previous stay at ICU in the past 180 days were independent risk factors for antimicrobial-resistant bacteremia in previously hospitalized patients.

Conclusion.—Previous hospitalization affects the antimicrobial susceptibility of subsequent bacteremia up to 360 days after hospital discharge. Presence of risk factors for antimicrobial-resistant bacteremia in previously hospitalized patients may help emergency physicians in selecting empirical antimicrobial agents and prompting infection control precautions.

▶ Dozens of articles have documented the adverse effects of initiation of inappropriate antimicrobial therapy on mortality and morbidity in serious infections. However, relatively few studies have examined the reasons for initiation of inappropriate therapy. Patients with recent previous antimicrobial exposure or immunocompromise are known to be at increased risk of inappropriate therapy because of an increased risk of resistant infections; so are patients with recent hospital admissions. However, the magnitude and duration of risk of infection with resistant infections in patients with recent hospital admissions have not been examined. This study helps to delineate those risks and demonstrates a progressive increase in risk from about 1% for admissions greater than a year in the past to >15% with relatively recent admissions. In addition to known previous isolation of a resistant organism, an intensive care unit (ICU) admission within 6 months is also independently associated with risk of bacteremia with a resistant organism. Intensivists will have to be aware of this kind of data to ensure appropriate antibiotic administration in high-risk patients.

A. Kumar, MD

6 Postoperative Management

Cardiovascular Surgery

Amiodarone Cost Effectiveness in Preventing Atrial Fibrillation After Coronary Artery Bypass Graft Surgery

Zebis LR, Christensen TD, Kristiansen IS, et al (Aarhus Univ Hosp, Skejby, Denmark; Univ of Southern Denmark, Odense; Univ of Oslo, Norway)
Ann Thorac Surg 85:28-33, 2008

Background.—The purpose of this study was to estimate the costs and health benefits of routinely administered postoperative amiodarone as prevention of atrial fibrillation for patients undergoing coronary artery bypass grafting (CABG) for stable angina.

Methods.—This cost-effectiveness study was based on a randomized, controlled, double-blind trial (the RASCABG study) using avoidance of atrial fibrillation as the measure of benefit at the Department of Cardiothoracic and Vascular Surgery, Aarhus University Hospital, Skejby, Denmark. Two hundred and fifty eligible consecutively enrolled CABG patients were included to receive either 300 mg amiodarone or placebo (5% aqueous dextrose solution) administered intravenously over 20 minutes followed by 600 mg amiodarone/placebo orally twice a day (8 AM and 8 PM) for the first 5 postoperative days.

Results.—In the amiodarone group, there were 14 cases of atrial fibrillation compared with 32 in the control group ($p < 0.01$) whereas there were no differences in the length of stay. The mean total cost per patient was €7,639 in the amiodarone group and €7,814 in the placebo group ($p < 0.01$).

Conclusions.—Routine use of postoperative prophylactic intravenous bolus and subsequent 5 days of oral amiodarone therapy after coronary artery bypass grafting reduces the risk of atrial fibrillation and decreases the total costs of care by €175 per patient (Table 4).

▶ Atrial fibrillation (AF) after cardiac surgery remains a significant postoperative complication and affects anywhere from 5% to 65% of patients depending on their risk factors. Although it is frequently a self-limited complication, it is

TABLE 4.—Average Cost (€) per Patient According to Treatment Arm With 95% Confidence Intervals (CI)

Mean [Patients] (95% CI)	Amiodarone Prophylaxis Group per Patient	Placebo Group per Patient
Amiodarone (prophylaxis)	15.25 [125 pts]	
Extra blood samples	2.64 [14 pts] (1.32–3.97)	6.04 [32 pts] (4.21–7.87)
Nurse and doctor (time)	2.21 [14 pts] (1.11–3.32)	5.06 [32 pts] (3.53–6.59)
Amiodarone infusion	0.57 [2 pts] (−0.23–1.38)	2.30 [8 pts] (0.74–3.86)
Radiology examinations	0.10 [1 pt] (−0.10–0.29)	0.30 [3 pts] (−0.04–0.63)
Direct current conversion	0.00 [0 pts]	0.65 [2 pts] (−0.26–1.57)
Bolus infusion initiating AF treatment	0.60 [6 pts] (0.13–1.08)	2.71 [27 pts] (1.79–3.63)
Oral treatment of diagnosed AF	0.60 [14 pts] (0.30–0.90)	1.38 [32 pts] (0.96–1.79)
Cost at the intensive care unit	1,460 (1,335–1,586)	1,578 (1,164–1,991)
Cost at the intermediate care unit	120 (31–209)	264 (116–411)
Cost of stay at Aarhus University Hospital, Skejby	4,187 (3,714–4,660)	4,384 (3,542–5,226)
Cost of stay at local hospital	1,849 (1,453–2,246)	1,570 (1,067–2,074)
Total cost	7,639 (7,636–7,643)	7,814 (7,808–7,820)
Difference	175 [$p < 0.01$] (168–182)	

AF = atrial fibrillation.
pts = patients.
(Reprinted from Zebis LR, Christensen TD, Kristiansen IS, et al. Amiodarone cost effectiveness in preventing atrial fibrillation after coronary artery bypass graft surgery. *Ann Thorac Surg.* 2008;85:28-33. Copyright 2008, with permission from The Society of Thoracic Surgeons.)

associated with increased morbidity, length of stay (LOS), and hospital costs. Many studies have explored both prevention and treatment interventions. Amiodarone prophylaxis has previously been shown to reduce the incidence of postoperative AF.[1,2] Most regimens have included preoperative dosing that is not always feasible as patients are referred for emergency surgery or may not be seen early enough preoperatively to implement such protocols. Zebis and colleagues previously reported their experience with a practical regimen in which amiodarone was initiated postoperatively. They performed a double-blind randomized clinical trial of 250 patients comparing amiodarone with placebo and showed a reduction in the incidence of both symptomatic and asymptomatic postoperative AF by 18% with a relative risk reduction of 14% (95% confidence interval [CI], 5.0%-24.0%) and a number needed to treat of 6.9 (95% CI, 4.2-20). Furthermore, 57% of patients in the amiodarone arm had asymptomatic episodes compared with only 16% in the placebo arm. The asymptomatic episodes were those that did not result in any clinical symptoms or require intervention and were detected on the daily morning electrocardiograms and not by continuous monitoring.

In this article they present their economic outcomes from this trial including cost and LOS. The cost analysis was performed from the payer perspective and included the cost for resources used for the procedure and any complications that might have resulted. The LOS analysis included time in the intermediate care unit, LOS in the hospital where the procedure was performed (Aarhus University Hospital, a tertiary care center), and LOS in their local hospital (where they returned for continued care after discharge from the tertiary center). Although the intervention resulted in a significant decreased risk of developing AF, there was no difference in LOS in any of the locations. However, they did find an associated decreased total cost per patient of €175 (Table 4) for patients in the treatment arm.

Although this study has limitations, it presents encouraging data supporting the use of a prophylactic regimen in the prevention of clinically evident/important AF using what they appropriately describe as a practical regimen. From the meta-analysis on the prevention of AF, there are many additional and important potential benefits from preventing AF. Although the authors may have underestimated the rate of AF because continuous cardiac monitoring was not used, they showed a statistically significant difference in the rates of what may cautiously be accepted as clinically relevant AF. It is unknown how important brief asymptomatic episodes, which might only be detected by continuous monitoring, are in relation to the complications of AF. If the longer or symptomatic episodes are more clinically relevant with regard to complications, then this postoperative regimen may offer significant benefit to patients. The lack of difference in LOS is interesting and similar to our local findings as part of a performance improvement initiative. Many other factors can affect the LOS, including bed availability and as the authors point out, subclinical AF episodes in addition to other possible complications or confounders could have a greater effect on LOS. Finally, although they showed a cost savings within their system, if there is no difference in LOS, this cost savings may not be realized in other centers.

E. A. Martinez, MD, MHS

References

1. Bagshaw SM, Galbraith PD, Mitchell LB, Sauve R, Exner DV, Ghali WA. Prophylactic amiodarone for prevention of atrial fibrillation after cardiac surgery: a meta-analysis. *Ann Thorac Surg.* 2006;82:1927-1937.
2. Daoud EG, Strickberger SA, Man KC, et al. Preoperative amiodarone as prophylaxis against atrial fibrillation after heart surgery. *N Engl J Med.* 1997;337:1785-1791.

Predictors and Early and Late Outcomes of Respiratory Failure in Contemporary Cardiac Surgery
Filsoufi F, Rahmanian PB, Castillo JG (Mount Sinai School of Medicine, NY)
Chest 133:713-721, 2008

Background.—Respiratory failure (RF) is a serious complication following heart surgery. The profile of patients referred for cardiac surgery has changed during the last decade, making prior investigations of RF after cardiac surgery less relevant to the current population. This study was designed to analyze the incidence, predictors of RF, and early and late outcomes following this complication in a large contemporary cardiac surgery population.

Methods.—We retrospectively analyzed prospectively collected data from the New York State Department of Health database including

5,798 patients undergoing cardiac surgery between January 1998 and December 2005. Patients with RF (intubation time ≥ 72 h) were compared to patients without RF.

Results.—The incidence of RF was 9.1% (n = 529). The highest incidence of RF was observed following combined valve/coronary artery bypass graft (14.8%) and aortic procedures (13.5%). Multivariate analysis revealed preoperative and operative predictors of RF such as renal failure (odds ratio [OR], 2.3), aortic procedures (OR, 2.6), hemodynamic instability (OR, 3.2), and intraaortic balloon pump (OR, 2.6). The mortality rate following RF was 15.5% (n = 82), compared to 2.4% (n = 126) in the no-RF group (p < 0.001). Kaplan-Meier survival curves showed significantly poorer survival among RF patients (p < 0.001) compared to the no-RF group.

Conclusion.—RF remains a serious and common complication following cardiac surgery, particularly in patients undergoing complex procedures. RF is associated with significant comorbidity, increased hospital mortality, and reduced long-term survival. Future research efforts should focus on a more precise identification of patients at risk and the development of new treatment modalities that would potentially prevent the occurrence of this complication.

▶ Respiratory failure following cardiac surgery is known to be associated with increased morbidity and mortality. The authors retrospectively analyzed data from the New York State Department of Health database to identify risk factors for respiratory failure (RF) in a contemporary cohort. The strength of this study is that it not only assessed early outcomes but long-term outcomes as well. In the multivariate analysis, multiple risk factors for the development of RF were identified. Those noted in the abstract are those associated with the highest odds of RF, but other statistically significant factors included—active endocarditis, congestive heart failure, reoperation, peripheral vascular disease, chronic obstructive pulmonary disease, age > 70 years, combined valve and coronary artery bypass graft (CABG) surgery, diabetes, ejection fraction ≤30%, and female gender. By univariate analysis, those patients who had RF were more likely to have postoperative complications which included stroke, myocardial infarction, renal failure requiring dialysis, deep sternal wound infection, a systemic infection, re-exploration for bleeding, gastrointestinal complications, increased length of stay, and a higher mortality. Among patients with RF, preoperative renal failure requiring dialysis, intra-aortic balloon pump insertion, postoperative renal failure requiring dialysis, and re-exploration for bleeding were all important predictors of mortality. Furthermore, the increased mortality associated with RF was consistent across European system for cardiac operative risk evaluation (EuroSCORE)[1] groups. Table 4, in the original article, shows that the contribution of RF to mortality in the highest risk group was less than that for the lowest risk group, implying that those in the highest risk category had other important contributors to their risk of death. An important contribution of this study is the significance in survival differences for those with and without RF.

Limitations of this trial are important to discuss. Although they showed an association of increased mortality with RF, we cannot conclude that the RF is the cause of this increased mortality but rather could be the result of a complication that resulted in RF or a marker of an unmeasured risk factor or confounding variable. By reporting the risk of mortality by EuroSCORE risk groups for patients with and without RF, they may have adequately accounted for the potential confounders, as this is conceptually similar to a propensity score comparison but not as rigorous. However, given the observational and retrospective nature of this study, this cannot be guaranteed. Of course, there would never be a trial that would randomize patients to planned ventilatory support for more than 72 hours and this level of evidence may be the strongest we will ever have. Despite these important limitations, this study highlights that the sequelae associated with postoperative RF are significant and that we need to better understand how to prevent RF and mitigate these sequelae.

E. A. Martinez, MD, MHS

Reference

1. Nashef SA, Roques F, Michel P, Gauducheau E, Lemeshow S, Salamon R. European system for cardiac operative risk evaluation (EuroSCORE). *Eur J Cardiothorac Surg.* 1999;16:9-13.

The effect of mannitol on renal function after cardiopulmonary bypass in patients with established renal dysfunction

Smith MNA, Best D, Sheppard SV, et al (Wessex Cardiothoracic Centre, Southampton, UK)
Anaesthesia 63:701-704, 2008

The usefulness of mannitol in the priming fluid for cardiopulmonary bypass is uncertain in patients with normal renal function, and has not been studied in patients with established renal dysfunction. We studied 50 patients with serum creatinine between 130 and 250 $\mu mol.l^{-1}$ having cardiac surgery. Patients were randomised to receive mannitol 0.5 $g.kg^{-1}$, or an equivalent volume of Hartmann's solution, in the bypass prime. There were no differences between the groups in plasma creatinine or change in creatinine from baseline, urine output, or fluid balance over the first three postoperative days. We conclude that mannitol has no effect on routine measures of renal function during cardiac surgery in patients with established renal dysfunction.

▶ Perioperative renal failure is associated with a significant increase in morbidity and mortality in patients undergoing cardiac surgical procedures. Depending on the definition used, approximately 3.53% of patients undergoing coronary artery bypass surgery develop renal failure.[1] Strategies to mitigate the risk of the progression of preoperative renal dysfunction or development of new renal dysfunction have been of long interest to those who care for cardiac surgical patients. To date, no therapy has provided a silver bullet. Two recent trials have shown that the use of *N*-acetylcysteine, which has shown significant promise for contrast-induced nephropathy,[2] does not decrease the risk of perioperative renal failure among cardiac surgical patients.[3,4] Mannitol, an osmotic diuretic, is frequently used to prime the cardiopulmonary bypass circuit with the goal of reducing the risk of perioperative renal dysfunction. However, there remains controversy as to whether mannitol has any impact on postoperative renal function in patients with or without preoperative renal dysfunction. Smith and colleagues sought to evaluate whether the use of mannitol had any protective effect on postoperative renal function. They previously reported their experience in patients with normal preoperative creatinine,[5] and this article addresses patients with established preoperative renal dysfunction. Unfortunately, mannitol did not alter the measured outcomes in either subset of patients. Based on their findings, the authors suggest that the routine use of mannitol in on-pump cardiac surgical procedures is unnecessary. Although this is most likely the case, the limitations of these 2 studies, the small sample sizes (40 patients with normal renal function and 50 patients with preoperative renal dysfunction) and the limitations of global measures of renal function (urine output, fluid balance, and creatinine), limit their impact on changing a long-standing practice. Potentially, the use of novel biomarkers specific for acute kidney injury will increase the sensitivity for the detection of renal injury in the future.[6] Either way, the search continues for interventions to prevent or mitigate deterioration in renal function in cardiac surgical patients, a critically important goal given its association with morbidity and mortality.

E. A. Martinez, MD, MHS

References

1. Shroyer AL, Coombs LP, Peterson ED, et al. The Society of Thoracic Surgeons: 30-day operative mortality and morbidity risk models. *Ann Thorac Surg.* 2003; 75:1856-1864.
2. Venkataraman R. Can we prevent acute kidney injury? *Critical Care Med.* 2008; 36(4 Suppl):S166-S171.
3. Adabag AS, Ishani A, Koneswaran S, et al. Utility of N-acetylcysteine to prevent acute kidney injury after cardiac surgery: a randomized controlled trial. *Am Heart J.* 2008;155:1143-1149.
4. Haase M, Haase-Fielitz A, Bagshaw SM, et al. Phase II, randomized, controlled trial of high-dose N-acetylcysteine in high-risk cardiac surgery patients. *Crit Care Med.* 2007;35:1324-1331.
5. Yallop KG, Sheppard SV, Smith DC. The effect of mannitol on renal function following cardio-pulmonary bypass in patients with normal pre-operative creatinine. *Anaesth.* 2008;63:576-582.
6. Boldt J, Wolf M. Identification of renal injury in cardiac surgery: the role of kidney-specific proteins. *J Cardiothorac Vasc Anesth.* 2008;22:122-132.

Preoperative apolipoprotein CI levels correlate positively with the proinflammatory response in patients experiencing endotoxemia following elective cardiac surgery
Schippers EF, Berbée JFP, van Disseldorp IM, et al (Leiden Univ Med Ctr, The Netherlands; et al)
Intensive Care Med 34:1492-1497, 2008

Objective.—Experimental models show that apolipoprotein CI (apoCI) binds and enhances the inflammatory response to endotoxin. We studied in patients undergoing cardiopulmonary bypass surgery (CPB) and experiencing endotoxemia during reperfusion whether plasma apoCI levels correlate with the inflammatory response and perioperative cytokine release.

Design.—Prospective, observational, clinical cohort study.

Setting.—Operating room (OR) and intensive care unit (ICU) of a university hospital.

Patients.—One hundred fifty-nine consecutive patients > 18 years of age (66% males ($n = 105$), median age 65 and 67 years for males and females, respectively) undergoing elective cardiothoracic surgery with cardiopulmonary bypass.

Interventions.—None.

Measurements.—Baseline apoCI, apoCIII, total cholesterol and triglyceride levels, and perioperative endotoxin and TNF-α levels were determined.

Results.—High preoperative plasma apoCI, but not apoCIII, levels were associated ($p < 0.05$) with increased perioperative levels of TNF-α in patients experiencing endotoxemia. This association was not observed in patients without endotoxemia.

Conclusion.—High plasma apoCI is positively related to proinflammatory response in patients experiencing endotoxemia and confirms the observations in animal models.

▶ Apolipoprotein CI (apoCI) has been shown to be a mediator of the host inflammatory response of macrophages in response to endotoxin from gram-negative bacterial cell walls. Previous studies have shown that serum endotoxin levels rise in response to splanchnic hypoperfusion during cardiopulmonary bypass (CPB). In addition, cardiac surgery is associated with varying degrees of a perioperative systemic inflammatory response syndrome (SIRS) regardless of endotoxin levels.[1] Schippers and colleagues hypothesized that apoCI significantly contributes to the perioperative inflammatory response in cardiac surgical patients who have endotoxemia. They performed an exploratory observational study of 150 patients undergoing elective surgery with CPB. Serum levels of apoCI, endotoxin, and tumor necrosis factor (TNF)-α were measured preoperatively, and at aortic unclamping, 30 min post reperfusion, and on admission to the intensive care unit (ICU). Significant correlations were found between apoCI and TNF-α among patients with elevated levels of endotoxin. This relationship was not significant among patients without endotoxemia. This study is strengthened by also assessing the association of TNF-α to other molecules with similar physical characteristics, apoCIII, total cholesterol, and triglycerides to demonstrate that this was not just an association with lipid or apolipoprotein levels. Although there was a correlation between cholesterol and TNF-α at times 2 and 3, this was not consistent.

They did not correlate levels of apoCI and TNF-α with clinical parameters of SIRS (oxygenation, vasopressor requirements), which would be interesting and give the reader an important perspective on what these findings mean clinically. The study was exploratory and we would expect such data to be reported in a future adequately powered trial in addition to a more robust evaluation of whether cholesterol does or does not consistently correlate with TNF-α levels. Because there are studies that have shown that high levels of elevated apoCI correlate with improved outcomes, it will be interesting to see if in a follow-up study this holds true for patients undergoing cardiac surgery and, more importantly, if this is a modifiable risk for both patients undergoing cardiac surgery and in patients with gram-negative sepsis.

E. A. Martinez, MD, MHS

Reference

1. Bouter H, Schippers EF, Luelmo SA, et al. No effect of preoperative selective gut decontamination on endotoxemia and cytokine activation during cardiopulmonary bypass: a randomized, placebo-controlled study. *Crit Care Med.* 2002;30:38-43.

Quality improvement program decreases mortality after cardiac surgery
Stamou SC, Camp SL, Stiegel RM, et al (Heart Inst Carolinas Med Ctr, Charlotte, NC)
J Thorac Cardiovasc Surg 136:494-499, 2008

Objective.—This study investigated the effects of a quality improvement program and goal-oriented, multidisciplinary protocols on mortality after cardiac surgery.

Methods.—Patients were divided into two groups: those undergoing surgery (coronary artery bypass grafting, isolated valve surgery, or coronary artery bypass grafting and valve surgery) after establishment of the multidisciplinary quality improvement program (January 2005–December 2006, n = 922) and those undergoing surgery before institution of the program (January 2002–December 2003, n = 1289). Logistic regression and propensity score analysis were used to adjust for imbalances in patients' preoperative characteristics.

Results.—Operative mortality was lower in the quality improvement group (2.6% vs 5.0%, $P < .01$). Unadjusted odds ratio was 0.5 (95% confidence interval 0.3–0.8, $P < .01$); propensity score–adjusted odds ratio was 0.6 (95% confidence interval 0.4–0.99, $P = .04$). In multivariable analysis, diabetes ($P < .01$), chronic renal insufficiency ($P = .05$), previous cardiovascular operation ($P = .04$), congestive heart failure ($P < .01$), unstable angina ($P < .01$), age older than 75 years ($P < .01$), prolonged pump time ($P < .01$), and prolonged operation ($P = .05$) emerged as independent predictors of higher mortality after cardiac surgery, whereas quality improvement program ($P < .01$) and male sex ($P = .03$) were associated with lower mortality. Mortality decline was less pronounced in patients with than without diabetes ($P = .04$).

Conclusion.—Application of goal-directed, multidisciplinary protocols and a quality improvement program were associated with lower mortality after cardiac surgery. This decline was less prominent in patients with diabetes, and focused quality improvement protocols may be required for this subset of patients (Fig 1).

▶ There are many well-established risk factors for mortality after cardiac surgery, including complexity of the procedure, age, gender, diabetes, and pre-existing renal failure to name a few. There also have been data that suggest that the procedure volume of the surgeon and hospital impacts outcomes, with resultant recommendation for selective referrals to high-volume centers for cardiac surgery.[1] Importantly, no studies have evaluated what aspects of care explain this potential difference in outcomes based on volume. Stamou and colleagues present the results of a pre-postobservational trial in which a quality improvement program (QIP) was introduced in a single center. They showed a decrease in the risk-adjusted mortality rate in the overall population after introduction of a QIP. The propensity score-adjusted odds ratio for mortality was 0.6 (95% confidence interval [CI] 0.4-0.99, $P = 0.04$), showing that post-QIP implementation mortality was decreased (Fig 1). This study offers important insight into factors that might explain the variations in outcomes among cardiac surgical centers, for example, the implementation of well-developed QIPs. Although it would be interesting to understand the impact of specific interventions,

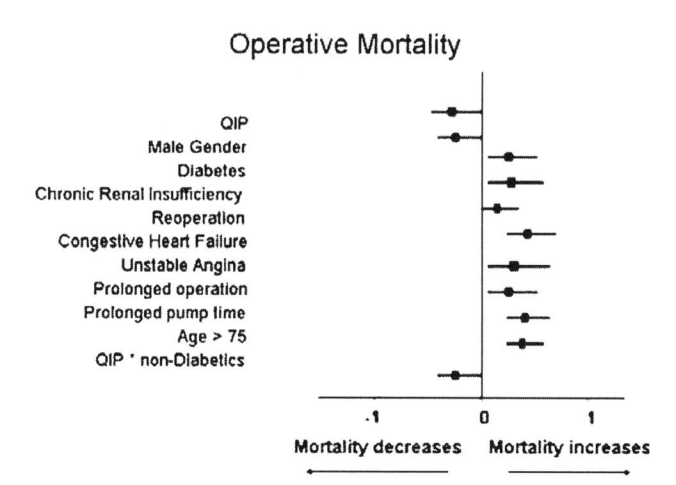

FIGURE 1.—Independent predictors of operative mortality after cardiac surgery (multivariable logistic regression analysis). *QIP*, Quality improvement program. (Reprinted from Stamou SC, Camp SL, Stiegel RM, et al. Quality improvement program decreases mortality after cardiac surgery. *J Thorac Cardiovasc Surg.* 2008;136:494-499, with permission from The American Association for Thoracic Surgery.)

such as implementation of a glycemic control protocol or use of postoperative chlorhexidine baths, this study demonstrates the potential impact of a comprehensive QIP and offers opportunities for all centers to make ongoing improvements in the care of cardiac surgical patients.

E. A. Martinez, MD, MHS

Reference

1. Birkmeyer JD, Finlayson EV, Birkmeyer CM. Volume standards for high-risk surgical procedures: potential benefits of the Leapfrog initiative. *Surgery.* 2001; 130:415-422.

Oxygenation and release of inflammatory mediators after off-pump compared with after on-pump coronary artery bypass surgery

Rasmussen BS, Laugesen H, Sollid J, et al (Aarhus Univ Hosp, Denmark; et al)
Acta Anaesthesiol Scand 51:1202-1210, 2007

Background.—In a previous study, we showed that oxygenation was impaired for up to 5 days after conventional coronary artery bypass grafting (CABG). As cardiopulmonary bypass (CPB) may have a detrimental effect on pulmonary function, we hypothesized that coronary revascularization grafting without the use of CPB (OPCAB) would affect post-operative oxygenation and release of inflammatory mediators less compared with CABG.

Methods.—Low-risk patients scheduled for elective coronary revascularization were randomly assigned to one of two groups (CABG, $n = 17$ or OPCAB, $n = 18$). Two parameters of oxygenation, shunt (%) and ventilation-perfusions mismatch, described as ΔPO_2 (kPa), were estimated for up to 5 days post-operatively. Systemic release of interleukin (IL)-6, -8 and -10, C-reactive protein (CRP) and neutrophils were measured in peripheral blood samples for up to 3 days post-operatively. The lungs participation in the cytokine response was evaluated from mixed venous blood samples taken within the first 16 h post-operatively.

Results.—OPCAB was followed by a higher shunt ($P = 0.047$), with no difference ($P = 0.47$) in the deterioration of ΔPO_2 between the groups. OPCAB was followed by an attenuated systemic release of IL-8 ($P = 0.041$) and IL-10 ($P = 0.006$), while the release of IL-6 ($P = 0.94$), CRP ($P = 0.121$) and neutrophils ($P = 0.078$) did not differ between the groups. Indications of an uptake of cytokines in the lungs were found after OPCAB.

Conclusions.—When comparing OPCAB with CABG, oxygenation was more affected and only part of the systemic inflammatory response was attenuated.

▶ There has been much interest in the potential benefits of off-pump coronary artery bypass (OPCAB) procedures compared with on-pump coronary artery bypass (CABG) procedures, and it remains uncertain whether OPCAB offers a true benefit over CABG. One of the key theoretical benefits of OPCAB is the decrease in the systemic inflammatory response that is initiated with exposure to the bypass circuit, hypothermia, and hemodilution[1] with consequent impact on oxygenation and lung function. Thus, Rasmussen and colleagues hypothesized that the OPCAB procedure would have less of a negative impact on oxygenation and be associated with a less marked release of inflammatory markers, because both are associated with the systemic inflammatory response. They randomized 35 low-risk patients to either OPCAB or CABG and assessed perioperative oxygenation and inflammatory markers for up to 5 days postoperatively. Surprisingly, they found that although oxygenation deteriorated in both groups, the OPCAB patients had worse oxygenation. This was caused by increased shunt rather than ventilation/perfusion (V/Q) mismatch as assessed by a 2-parameter model of gas exchange, and there was no difference in duration of intubation. They suggested that this shunt difference may be a result of atelectasis, possibly because of the lack of a recruitment protocol, lower intraop positive end-expiratory pressure (PEEP), and Trendelenburg positioning. OPCAB attenuated the plasma increase in 2 cytokines, proinflammatory interleukin (IL)-8 and anti-inflammatory IL-10, without differences seen in IL-6, C-reactive protein (CRP), or neutrophils. In addition, there was a statistically significant difference in the pulmonary processing of the 3 cytokines, with the OPCAB group demonstrating pulmonary uptake while the CABG group showed less uptake and pulmonary production. As is frequently the case, these plasma cytokine results are difficult to interpret, but the hypothesized global reduction in inflammatory markers with OPCAB surgery was not observed. Despite the limitations of relatively small sample size, the inclusion of low-risk patients, and the use of plasma cytokines to infer pulmonary processes, this well-conducted randomized study is able to conclude that defects in postoperative oxygenation and systemic inflammatory responses are not restricted to the use of cardiopulmonary bypass (CPB), and that attention regarding postoperative oxygenation should be focused on optimal ventilation and lung recruitment strategies in the OR and intensive care unit (ICU). Further light on the potential advantages of OPCAB surgery will require larger trials and possibly more sensitive measures of organ-level inflammatory effects.

E. A. Martinez, MD, MHS

Reference

1. Laffey JG, Boylan JF, Cheng DC. The systemic inflammatory response to cardiac surgery: implications for the anesthesiologist. *Anesthesiology.* 2002;97:215-252.

Pulse Pressure Is an Age-Independent Predictor of Stroke Development After Cardiac Surgery
Benjo A, Thompson RE, Fine D, et al (Johns Hopkins Med Institutions, Baltimore, MD; Bloomberg School of Public Health, Baltimore, MD)
Hypertension 50:630-635, 2007

Chronologic age is a strong predictor of adverse outcomes after cardiac surgery. The variability in age-related cardiovascular changes suggests that age may not be the most accurate predictor of adverse perioperative outcomes. Vascular stiffness has emerged as an important surrogate of vascular aging. In a retrospective review, we investigated the value of vascular stiffness, as assessed by brachial pulse pressure (PP) measurements, in predicting stroke in 703 patients (63.4% men and 36.6% women). Patients were followed for 348 ± 215 days after cardiac surgery. We used a multivariable logistic model and unadjusted and adjusted Cox proportional-hazard models to assess the probability of stroke and the hazards of stroke over time. Stroke patients had a significantly higher PP (81.2 mm Hg versus 64.5 mm Hg; $P=0.0006$). In the logistic regression model, PP was an independent predictor of stroke development (unadjusted odds ratio: 1.35; 95% CI: 1.13 to 1.62, for every 10-mm Hg increase in PP; $P=0.001$). In the unadjusted and adjusted Cox models, PP again predicted stroke (hazard ratio: 1.32; 95% CI: 1.12 to 1.57; hazard ratio: 2.62; 95% CI: 1.49 to 4.60, respectively; $P=0.001$ for both) for every 10 mm Hg increase in PP. Age, gender, and diabetes were not independent predictors of stroke. Ejection fraction was inversely related to stroke in the adjusted model. Kaplan–Meier estimates and corresponding log-rank test indicated that the probability of stroke-free survival function was significantly lower ($P=0.0067$) in patients with PP >72 mm Hg versus <72 mm Hg. This analysis suggests that indices of vascular stiffness could be important predictors of neurologic complications.

▶ Stroke following cardiac surgical procedures remains a significant complication and is associated with increased mortality despite improvements in the perioperative care of such patients. Age remains an important risk factor for stroke and for other morbid events following cardiac surgery. Importantly, there are increasing data supporting that age is also associated with vascular changes that are potentially modifiable. These age-related vascular changes are manifested as increased vascular stiffness. Vascular stiffness has previously been shown to be an independent risk factor for cardiovascular disease.[1,2] Younger and/or nondiseased vasculature is notable for being compliant. This translates into a characteristic transmission pattern of the arterial waveform. Benjo et al describe that "in compliant vessels, the reflected wave returns to the central circulation during diastole augmenting diastolic myocardial perfusion. In a stiff vasculature, this reflected wave returns to the central circulation during systole." Therefore, vascular stiffness is noted by an elevated systolic blood pressure, pulse pressure (PP), or pulse wave velocity.

The authors of this observational retrospective cohort study proposed that a measure of vascular stiffness would be an independent risk factor for a stroke following cardiac surgery. For this analysis, stroke was defined as a "new, nonreversible focal neurologic deficit, diagnosed clinically by a neurologist with or without confirmation by brain imaging." They used the peripheral PP as assessed at the brachial artery using oscillometry (eg, standard blood pressure assessment in an upper extremity) as their independent predictor. An adjusted logistic regression was used to calculate the odds ratio of stroke for independent variables which had a $P \leq .10$ in the unadjusted analysis. They showed that stroke patients had a higher PP than those who did not suffer a perioperative stroke with a mean PP of 81.2 mmHg versus 64.5 mmHg in patients without a stroke ($P = .0006$). The adjusted odds of having a stroke were 2.62, or more than double, for each increase in PP of 10 mm Hg. In other words, a patient with a PP of 85 mm Hg (180/95 mm Hg) had 2-1/2 times increased odds of stroke compared with somebody with a PP of 75 mm Hg (180/105). The unadjusted probability of having a perioperative stroke is shown in Fig 1 in the original article. The authors also present a Kaplan-Meier curve (Fig 2 in the original article) demonstrating stroke-free survival with and without an elevated PP of 72 mm Hg as determined by a receiver-operator curve.

This well-done retrospective observational study extends the previous literature, which has shown an association with elevated PP and cardiovascular outcomes to the cardiac surgical patient population. This important study gives insight into the variation of the risk of stroke, which is associated with age, and offers a physiological pathway that might explain the association of age with stroke. Importantly, it offers a potentially reversible risk factor, unlike age in and of itself. An important limitation of this study is that noninvasive measures of peripheral (brachial) blood pressure monitoring were used as indirect measures of central vascular stiffness as opposed to more direct indices (eg, pulse wave velocity).[3] However, this does not limit the importance of this study, which has shown that PP is an independent risk factor for stroke following cardiac surgery. Of course, the key will be whether this risk is modifiable.

E. A. Martinez, MD, MHS

References

1. Sutton-Tyrrell K, Najjar SS, Boudreau RM, Venkitachalam L, et al. for the Health ABC Study. Elevated aortic pulse wave velocity, a marker of arterial stiffness, predicts cardiovascular events in well-functioning older adults. *Circulation.* 2005;111:3384-3390.
2. Mattace-Raso FUS, van der Cammen TJM, Hofman A, et al. Arterial stiffness and risk of coronary heart disease and stroke. The Rotterdam Study. *Circulation.* 2006; 113:657-663.
3. Safar ME, Levy BI, Struijker-Boudier H. Current perspectives on arterial stiffness and pulse pressure in hypertension and cardiovascular diseases. *Circulation.* 2003; 107:2864-2869.

Other

Negative Pressure Wound Therapy. A Vacuum of Evidence?
Gregor S, Maegele M, Sauerland S, et al (Univ of Witten/Herdecke, Cologne, Germany)
Arch Surg 143:189-196, 2008

Objective.—To systematically examine the clinical effectiveness and safety of negative pressure wound therapy (NPWT) compared with conventional wound therapy.

Data Sources.—MEDLINE, EMBASE, CINAHL, and the Cochrane Library were searched. Manufacturers were contacted, and trial registries were screened.

Study Selection.—Randomized controlled trials (RCTs) and non-RCTs comparing NPWT and conventional therapy for acute or chronic wounds were included in this review. The main outcomes of interest were wound-healing variables. After screening 255 full-text articles, 17 studies remained. In addition, 19 unpublished trials were found, of which 5 had been prematurely terminated.

Data Extraction.—Two reviewers independently extracted data and assessed methodologic quality in a standardized manner.

Data Synthesis.—Seven RCTs (n = 324) and 10 non-RCTs (n = 278) met the inclusion criteria. The overall methodologic quality of the trials was poor. Significant differences in favor of NPWT for time to wound closure or incidence of wound closure were shown in 2 of 5 RCTs and 2 of 4 non-RCTs. A meta-analysis of changes in wound size that included 4 RCTs and 2 non-RCTs favored NPWT (standardized mean difference: RCTs, −0.57; non-RCTs, −1.30).

Conclusions.—Although there is some indication that NPWT may improve wound healing, the body of evidence available is insufficient to clearly prove an additional clinical benefit of NPWT. The large number of prematurely terminated and unpublished trials is reason for concern.

▶ Negative pressure wound therapy (NPWT) was developed in the early 1990s. This therapy consists of a foam dressing covered with an adhesive drape to which a vacuum pump is attached creating intermittent or continuous pressure. Positive effects have been demonstrated in the basic science laboratory and case series suggest widespread applicability of this technology in various clinical settings.[1,2] Remarkably, in this meta-analysis, only 600 patients were found in evaluable trials that included both randomized controlled studies and nonrandomized controlled studies. There is a dramatic difference from the widespread use of this technology in clinical practice. NPWT, as the authors note, is innovative and commercially successful. It is thought to facilitate wound care, particularly in patients with large or heavily secreting wounds.[3] Clearly, conventional dressings require more frequent changing that may result in increases in nursing interventions, patient discomfort, and length of stay. However, because of costs associated with NPWT, overall wound treatment costs are similar to older, more labor-intensive methods. NPWT is reported to be safe and applicable in the ambulatory setting. This critical review of the data, however, does not allow for consistent optimistic recommendations. In light of significant cost and a paucity of rigorous evidence, selective application of NPWT with careful review of outcomes is warranted.

D. J. Dries, MSE, MD

References

1. Morykwas MJ, Argenta LC, Shelton-Brown EI, McGuirt W. Vacuum-assisted closure: a new method for wound control and treatment: animal studies and basic foundation. *Ann Plast Surg.* 1997;38:553-562.
2. Morykwas MJ, Faler BJ, Pearce DJ, Argenta LC. Effects of varying levels of subatmospheric pressure on the rate of granulation tissue formation in experimental wounds in swine. *Ann Plast Surg.* 2001;47:547-551.
3. Maegele M, Gregor S, Steinhausen E, et al. The long-distance tertiary air transfer and care of tsunami victims: injury pattern and microbiological and psychological aspects. *Crit Care Med.* 2005;33:1136-1140.

Restrictive red blood cell transfusion: not just for the stable intensive care unit patient
Wendy WL, Hemmila MR, Maggio PM, et al (Univ of Michigan Health System, Ann Arbor, MI; et al)
Am J Surg 195:803-806, 2008

Background.—Multiple studies report that patients receiving red blood cell (RBC) transfusion in the intensive care unit (ICU) are more likely to experience complications. Despite these findings, surgical patients are frequently transfused for operative procedures, trauma, and burns. We hypothesized that a RBC transfusion guideline would safely decrease our use of RBC transfusions in the ICU and lower the hematocrit at which our trauma and burn patients were transfused, both in the stable and symptomatic patient.

Methods.—For each episode of RBC transfusion, the pretransfusion vital signs and reasons for transfusion were recorded prospectively from August 2003 through April 2004. Before institution of the transfusion guideline, which stressed withholding transfusion for hematocrit over 23 in asymptomatic patients, intensive education of all caregivers occurred. Data from all transfusions during 2005 were also reviewed for long-term compliance with the guideline.

Results.—Eighty-two of 316 ICU patients (26%) had 315 RBC transfusion events during the initial study period. Mean transfusion hematocrits decreased from 26.6 ± 4.7 to 23.9 ± 2.6 ($P < .0003$) for all patients. For the follow-up period in 2005, 94 of 523 patients (18%) were transfused in the ICU at a mean transfusion hematocrit of 24.1 for symptomatic ($P < .0001$) and 22.5 for asymptomatic patients ($P < .0001$). Low hematocrit was the most frequently cited reason for transfusion for all patients in the first part of the study, whereas hemodynamic instability (n = 91 events) and perioperative losses (n = 49 events) ranked highest for symptomatic patients.

Conclusion.—A transfusion guideline accompanied by intensive education is effective in reducing RBC transfusions in a trauma-burn ICU. A lower hematocrit was well tolerated in both the symptomatic and asymptomatic groups of surgical patients. With education and follow-up, the changes in transfusion practices were durable and affected transfusion practices for both asymptomatic and symptomatic patients.

▶ As with other populations of critically ill patients, a body of literature has been evolving that supports the limitation of transfusion of packed red blood cells (PRBC) in trauma and burn patients, despite the historical assumptions that these patients require aggressive resuscitation with such products. In this study, the investigators evaluated the adherence to and impact of a restrictive transfusion strategy after the institution of a series of transfusion guidelines in a combined trauma-burn ICU. Adherence to the guidelines was good and overall use of PRBC declined significantly after their institution, along with an associated decline in ICU and hospital lengths of stay and a strong trend toward a decrease in mortality that did not reach statistical significance. The allowed indications for transfusion in the guidelines used in this unit are perhaps open to debate. The numerical threshold for transfusion was established at a hematocrit of 23%. Transfusion at a hematocrit above this level was allowed for symptomatic patients, with symptoms defined as including the following: hypotension, use of pressor support, poor oxygenation despite maximization of ventilator mechanics, angina, and evidence of acute myocardial ischemia. It is questionable as to whether some of the patients who may have received PRBC based on these indications may have actually required or benefited from such an intervention, and what effect their assignment to the restrictive group may have had on the outcomes of the study, had more specific indications for transfusion been required. As the authors specifically point out in their discussion, they have no data that transfusion improved oxygenation or pulmonary function in their ventilated patients. Also, a significant body of literature which has developed after the period during which these data were collected has questioned the use of routine transfusion of PRBC even in active coronary ischemia, at least when hemoglobin is > 8 g/dL (hematocrit about 24%). Overall, however, these data continue to add further support to the idea that restrictive use of PRBC is at least not harmful and perhaps beneficial to a broad array of critically ill patients, including those suffering from significant injury.

D. R. Gerber, DO

7 Sepsis/Septic Shock

Isolated and reversible impairment of ventricular relaxation in patients with septic shock
Bouhemad B, Nicolas-Robin A, Arbelot C, et al (Univ Pierre et Marie Curie, Paris, France)
Crit Care Med 36:766-774, 2008

Objective.—Many patients with septic shock and increased cardiac troponin I (cTnI) do not exhibit significant left ventricular systolic dysfunction. We hypothesized that an isolated and reversible impairment of ventricular relaxation may be associated with the increase in cTnI.

Design.—Prospective, observational study.

Setting.—Surgical intensive care unit in a university hospital.

Patients.—Total of 54 patients with septic shock.

Interventions.—Fractional area change, early diastolic velocity of mitral annulus, flow propagation velocity of early diastolic mitral inflow, cTnI, tumor necrosis factor-α, interleukin (IL)-6, -1β, -8, and -10 were measured at days 1, 2, 3, 4, 7, and 10 after onset of septic shock. Patients were classified into three groups: normal cTnI (group 1), increased cTnI and fractional area change <50% (group 2), and increased cTnI and fractional area change >50% (group 3).

Measurements and Main Results.—A total of 22 patients had an increase in cTnI, 11 with both systolic and diastolic dysfunctions and 11 with isolated impairment of left ventricular relaxation. At day 1, early diastolic velocity of mitral annulus and flow propagation velocity of early diastolic mitral inflow were significantly lower and tumor necrosis factor-α, IL-8, and IL-10 significantly higher in groups 2 and 3 compared with group 1. With resolution of septic shock, early diastolic velocity of mitral annulus and flow propagation velocity of early diastolic mitral inflow measured in patients of groups 2 and 3 returned progressively to values observed in group 1, with a parallel normalization of tumor necrosis factor-α, IL-8, and IL-10.

Conclusions.—Isolated and reversible impairment of left ventricular relaxation, associated with transient increases in cTnI, tumor necrosis factor-α, IL-8, and IL-10, was observed in 20% of patients with septic shock.

▶ These investigators were able to identify diastolic dysfunction during septic shock with improvement and reversal with resolution of shock. They also showed correlation of troponin elevation with cardiac dysfunction and point to diastolic dysfunction alone as a potential cause of elevated troponin.

Drugs that target diastolic dysfunction without interfering with systolic function, such as levosimendan, might be of value in septic shock.

R. P. Dellinger, MD

Liberal vs. conservative vasopressor use to maintain mean arterial blood pressure during resuscitation of septic shock: an observational study
Subramanian S, Yilmaz M, Rehman A, et al (Mayo Clinic, Rochester, MN; et al)
Intensive Care Med 34:157-162, 2008

Objective.—The optimal role of vasopressor therapy in septic shock is not known. We hypothesized that the variability in the use of vasopressors to treat hypotension is associated with subsequent organ failures.

Design.—Retrospective observational single-center cohort study.

Setting.—Tertiary care hospital.

Patients and Participants.—Consecutive patients with septic shock.

Measurement and Results.—Ninety-five patients were enrolled. Serial blood pressure recordings and vasopressor use were collected during the first 12 h of septic shock. Median duration of hypotension that was not treated with vasopressors was 1.37 h (interquartile range [IQR] 0.62–2.66). Based on the observed variability, we evaluated liberal (duration of untreated hypotension < median) vs. conservative (duration of untreated hypotensionn > median) vasopressor therapy. Compared with patients who received conservative vasopressor therapy, patients treated liberally had similar baseline organ impairment [median Sequential Organ Failure Assessment (SOFA) score 8 vs. 8, $p = 0.438$] were more likely to be younger (median age 70 vs. 77 years, $p = 0.049$), to require ventilator support (78 vs. 49%, $p < 0.001$), and to have progression of organ failures after 24 h (59 vs. 37%, $p = 0.032$). When adjusted for age and mechanical ventilation, early therapy aimed at achieving global tissue perfusion [odds ratio (OR) 0.33, 95% confidence interval (CI 0.11–0.88), and early adequate antibiotic therapy (OR 0.27, 95% CI 0.09–0.76), but not liberal vasopressor use (OR 2.13, 95% CI 0.80–5.84), prevented progression of organ failures.

Conclusions.—In our retrospective study, early adequate antibiotics and achieving adequate global perfusion, but not liberal vasopressor therapy, were associated with improved organ failures after septic shock. Clinical trials which compare conservative vs. liberal vasopressor therapy are warranted (Fig 1).

▶ Current guidelines for hemodynamic support in patients with septic shock recommend maintaining a mean arterial pressure (MAP) < 65 mm Hg to ensure optimal organ perfusion. The therapeutic tools used to achieve this goal are fluids (crystalloids or colloids) and vasopressors. Some experts have cautioned regarding potential detrimental effects caused by aggressive use of vasopressor drugs before adequate fluid resuscitation and optimization of intravascular volumes. Others have argued that correction of blood pressure is most

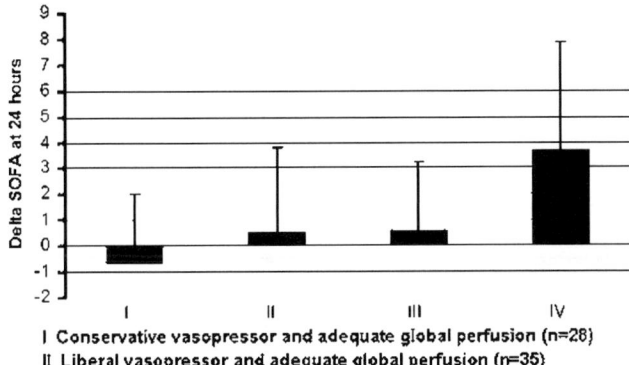

FIGURE 1.—Change in SOFA at 24 h stratified by fluid resuscitation and vasopressor use ($p = 0.019$): I Conservative vasopressor and adequate global perfusion ($n = 28$); II liberal vasopressor and adequate global perfusion ($n = 35$); III conservative vasopressor and inadequate global perfusion ($n = 21$); IV liberal vasopressor and inadequate global perfusion ($n = 11$). Error bars represent standard deviations. (Reprinted from Subramanian S, Yilmaz M, Rehman A, et al. Liberal vs. conservative vasopressor use to maintain mean arterial blood pressure during resuscitation of septic shock: an observational study. Intensive Care Med. 2008;34:157-162, with kind permission from Springer Science+Business Media.)

important and that, if needed, early concomitant use of vasopressors as fluids are being administered is preferred. Studies have shown the importance of early goal-directed resuscitation as a general strategy that favorably impacts outcomes. However, the best timing of vasopressor use in relation to other supportive methods remains to be elucidated. Thus, for the clinician at the patient's bedside, determining the best time to initiate vasopressor support remains extremely difficult.

In this retrospective observational study, the authors evaluated the use of vasopressors during the first 12 hours of resuscitation in patients with septic shock. They observed significant variability in the duration of hypotension that was not treated with vasopressors. Based on the median duration of hypotension not treated with vasopressors the authors divided the patient in 2 groups: liberal vasopressor use (duration of hypotension < median) and conservative vasopressor use (duration of hypotension > median). Patients who received liberal vasopressor therapy were younger, treated more aggressively (earlier mechanical ventilation), and more likely to have progression of organ failures after 24 hours compared with those who received conservative vasopressor therapy. When adjusted for age and mechanical ventilation, factors associated with decreased progression of organ failure were early therapy aimed at achieving global tissue perfusion and early adequate antibiotic therapy. Liberal vasopressor use was not an independent factor associated with prevention of organ failure progression. Perhaps most interesting are the findings related to changes in organ failure (Sequential Organ Failure Assessment [SOFA] at 24 h) stratified by fluid resuscitation and vasopressor use (Fig 1). This analysis suggests that conservative vasopressor use with adequate global perfusion is best, and that liberal vasopressor use with inadequate global perfusion is worse.

Although this study addresses an important clinical question, because of its limitations it is unable to provide a definitive answer. Furthermore, it is difficult to sort out if liberal vasopressor use was determined by level of aggressiveness of treating intensivist or by perceived acuity of patients. In any event it does pose very interesting questions regarding the optimal timing and threshold to initiate vasopressor support in patients with septic shock.

S. Zanotti, MD

Hydrocortisone Therapy for Patients with Septic Shock
Sprung CL, Annane D, Keh D, et al (Hadassah Hebrew Univ Med Ctr, Jerusalem, Israel; Univ of Versailles, Garches, France; Charité Universitätsmedizin Berlin; et al)
New Engl J Med 358:111-124, 2008

Background.—Hydrocortisone is widely used in patients with septic shock even though a survival benefit has been reported only in patients who remained hypotensive after fluid and vasopressor resuscitation and whose plasma cortisol levels did not rise appropriately after the administration of corticotropin.

Methods.—In this multicenter, randomized, double-blind, placebo-controlled trial, we assigned 251 patients to receive 50 mg of intravenous hydrocortisone and 248 patients to receive placebo every 6 hours for 5 days; the dose was then tapered during a 6-day period. At 28 days, the primary outcome was death among patients who did not have a response to a corticotropin test.

Results.—Of the 499 patients in the study, 233 (46.7%) did not have a response to corticotropin (125 in the hydrocortisone group and 108 in the placebo group). At 28 days, there was no significant difference in mortality between patients in the two study groups who did not have a response to corticotropin (39.2% in the hydrocortisone group and 36.1% in the placebo group, $P=0.69$) or between those who had a response to corticotropin (28.8% in the hydrocortisone group and 28.7% in the placebo group, $P=1.00$). At 28 days, 86 of 251 patients in the hydrocortisone group (34.3%) and 78 of 248 patients in the placebo group (31.5%) had died ($P=0.51$). In the hydrocortisone group, shock was reversed more quickly than in the placebo group. However, there were more episodes of superinfection, including new sepsis and septic shock.

Conclusions.—Hydrocortisone did not improve survival or reversal of shock in patients with septic shock, either overall or in patients who did not have a response to corticotropin, although hydrocortisone hastened reversal of shock in patients in whom shock was reversed. (ClinicalTrials.gov number, NCT00147004.)

▶ The role of corticosteroids in sepsis has been the subject of controversy and discussion for several decades. Initial attempts to blunt the inflammatory response in sepsis by using supraphysiologic doses of corticosteroids fell out of favor after large randomized studies in the late 1980s showed no benefit and in some cases suggested worse outcomes for patients treated with corticosteroids. In the late 1990s a resurgence of corticosteroid use in sepsis was based on the concept of relative adrenal insufficiency and the potential benefit of physiologic doses of corticosteroids (ie, 200-300 mg of hydrocortisone/day). The rationale for therapy with corticosteroids at physiologic doses originated from observations that patients with septic shock who had a reduced response to corticotropin stimulation (increase in plasma cortisol $> 9\,\mu g/dL$) had higher mortality.[1] In addition, small studies demonstrated decrease vasopressor requirement in patients receiving physiologic doses of hydrocortisone.[2] Results of a clinical trail conducted by Annane and collaborators suggested improved 28-day mortality in patients with septic shock who did not respond to corticotropin stimulation and received 7 days of hydrocortisone plus fludrocortisone.[3] Despite growing concerns with the reliability of the corticotropin stimulation test in identifying septic patients with potential adrenal dysfunction, the positive clinical data led to guideline recommendations supporting the use of corticosteroids at physiologic doses in patients with septic shock. Many experts argued that the recommendation for the use of corticosteroids in septic shock patients was heavily based on the results of 1 trial, the Annane trial.[3] Furthermore, these experts contended that this particular trial presented some limitations and that a larger multicenter trial was justified to validate its results.

The Corticosteroid Therapy of Septic Shock (CORTICUS) study was designed to further elucidate the proper role of hydrocortisone in patients with septic shock. This multicenter trial randomized patients with septic shock that remained hypotensive or required treatment with vasopressors for at least 1 hour after adequate fluid resuscitation. Initially, patients were required to be randomized within the first 24 hours of septic shock, later this window was expanded to 72 hours. Patients received either hydrocortisone (200 mg/d) or placebo for 5 days; they then received a tapered dose of hydrocortisone/placebo for 6 days, after which the drug was stopped. Slow recruitment, greatly because of widespread use of hydrocortisone in the clinical setting, lead to the trial stopping short of its projected number of patients (500 instead of the initially planned 800). The 2 groups were well-matched at baseline. The use of open-label corticosteroids and other supportive treatments was similar in both groups. The primary endpoint of death at 28 days was not significantly different between the treatment group and the placebo group. Furthermore, when patients were stratified based on their response to the corticotropin stimulation test no difference in 28-day mortality was observed. Of interest was the finding that shock was reversed more rapidly in patients receiving hydrocortisone, but this was not associated with improved mortality.

Where do these results leave us today with respect to the use of hydrocortisone in septic shock? First, we could discuss potential explanations to these results in contrast to what was becoming common practice. Differences between the CORTICUS study and the Annane study include the following: (1) patients were sicker in the Annane study (higher control group mortality); (2) were enrolled earlier and after failed hemodynamic support measures (blood pressure < 90 mm Hg after 1 h of fluids and vasopressors); and (3) patients received fludrocortisone in addition to hydrocortisone only in the Annane trial. Furthermore, the CORTICUS study because of a lower than expected mortality in the control group and decreased number of enrolled patients in relation to initial projection was less able to detect a significant difference in mortality. The 95% confidence interval for relative risk of death (0.84-1.41) is not inconsistent with the overall point estimate of the Annane study (0.89). It becomes difficult in view of the CORTICUS trial results to support widespread use of hydrocortisone in septic shock. However, it still remains unclear if certain patients with septic shock, perhaps patients that resemble the patients enrolled in the Annane study, could benefit from corticosteroids. Unfortunately the CORTICUS study was unable to define the role of corticosteroids in septic shock. However, it still provides valuable information and serves as a strong reminder that few critical care practices are based on irrefutable evidence. Even what becomes common practice and recommended by guidelines should be subject to critical appraisal and large clinical trials.

S. Zanotti, MD

References

1. Annane D, Sebille V, Troche G, et al. A 3-level prognostic classification in septic shock based on cortisol levels and cortisol response to corticotropin. *JAMA*. 2000;283:1038-1045.
2. Briegel J, Forst H, Haller M, et al. Stress doses of hydrocortisone reverse hyperdynamic septic shock: a prospective, randomized, double-blind, single-center study. *Crit Care Med*. 1999;27:723-732.
3. Annane D, Sebille V, Charpentier C, et al. Effect of treatment with low doses of hydrocortisone and fludrocortisone on mortality in patients with septic shock. *JAMA*. 2002;288:862-871.

Use of Procalcitonin to Shorten Antibiotic Treatment Duration in Septic Patients: A Randomized Trial

Nobre V, Harbarth S, Graf J-D, et al (Univ Hosps of Geneva, Switzerland)
Am J Respir Crit Care Med 177:498-505, 2008

Rationale.—The duration of antibiotic therapy in critically ill patients with sepsis can result in antibiotic overuse, increasing the risk of developing bacterial resistance.

Objectives.—To test the hypothesis that an algorithm based on serial measurements of procalcitonin (PCT) allows reduction in the duration of antibiotic therapy compared with empirical rules, and does not result in more adverse outcomes in patients with severe sepsis and septic shock.

Methods.—In patients randomly assigned to the intervention group, antibiotics were stopped when PCT levels had decreased 90% or more from the initial value (if clinicians agreed) but not before Day 3 (if baseline PCT levels were <1 µg/L) or Day 5 (if baseline PCT levels were ≥1 µg/L). In control patients, clinicians decided on the duration of antibiotic therapy based on empirical rules.

Measurements and Main Results.—Patients assigned to the PCT group had 3.5-day shorter median duration of antibiotic therapy for the first episode of infection than control subjects (intention-to-treat, n = 79, $P = 0.15$). In patients in whom a decision could be taken based on serial PCT measurements, PCT guidance resulted in a 4-day reduction in the duration of antibiotic therapy (per protocol, n = 68, $P = 0.003$) and a smaller overall antibiotic exposure ($P = 0.0002$). A similar mortality and recurrence of the primary infection were observed in PCT and control groups. A 2-day shorter intensive care unit stay was also observed in patients assigned to the PCT group ($P = 0.03$).

Conclusions.—Our results suggest that a protocol based on serial PCT measurement allows reducing antibiotic treatment duration and exposure in patients with severe sepsis and septic shock without apparent harm (Fig 2).

▶ Current clinical practice in severe sepsis and septic shock dictates empiric rules on antibiotic length of treatment. These rules are often arbitrary and range from 10 to 14 or more days of antibiotic treatment. It appears reasonable to believe that the appropriate length of antibiotic treatment might be different among patients

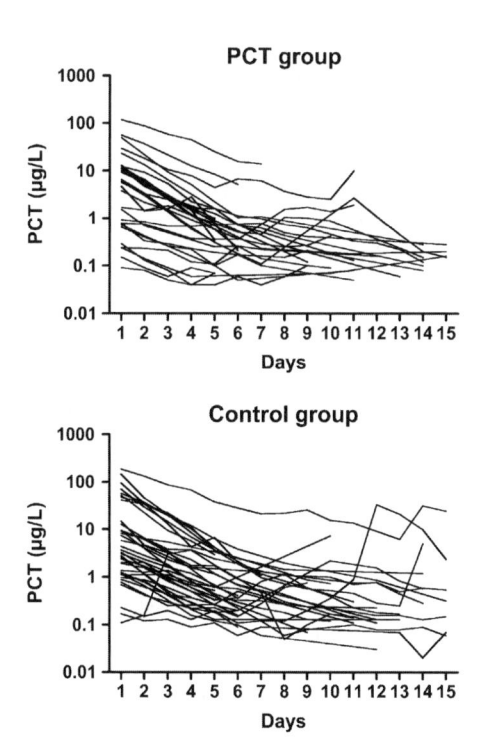

FIGURE 2.—Plasma procalcitonin (PCT) levels over time in patients from the PCT group (n = 31) *(A)* and in control subjects (n = 37) *(B)*, perprotocol analysis. (Reprinted from Nobre V, Harbarth S, Graf J-D, et al. Use of procalcitonin to shorten antibiotic treatment duration in septic patients: a randomized trial. *Am J Respir Crit Care Med.* 2008;177:498-505, Official Journal of the American Thoracic Society, Copyright of the American Thoracic Society.)

based on multiple factors such as patient's comorbidities, site of infection, and virulence of causative organisms. Furthermore, prolonged antibiotic courses can be associated with undesired consequences (ie, increased cost, increased antibiotic pressure leading to resistant organisms and, finally, higher risk of adverse effects from the antibiotics themselves). If one considers these factors, it becomes evident that an objective rule, capable of tailoring antibiotic length of treatment to individual clinical situations, would be extremely beneficial.

In this study, the authors evaluated the use of an objective rule based on serial plasma procalcitonin (PCT) levels to shorten duration of antibiotics in severe sepsis and septic shock patients. Patients were randomized to either the PCT group or the control group. PCT levels were measured in all patients (Fig 2). In the PCT group, antibiotics where stopped when the PCT level dropped by 90%. In the control group, PCT levels were kept blinded from apostrophe treating physicians and antibiotics were stopped at the treating physicians' discretion based on empiric rules. Using a PCT plasma level-based algorithm, the authors were able to significantly shorten the duration of antibiotic therapy in patients with severe sepsis and septic shock. This was accomplished without an apparent increase in mortality and with the added benefit of a significant decrease of ICU/hospital length of stay.

This study presents some limitations that are important to consider. First, it is a single center study and had various exclusion criteria, which make its results more difficult to generalize to ICU patients in other clinical settings. Second, the size of the study probably precludes definitive assessment of the impact a PCT-based algorithm could have on mortality. Despite these limitations, the results of this study are extremely positive and very encouraging. These results support the potential role of serial PCT plasma levels as a powerful tool to optimize the duration of antibiotic treatment in patients with severe sepsis and septic shock. A multicenter randomized trial with a larger number of patients should be conducted to validate these findings.

S. Zanotti, MD

Cardiac morphological and functional changes during early septic shock: a transesophageal echocardiographic study
Etchecopar-Chevreuil C, François B, Clavel M, et al (Medical-Surgical Intensive Care Unit, Limoges Cedex, France; et al)
Intensive Care Med 34:250-256, 2008

Objective.—The objective was to prospectively evaluate cardiac morphological and functional changes using transesophageal echocardiography (TEE) during early septic shock.

Design.—Prospective, observational study.

Setting.—Medical-surgical intensive care unit of a teaching hospital.

Patients and Participants.—Ventilated patients with septic shock, sinus rhythm and no cardiac disease underwent TEE within 12 h of admission (Day 0), after stabilization of hemodynamics by fluid loading (median volume: 4.9 l [lower and upper quartiles: 3.7–9.6 l]) and vasopressor therapy, and after vasopressors were stopped (Day n).

Measurements and Results.—Thirty-five patients were studied (median age: 60 years [range 44–68]; SAPS II: 53 [46–62]; SOFA score: 9 [8–11]) and 9 of them (26%) died while on vasopressors. None of the patients exhibited TEE findings of cardiac preload dependence. Between Day 0 and Day n (7 days [range 6–9]), mean left ventricular (LV) ejection fraction (EF) increased (47 ± 20 vs. 57 ± 14%: $p < 0.05$), whereas mean LV end-diastolic volume decreased (97 ± 25 vs. 75 ± 20 ml: $p < 0.0001$). Out of 16 patients (46%) with LV systolic dysfunction on Day 0, 12 had normal LVEF on Day n and 4 patients fully recovered by Day 28. Only 4 women had LV dilatation (range, LV end-diastolic volume: 110–148 ml) on Day 0, but none on Day n. Doppler tissue imaging identified an LV diastolic dysfunction in 7 patients (20%) on Day 0 (3 with normal LVEF), which resolved on Day n.

Conclusions.—This study confirms that LV systolic and diastolic dysfunctions are frequent, but LV dilatation is uncommon in fluid-loaded septic patients on vasopressors. All abnormalities regressed in survivors, regardless of their severity.

Descriptors.—Shock: clinical studies (38), Cardiovascular monitoring (34).

▶ Left ventricular contractile dysfunction is observed in a significant proportion of patients with septic shock. The cardiac dysfunction is usually transient and reversible. This study by Etchecopar-Chevreuil et al demonstrated systolic dysfunction in as much as 50% of patients studied and diastolic dysfunction in about 20%. This study is significant for at least 2 reasons.

Firstly, the high incidence of myocardial contractile dysfunction means that for a large proportion of septic patients requiring resuscitation, the cardiac pressure-volume relationships are altered. This means that resuscitation based on static pressure end-points may not be as helpful, but may even be harmful. It makes the case for a functional approach to hemodynamic management in these patients.

Secondly, I believe studies like these help state the urgent need for focused echocardiographic training and certification for critical care physicians. Echocardiography remains the only imaging modality at the bedside that can provide real-time information on cardiac function. Most intensivists remain unfamiliar with the use of echocardiography and there are very few training opportunities adapted for intensivists.

The issues raised by this study are both timely and pertinent. These are issues that should change the way we practice critical care at the bedside. It is in the best interests of our patients.

O. Okorie, MD
C. Bekes, MD

Cardiac morphological and functional changes during early septic shock: a transesophageal echocardiographic study

Etchecopar-Chevreuil C, François B, Clavel M, et al (Dupuytren Teaching Hosp, Limoges Cedex, France)
Intensive Care Med 34:250-256, 2008

Objective.—The objective was to prospectively evaluate cardiac morphological and functional changes using transesophageal echocardiography (TEE) during early septic shock.

Design.—Prospective, observational study.

Setting.—Medical-surgical intensive care unit of a teaching hospital.

Patients and Participants.—Ventilated patients with septic shock, sinus rhythm and no cardiac disease underwent TEE within 12 h of admission (Day 0), after stabilization of hemodynamics by fluid loading (median volume: 4.9l [lower and upper quartiles: 3.7–9.6l]) and vasopressor therapy, and after vasopressors were stopped (Day n).

Measurements and Results.—Thirty-five patients were studied (median age: 60 years [range 44–68]; SAPS II: 53 [46–62]; SOFA score: 9 [8–11]) and 9 of them (26%) died while on vasopressors. None of the patients exhibited TEE findings of cardiac preload dependence. Between Day 0 and Day n (7 days [range 6–9]), mean left ventricular (LV) ejection fraction (EF) increased (47 ± 20 vs. 57 ± 14%: $p < 0.05$), whereas mean LV end-diastolic volume decreased (97 ± 25 vs. 75 ± 20ml: $p < 0.0001$). Out of 16 patients (46%) with LV systolic dysfunction on Day 0, 12

TABLE 1.—Patients' Characteristics During The Early Phase (Within 12 H) Of Septic Shock After Fluid Loading And Initiation Of Vasopressor Therapy (Day 0) And After The Interruption Of Vasoactive Drugs (Day n)

Parameters	Day 0 ($n = 35$) ICU death ($n = 9$)	Day 0 ($n = 35$) ICU discharge ($n = 26$)	Day n ($n = 26$)
Age (years)	68 (56–78)	54 (43–67)	–
Male	5	14	–
Heart rate (bpm)	124 (114–142)	114 (101–133)	95 (81–100)**
Systolic blood pressure (mmHg)	112 (103–126)	120 (114–126)	121 (115–128)
Mean blood pressure (mmHg)	82 (79–86)	84 (80–91)	86 (82–92)
Fluid resuscitation (l)	5.0 (4.0–7.0)	5.0 (3.5–8.0)	–
Vasopressors (μg/kg/min)			
Norepinephrine	0.41 (0.30–0.51)	0.21 (0.09–0.33)*	–
Epinephrine	0.41 (0.19–0.52)	0.21 (0.11–0.37)	–
Tidal volume (ml/kg)	7.1 (6.3–9.4)	7.7 (7.2–8.4)	8.0 (7.0–9.0)
PaO_2/F_IO_2	172 (94–257)	233 (160–252)	267 (233–292)**
Arterial lactates (mmol/l)	10.4 (8.7–16.9)	6.0 (3.8–7.7)*	1.7 (1.2–2.2)**
SOFA	12 (11–13)	9 (7–10)*	3 (2–5)**

Data are expressed as medians and numbers in parentheses are lower and upper quartiles
*$p < 0.05$ compared with deceased patients
**$p < 0.05$ compared with survivors on Day 0

(Reprinted from Etchecopar-Chevreuil C, François B, Clavel M, et al. Cardiac morphological and functional changes during early septic shock: a transesophageal echocardiographic study. *Intensive Care Med.* 2008;34:250-256, with kind permission from Springer Science+Business Media: *Intensive Care Medicine*.)

TABLE 2.—Transesophageal Echocardiography (TEE) Parameters Measured Within 12 h of Septic Shock After Fluid Loading And Initiation Of Vasopressor Therapy (Day 0) and After The Interruption Of Vasoactive Drugs (Day n)

TEE parameters	Day 0 ($n=35$) ICU death ($n=9$)	ICU discharge ($n=26$)	Day n ($n=26$)
SVC collapsibility index (%)	13 (6–16)	14 (9–22)	14 (9–19)
Respiratory variations of aortic Doppler velocity (%)	3 (2–4)	4 (2–6)	4 (3–6)
LVEF, modified Simpson's rule (%)	51 (18–57)	50 (34–62)	58 (54–64)
LVEF, four-chamber area-length (%)	52 (20–59)	51 (33–63)	58 (54–65)
LV stroke volume (ml)	41 (34–55)	53 (47–69)	64 (56–74)*
LV end-diastolic volume, modified Simpson's rule (ml)	104 (80–113)	95 (76–110)	76 (65–94)*
LV end-diastolic volume, four-chamber area-length (ml)	102 (83–117)	99 (79–114)	80 (66–96)*
Ea lateral mitral ring (cm/s)	12.0 (11.1–13.4)	11.4 (9.1–16.0)	11.1 (10.2–12.5)

Data are expressed as medians and numbers in parentheses are 95% confidence intervals
TEE, transesophageal echocardiography; SVC, superior vena cava; LV, left ventricle; EF, ejection fraction; Vp, early diastolic blood flow propagation velocity; Ea, early diastolic tissue Doppler imaging velocity of the lateral mitral ring
*$p < 0.05$ compared with survivors on Day 0
(Reprinted with permission from Etchecopar-Chevreuil C, François B, Clavel M, et al. Cardiac morphological and functional changes during early septic shock: a transesophageal echocardiographic study. *Intensive Care Med*. 2008;34:250-256, with kind permission from Springer Science+Business Media: *Intensive Care Medicine*.)

had normal LVEF on Day n and 4 patients fully recovered by Day 28. Only 4 women had LV dilatation (range, LV end-diastolic volume: 110–148 ml) on Day 0, but none on Day n. Doppler tissue imaging identified an LV diastolic dysfunction in 7 patients (20%) on Day 0 (3 with normal LVEF), which resolved on Day n.

Conclusions.—This study confirms that LV systolic and diastolic dysfunctions are frequent, but LV dilatation is uncommon in fluid-loaded septic patients on vasopressors. All abnormalities regressed in survivors, regardless of their severity.

Descriptors.—Shock: clinical studies (38), Cardiovascular monitoring (34) (Tables 1 and 2).

▶ This study (a) further validates decreased contractility in patients with septic shock, (b) points to the potential importance of diastolic dysfunction, and (c) questions the frequency of left ventricular (LV) dilatation. LV dilatation has been proposed in the past as a mechanism by which the heart compensates for septic shock, that is, taking advantage of the Starling principle by producing increased contractile force for any given contractile state by stretching of the myocardial fiber at end diastole. Drugs that target diastolic dysfunction without interfering with systolic function (such as levosimendan) might be of value in septic shock.

R. P. Dellinger, MD

Actual incidence of global left ventricular hypokinesia in adult septic shock

Vieillard-Baron A, Caille V, Charron C, et al (Univ Hosp Ambroise Paré, Boulogne Cedex, France)
Crit Care Med 36:1701-1706, 2008

Rationale and Objective.—To evaluate the actual incidence of global left ventricular hypokinesia in septic shock.

Method.—All mechanically ventilated patients treated for an episode of septic shock in our unit were studied by transesophageal echocardiography, at least once a day, during the first 3 days of hemodynamic support. In patients who recovered, echocardiography was repeated after weaning from vasoactive agents. Main measurements were obtained from the software of the apparatus. Global left ventricular hypokinesia was defined as a left ventricular ejection fraction of <45%.

Measurements and Main Results.—During a 3-yr period (January 2004 through December 2006), 67 patients free from previous cardiac disease, and who survived for >48 hrs, were repeatedly studied. Global left ventricular hypokinesia was observed in 26 of these 67 patients at admission (primary hypokinesia) and in 14 after 24 or 48 hrs of hemodynamic support by norepinephrine (secondary hypokinesia), leading to an overall hypokinesia rate of 60%. Left ventricular hypokinesia was partially corrected by dobutamine, added to a reduced dosage of norepinephrine, or by epinephrine. This reversible acute left ventricular dysfunction was not associated with a worse prognosis.

Conclusion.—Global left ventricular hypokinesia is very frequent in adult septic shock and could be unmasked, in some patients, by norepinephrine treatment. Left ventricular hypokinesia is usually corrected by addition of an inotropic agent to the hemodynamic support.

▶ This study allows characterization of the frequency of septic shock patients with systolic dysfunction at the time of presentation as well as those who develop it over the first 3 days of hemodynamic support. Because of the variable courses of patients with septic shock, over time (improvement vs no change vs worsening) it is important to recognize the potential for inotropic therapy to initially be of value or become of value in hypoperfused septic patients. This finding also supports the use of a combined inotrope/vasopressin in most patients with septic shock.

R. P. Dellinger, MD

Are Blood Transfusions Associated with Greater Mortality Rates? Results of the Sepsis Occurrence in Acutely Ill Patients Study
Vincent J-L, Sakr Y, Sprung C, et al (Free Univ of Brussels, Belgium; Friedrich-Schiller-Univ, Jena, Germany; Hadassah Hebrew Univ Med Ctr, Jerusalem, Israel; et al)
Anesthesiology 108:31-39, 2008

Background.—Studies have suggested worse outcomes in transfused patients and improved outcomes in patients managed with restricted blood transfusion strategies. The authors investigated the relation of blood transfusion to mortality in European intensive care units (ICUs).

Methods.—The Sepsis Occurrence in Acutely Ill Patients study was a multicenter, observational study that included all adult patients admitted to 198 European ICUs between May 1 and May 15, 2002 and followed them until death, until hospital discharge, or for 60 days. Patients were classified depending on whether they had received a blood transfusion at any time during their ICU stay.

Results.—Of 3,147 patients, 1,040 (33.0%) received a blood transfusion. These patients were older (mean age, 62 *vs.* 60 yr; $P = 0.035$) and were more likely to have liver cirrhosis or hematologic cancer, to be a surgical admission, and to have sepsis. They had a longer duration of ICU stay (5.9 *vs.* 2.5 days; $P < 0.001$) and a higher ICU mortality rate (23.0 *vs.* 16.3%; $P < 0.001$) but were also more severely ill on admission (Simplified Acute Physiology Score II, 40.2 *vs.* 34.7; $P < 0.001$; Sequential Organ Failure Assessment score, 6.5 *vs.* 4.5; $P < 0.001$). There was a direct relation between the number of blood transfusions and the mortality rate, but in multivariate analysis, blood transfusion was not significantly associated with a worse mortality rate. Moreover, in 821 pairs matched according to a propensity score, there was a higher 30-day survival rate in the transfusion group than in the other patients ($P = 0.004$).

Conclusion.—This observational study does not support the view that blood transfusions are associated with increased mortality rates in acutely ill patients.

▶ Over the last decade or so, an increasing body of literature has been developed supporting the position that limitation of red blood cell transfusion is safe and, perhaps, even beneficial in a diverse array of critically ill patients. This is the first large scale study to offer contradictory findings in this area, and appears to breathe new life into the question of whether a more liberal transfusion strategy may be beneficial in critically ill patients. Despite the fact that the patients in the transfusion group were sicker as measured by a variety of parameters, as documented in Table 2 in the original article, and had worse outcomes (ICU and hospital mortality, ICU and hospital length of stay) overall, when subjected to a detailed analysis by propensity score, the authors determined that transfusion actually conferred a decreased 30-day risk of death. Although these results are intriguing, they must be interpreted with caution. Surprisingly, although presumably lower in the transfusion group, neither hemoglobin nor hematocrit values were noted in this report. In addition, as pointed out in the accompanying editorial by Nuttall and Houle[1], the use of propensity scores has become popular in recent years as a means of reducing the impact of treatment selection bias in observational studies. However, the use of such methodologies has its own limitations as these authors point out, including an inability to balance unmeasured characteristics in the populations being studied, among other problems, ultimately resulting in what they describe as a "black box" feeling about this process. Nevertheless, this data suggest that it is reasonable to re-evaluate the results of the Transfusion Requirements in Critical Care (TRICC) trial with a new prospective randomized trial, particularly in light of the widespread use of leukodepletion in the preparation of red cells before transfusion in contemporary practice.

D. R. Gerber, DO

Reference

1. Nuttall GA, Houle TT. Liars, damn liars, and propensity scores. *Anesthesiology.* 2008;108:3-4.

8 Metabolism/ Gastrointestinal/ Nutrition/ Hematology-Oncology

A prospective study on adrenal cortex responses and outcome prediction in acute critical illness: results from a large cohort of 203 mixed ICU patients
Dimopoulou I, Stamoulis K, Ilias I, et al (Univ of Athens, Greece; Elena Venizelou Hosp, Athens, Greece; et al)
Intensive Care Med 33:2116-2121, 2007

Objective.—To assess whether adrenal cortex hormones predict ICU mortality in acute, mixed, critically ill patients.

Design and Setting.—Prospective study in consecutive intensive care patients in the general ICU of a teaching hospital.

Patients.—203 severely ill patients with multiple trauma ($n = 93$), medical ($n = 57$), or surgical ($n = 53$) critical states.

Measurements and Results.—Within 24 h of admission in the ICU a morning blood sample was obtained to measure baseline cortisol, corticotropin (ACTH), and dehydropiandrosterone sulfate (DHEAS). Subsequently a low-dose (1 µg) ACTH test was performed to determine stimulated cortisol. The incremental rise in cortisol was defined as stimulated minus baseline cortisol. Overall, 149 patients survived and 54 died. Nonsurvivors were older and in a more severe critical state, as reflected by higher SOFA and APACHE II scores. Nonsurvivors had a lower incremental rise in cortisol (5.0 vs. 8.3 µg/dl and lower DHEAS (1065 vs. 1642 ng/ml) than survivors. The two groups had similar baseline and stimulated cortisol. Multivariate logistic regression analysis revealed that age (odds ratio 1.02), SOFA score (1.36), and the incremental rise in cortisol (0.88) were independent predictors for poor outcome.

Conclusions.—In general ICU patients a blunted cortisol response to ACTH within 24 h of admission is an independent predictor for poor

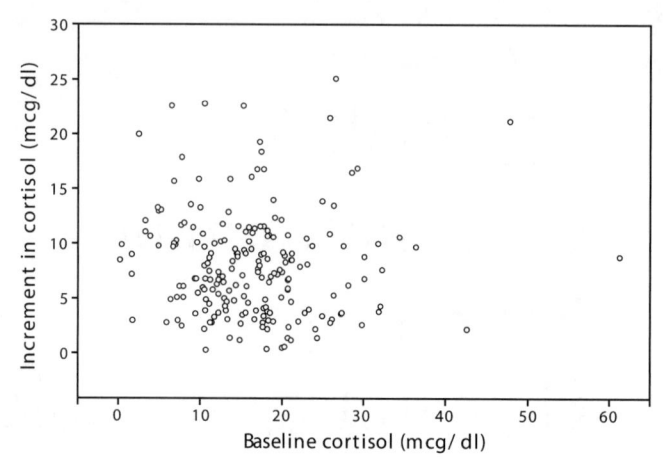

FIGURE 2.—Distribution of baseline cortisol in relation to the increment in cortisol. (Reprinted from Dimopoulou I, Stamoulis K, Ilias I, et al. A prospective study on adrenal cortex responses and outcome prediction in acute critical illness: results from a large cohort of 203 mixed ICU patients. *Intensive Care Med*. 2007;33:2116-2121, with kind permission from Springer Science+Business Media: *Intensive Care Medicine*.)

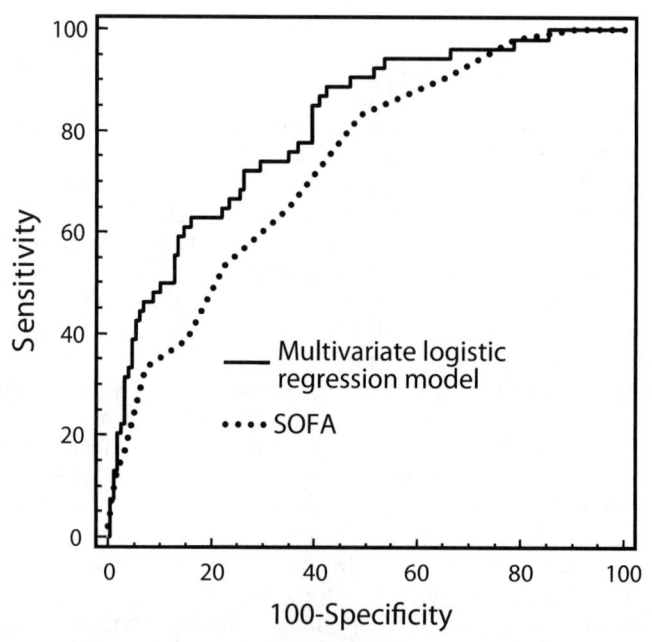

FIGURE 3.—ROC plot for the final multivariate logistic regression model vs. SOFA score alone. (Reprinted from Dimopoulou I, Stamoulis K, Ilias I, et al. A prospective study on adrenal cortex responses and outcome prediction in acute critical illness: results from a large cohort of 203 mixed ICU patients. *Intensive Care Med*. 2007;33:2116-2121, with kind permission from Springer Science+Business Media: *Intensive Care Medicine*.)

outcome. In contrast, baseline cortisol or adrenal androgens are not of prognostic significance (Figs 2 and 3).

▶ This study was conducted on a specific subset of ICU admissions, those requiring ventilatory support. It is important to interpret the results of this study in that light. The study measures total cortisol and not free cortisol concentrations and so does little to resolve any of that ongoing controversy. Furthermore, the conclusions require a different type of data analysis that was performed. Because pre stimulation values can have an impact on the post stimulation values, longitudinal data analysis or its equivalent is warranted. My final concern centers around the fact that ICU admission is not the same point in the time course of illness for all patients who present to the unit and, thus, although admission is an easy time point, it may obfuscate some findings. This article adds some to the understanding of adrenal status and critical illness across a broader population than previously evaluated. Furthermore, as can be seen in Fig 2, some correlation between basal levels and subsequent incremental change in cortisol concentrations exists, although no r value was provided. Fig 3 shows an appropriate receiver operating characteristic (ROC) of 0.807 for the model.

T. Dorman, MD

Accuracy of bedside capillary blood glucose measurements in critically ill patients

Critchell CD, Savarese V, Callahan A, et al (Thomas Jefferson Univ, Philadelphia, PA)
Intensive Care Med 33:2079-2084, 2007

Objective.—To compare the accuracy of fingerstick with laboratory venous plasma glucose measurements (laboratory glucose) in medical ICU patients and to determine the factors which interfere with the accuracy of fingerstick measurements.

Participants.—The study included 80 consecutive patients aged 58 ± 7 years, BMI 29.5 ± 9.0, and APACHE II score 15 ± 6 (277 simultaneous paired measurements).

Measurements.—This prospective observational study compared fingerstick measurements to simultaneously sampled laboratory glucose once a day in patients in our medical ICU (twice daily if on an insulin infusion). Data recorded included patient demographics, admission diagnoses, APACHE II score, BMI, daily hematocrit, arterial blood gasses, chemistry results, concomitant medications (including vasopressors and corticosteroids), and upper extremity edema. Accuracy was defined as the percentage of paired values not in accord (> 15 mg dl^{-1} / 0.83 mmol^{-1} l^{-1} difference for laboratory values < 75 mg dl^{-1} / 4.12 mmol^{-1} l^{-1} and > 20% difference for laboratory values ≥ 75 mg/dl). Outliers (blood glucose difference > 100 mg dl^{-1} / 5.56 mmol^{-1} l^{-1}) were excluded from the correlation and distribution analyses.

Results.—Mean fingerstick glucose was 129 ± 45 mg/dl (7.2 ± 2.5 mmol/l) and mean laboratory glucose 123 ± 44 mg/dl (6.8 ± 2.4 mmol/l). The correlation coefficient between the two values was 0.9110 (Clinical and Laboratory Standards Institute threshold 0.9751). The mean difference (bias) between the two methods was 8.6 ± 18.6 mg/dl (0.48 ± 1.0 mmol/l) and limits of agreement +45.8 and −28.6 mg/dl (+2.5 and −1.6 mmol/l). Fifty-three (19%) paired measurements in 22 patients were not in accord (CLSI threshold ≤ 5%). In 44 (83%) of these paired measurements fingerstick glucose was greater than laboratory glucose.

Conclusions.—The findings suggest that capillary blood glucose as measured by fingerstick is inaccurate in critically ill ICU patients and does not meet the CLSI standard. It is unclear whether the sampling method, device used, or both contributed to this inaccuracy. The wide limits of agreement suggest that fingerstick measurements should be used with great caution in protocols of tight glycemic control (Fig 2).

▶ Intensive insulin therapy for critically ill patients has been considered the standard of practice since the publication of Van den Berghe et al.[1] Critchell et al question the accuracy of bedside blood glucose measurements in critically ill patients and they offer multiple hypotheses as to why blood glucometers may not be accurate in intensive care units. This is not the first work to question the accuracy of bedside blood glucometers in intensive care units, but instead it adds to the growing body of literature citing their inaccuracy. The known

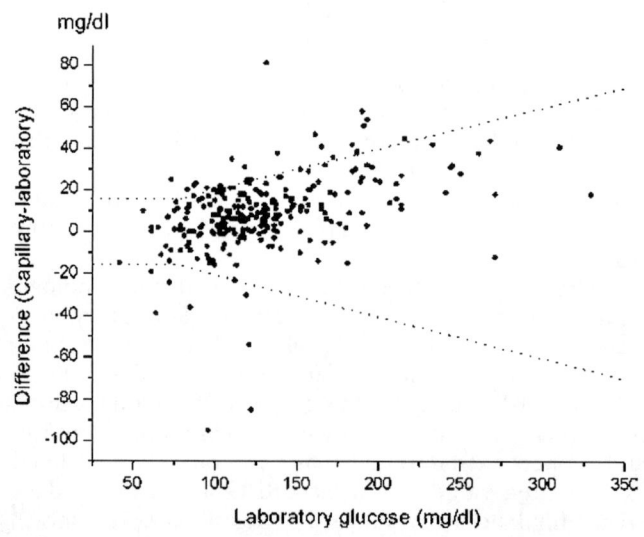

FIGURE 2.—Plot of laboratory glucose and difference (fingerstick minus laboratory glucose) with accuracy thresholds as defined by the CLSI. (Reprinted from Critchell CD, Savarese V, Callahan A, et al. Accuracy of bedside capillary blood glucose measurements in critically ill patients. *Intensive Care Med.* 2007;33:2079-2084, with kind permission from Springer Science+Business Media: *Intensive Care Medicine.*)

increase in mortality in patients with hypoglycemia and the inability of a sedated, ventilated patient to demonstrate the signs of hypoglycemia make this topic salient to critical care practitioners. The importance of this study is that it is prospective and it demonstrates what smaller retrospective studies have implied.[2] They also cite that approximately 50% of their patients had either upper extremity edema or vasopressor requirements which could be a cause of inaccurate bedside blood glucose readings due to the quality of blood obtained. The study did have significant limitations as only 1 type of glucometer was tested, no patient had a blood glucose less than 40 mg/dL, and there was a wide variation in the standard deviation of the patient's glucose readings. This study questions the accuracy of blood glucose in critically ill patients on vasopressors and with upper extremity edema; therefore, in these patients it may be judicious to check blood sugars through central venous or arterial lines. In the short term, it also may require practitioners to increase the lower limits of their intensive insulin therapy scale to avoid potential hypoglycemic episodes. It makes an individual practitioner question whether patients with decreased cognitive skills after an intensive care unit stay may have been adversely affected by too tight of glycemic control (due to inaccurate laboratory data).

N. Puri, MD
C. Bekes, MD

References

1. Van den Berghe G, Wilmer A, Hermans G, et al. Intensive insulin therapy in the medical ICU. *N Engl J Med.* 2006;354:449-461.
2. Finkielman JD, Oyen L, Afessa B. Agreement between beside blood and plasma glucose measurements in the ICU Setting. *Chest.* 2005;127:1749-1751.

Accuracy of Bedside Glucometry in Critically Ill Patients: Influence of Clinical Characteristics and Perfusion Index
Desachy A, Vuagnat AC, Ghazali AD, et al (Centre Hospitalier Général, Angoulême, France)
Mayo Clin Proc 83:400-405, 2008

Objectives.—To determine the accuracy of bedside glucose strip assay on capillary blood and on whole blood and to identify factors predictive of discrepancies with the laboratory method.

Patients and Methods.—We conducted a prospective 3-month (July 1–September 30, 2003) study in 85 consecutive patients who required blood glucose monitoring. Values obtained with a glucose test strip on capillary blood and on whole blood were compared with those obtained in the laboratory during serial blood sampling (up to 4 samples per patient). The test strip values were considered to disagree significantly with the laboratory values when the difference exceeded 20%. Clinical and biological parameters and the perfusion index, based on percutaneous oxygen saturation monitoring, were recorded when each sample was obtained.

Results.—Capillary glucose values conflicted with laboratory reference values in 15% of samples. A low perfusion index was predictive of conflicting values ($P=.04$). Seven percent of values obtained with glucose strip on whole-blood samples conflicted with laboratory reference values; factors associated with these discrepancies were mean arterial hypotension ($P=.007$) and generalized mottling ($P=.04$).

Conclusion.—Bedside blood glucose values must be interpreted with care in critically ill patients. A low perfusion index, reflecting peripheral hypoperfusion, is associated with poor glucose strip performance. Bedside measurements in whole blood seem to be most reliable, except in patients with arterial hypotension and generalized mottling (Figs 1 and 2).

▶ Achieving glucose control goals and the avoidance of hypoglycemic complications are predicated on the ability to accurately measure the blood glucose. Bedside testing with reagent strips, usually on capillary blood, is one of the most common laboratory measurements performed in the ICU, and results frequently influence therapy. This article demonstrates that in critically ill patients, bedside measurements on both capillary and whole blood may vary from laboratory methods by a potentially clinically significant amount (see Fig 1). Bedside whole-blood measurements correlated with laboratory measurements better than capillary blood (see Fig 2). Indicators of shock were significantly associated with variance from the laboratory standard. Interestingly, for measurements that varied from the standard, the direction of variance was not predictable.

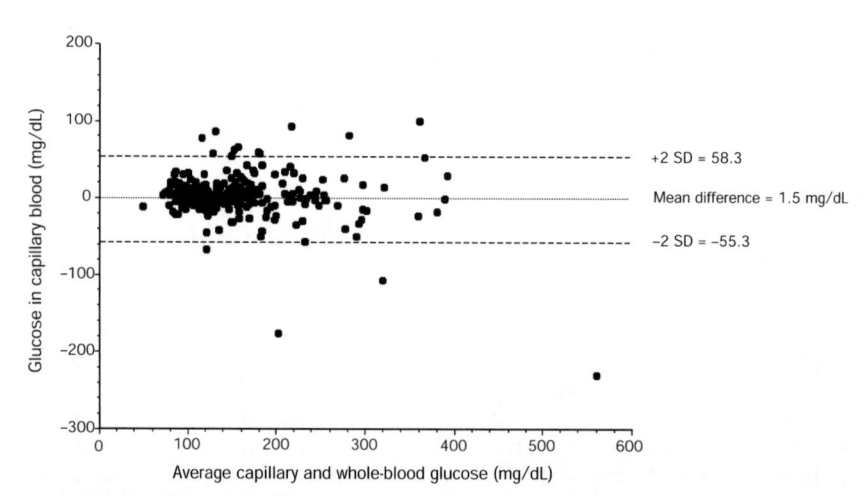

FIGURE 1.—Bland-Altman plot for agreement between capillary glucose values (test strip method) and laboratory blood glucose levels. SI conversion factor: To convert glucose value to mmol/L, multiply by 0.0555. (Reprinted from Desachy A, Vuagnat AC, Ghazali AD, et al. Accuracy of bedside glucometry in critically ill patients: influence of clinical characteristics and perfusion index. *Mayo Clin Proc.* 2008;83:400-405, with permission from Dowden Health Media.)

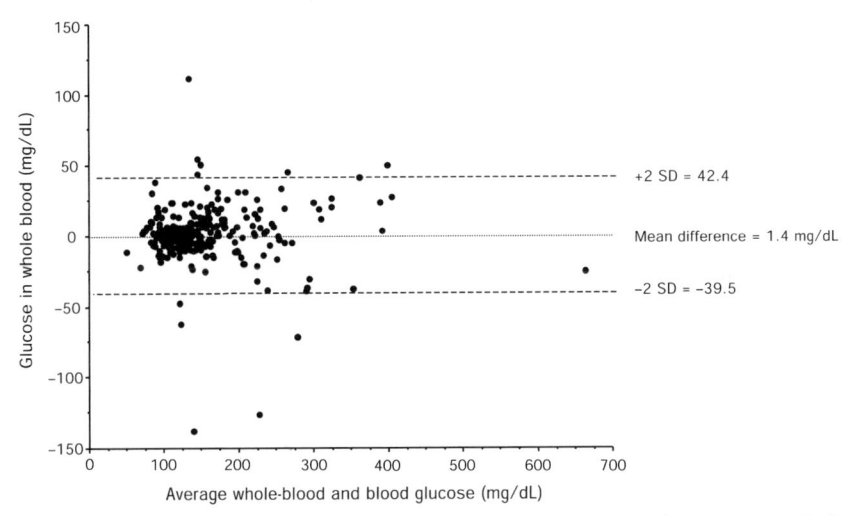

FIGURE 2.—Bland-Altman plot for agreement between whole-blood glucose values (test strip method) and laboratory blood glucose levels. SI conversion factor: To convert glucose value to mmol/L, multiply by 0.0555. (Reprinted from Desachy A, Vuagnat AC, Ghazali AD, et al. Accuracy of bedside glucometry in critically ill patients: influence of clinical characteristics and perfusion index. *Mayo Clin Proc.* 2008;83:400-405, with permission from Dowden Health Media.)

Unless all glucose measurements are to be made by the laboratory method, which is impractical, clinicians should interpret bedside determinations with caution. Bedside glucose measurements should be made on whole blood when practical. Clinicians should be aware that poor peripheral perfusion may decrease the reliability of bedside testing and that, when erroneous readings occur, they may be either higher or lower than laboratory values.

T. Lonergan, MD
C. Bekes, MD

Early versus late intravenous insulin administration in critically ill patients
Honiden S, Schultz A, Im SA (Yale Univ School of Medicine, New Haven, CT; Mount Sinai School of Medicine, NY; et al)
Intensive Care Med 34:881-887, 2008

Objective.—To investigate whether timing of intensive insulin therapy (IIT) after intensive care unit (ICU) admission influences outcome.

Design and Setting.—Single-center prospective cohort study in the 14-bed medical ICU of a 1,171-bed tertiary teaching hospital.

Patients.—The study included 127 patients started on ITT within 48 h of ICU admission (early group) and 51 started on ITT thereafter (late group); the groups did not differ in age, gender, race, BMI, APACHE III, ICU steroid use, admission diagnosis, or underlying comorbidities.

Mortality by Insulin Timing

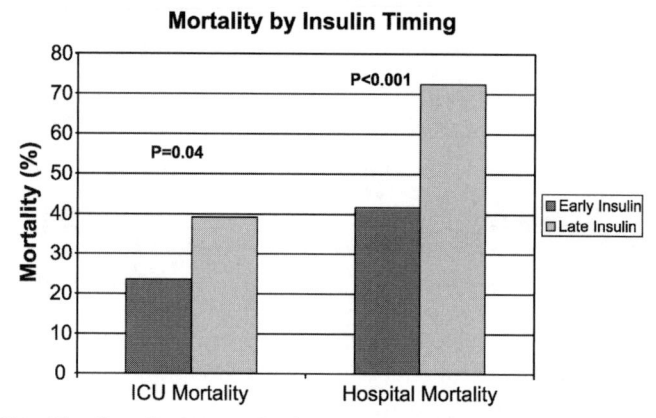

FIGURE 1.—The effect of intensive insulin therapy on ICU and hospital mortality according to timing of insulin. (Reprinted from Honiden S, Schultz A, Im SA, et al. Early versus late intravenous insulin administration in critically ill patients. *Intensive Care Med.* 2008;34:881-887, with kind permissiom from Springer Science+Business Media, Copyright 2008.)

Measurements and Results.—The early group had more ventilator-free days in the first 28 days after ICU admission (median 12 days, IQR 0-24, vs. 1 day, 0-11), shorter ICU stay (6 days, IQR 3-11, vs. 11 days, vs. 7-17), shorter hospital stay (15 days, IQR 9-30, vs. 25 days, 13-43), lower ICU mortality (OR 0.48), and lower hospital mortality (OR 0.27). On multivariate analysis, early therapy was still associated with decreased hospital mortality (OR_{adj} 0.29). The strength and direction of association favoring early IIT was consistent after propensity score modeling regardless of method used for analysis.

Conclusions.—Early IIT was associated with better outcomes. Our results raise questions about the assumption that delayed administration of IIT has the same benefit as early therapy. A randomized study is needed to determine the optimal timing of therapy (Fig 1).

▶ Glucose control has become a standard practice in the ICU, but concerns for hypoglycemia have also informed the discussion about intensive insulin therapy (IIT) protocols. In this small, prospective cohort study of 178 patients, the authors address the impact of the timing of initiation of IIT. Their data support the conclusion that earlier IIT (within the first 48 hours) is associated with better outcomes as measured by a number of markers, including 28-day mortality (Fig 1). Patients in the earlier IIT group tended to have greater degrees of hyperglycemia. Interestingly, they also report that there was no difference in hospital mortality between all patients treated with IIT and 30 patients who were hyperglycemic, but did not have IIT initiated (43% versus 49%, $P = .9$). Also, the number and severity of hypoglycemic events in either group were not reported. Thus, although this study lends support to the idea of earlier IIT, further larger studies are needed to better define the optimal timing of IIT.

T. Lonergan, MD
C. Bekes, MD

Hyperglycemia as a Predictor of In-Hospital Mortality in Elderly Patients without Diabetes Mellitus Admitted to a Sub-Intensive Care Unit

Sleiman I, Morandi A, Sabatini T, et al (Poliambulanza Hosp, Brescia, Italy; et al)
J Am Geriatr Soc 56:1106-1110, 2008

Objectives.—To investigate the association between hyperglycemia and in-hospital and 45-day mortality in acutely ill elderly patients.

Design.—Retrospective cohort.

Setting.—Hospital medical patients admitted to a sub-intensive care unit (sub-ICU) for elderly patients, which is a level of care between ordinary wards and intensive care.

Participants.—One thousand two hundred twenty-nine patients (mean age 79.6 ± 8.4) admitted to the sub-ICU from January 2003 to January 2006. Forty patients with acute myocardial infarction and 34 patients with extreme fasting glucose values (<60 or >500 mg/dL) were excluded. Eight hundred twenty-two patients without a history of diabetes mellitus (DM) and 333 patients with a diagnosis of DM were selected and subdivided into three categories according to serum fasting blood glucose: 60 to 126 mg/dL (Group A), 127 to 180 mg/dL (Group B), and 181 to 500 mg/dL (Group C).

Measurements.—Age, sex, mental and functional status, Acute Physiology Score, comorbid conditions, serum albumin, serum cholesterol, fasting serum glucose, and length of stay. In-hospital mortality was the primary outcome, and 45-day mortality was the secondary outcome.

Results.—Total in-hospital mortality was 14.5%. In patients with and without DM, mortality was 8.8% and 11.3%, respectively, in Group A; 13.6% and 17.3% in Group B, and 12.6% and 34.3% in Group C. After controlling for confounders, newly recognized hyperglycemia (>181 mg/dL) was independently associated with in-hospital mortality (adjusted odds ratio = 2.7, 95% confidence interval = 1.6–4.8). Forty-five-day mortality in newly recognized hyperglycemic patients was 17.5%, 25.7%, and 42% in Groups A, B, and C, respectively, whereas it was 21.2% in patients with DM.

Conclusion.—In elderly patients, newly recognized hyperglycemia was associated with a higher mortality rate than in those with a prior history of DM. These data suggest that further randomized clinical trials are needed to assess the efficacy and the risk of a target glucose of greater than 180 mg/dL.

▶ Acutely ill patients are often noted to have elevated blood glucose levels. The concept of stress-related hyperglycemia has been known for over 3 centuries. Thomas Willis in 1689 noted that stress preceded the development of elevated blood glucose in many patients.[1] Similar observations were made by French physiologist Claude Bernard and the father of modern medicine, Sir William Osler.[2,3]

This "diabetes of injury" or stress-related hyperglycemia was accepted as the adaptive metabolic response to severe stress. It was also presumed to be beneficial and important for survival, or at least benign. Osler distinguished "true diabetes," which he associated with a poorer prognosis from the transient glycosuria seen in persons who have undergone a severe stressful event and had a better prognosis. Inconsistencies in this view began to emerge in the later half of the 20th century and subsequent work shed light on the negative consequences of high glucose levels including abnormal immune function, increased infection rate, and hemodynamic and electromyocardial impairment.

Although the landmark study of intensive insulin therapy conducted by Van den Berghe and colleagues[4] ushered in an era of intensive glucose control in critically ill patients, subsequent studies instituting tight glycemic control in critically ill patients showed high rates of hypoglycemia and failed to show the same benefits.[5]

The results of the study by Drs Sleiman et al are consistent with what is known regarding the effects of hyperglycemia in acutely ill subjects. It is a welcome addition to the body of knowledge on the subject and provides further rationale for work to clarify who should receive intensive glucose control and how tight it should be.

O. Okorie, MD
C. Bekes, MD

References

1. Willis T. *Pharmaceutice Rationalis: Or the Exercitation of the Operation of Medicines in Humane Bodies. The Works of Thomas Willis.* London, UK: Dring, Harper & Leigh; 1679.
2. Bernard C. *Lecons de physiologie experimentale applique a la medicine.* Vol 1. Paris, France: Balliere; 1885:296-313.
3. Osler W. *The Principles and Practice of Medicine.* New York, NY: Appleton; 1892.
4. Van den Berghe G, Wouters P, Weekers F, et al. Intensive insulin therapy in the critically ill patients. *N Engl J Med.* 2001;345:1359-1367.
5. Brunkhorst FM, Kuhnt E, Engel C. Intensive insulin therapy in patient with severe sepsis and septic shock is associated with an increased rate of hypoglycemia: results from a randomized multicenter study (VISEP). *Infection.* 2005;33:19.

Risk Factors Associated With Adrenal Insufficiency in Severely Injured Burn Patients
Reiff DA, Harkins CL, McGwin G Jr, (Univ of Alabama at Birmingham, Alabama)
J Burn Care Res 28:854-858, 2007

Acute adrenal insufficiency (AI) is an uncommon disorder among critically ill burn patients, which can often go unrecognized. The goal of the current study is to identify risk factors for AI among patients who have sustained severe thermal injury. A case–control study was conducted among all adult patients admitted to the intensive care unit of the University of Alabama at Birmingham Burn Center during a 7-year period

(1997–2003). All burn patients who developed AI were selected as cases (n = 26), and a random sample of those ICU patients who did not develop AI were selected as controls (n = 56). Two variables demonstrated significant independent associations with the risk of AI. Patients who developed AI were older than controls (50 vs. 46 years, respectively) and suffered a significantly greater area of thermal injury when compared with controls (mean percentage of total body surface area burned for cases and controls 45.5% and 25.4%, respectively). Over half (59.1%) of the patients with AI died compared with only 14.6% of controls ($P < 0.0001$). The development of AI appears to be associated with a greater TBSA burn and older age. After severe thermal injury, the diagnosis of AI substantially increases the risk of death. A better understanding of factors that predispose burn patients to AI may aid in earlier diagnosis, initiation of therapy, and improved outcomes.

▶ Acute adrenal insufficiency has not been carefully evaluated in critically ill burn patients.[1] One study reviewed in this article cites an incidence of approximately 0.12%. This rate is not radically different than that seen in other critically ill surgical patients, however, in subpopulations, which have been more closely studied, the frequency of this problem is reported to be higher. It is important to note that this is a case-control study. Thus, this data cannot be examined to better understand the incidence of adrenal insufficiency in the setting of burn injury. Two simple clinical observations are made. Patients with large injury and advanced age are at increased risk for adrenal insufficiency. It is also important to note that these authors did not confirm the diagnosis of adrenal insufficiency without a low random cortisol level and a diagnostic cosyntropin stimulation test. Thus, some investigators would suggest failure to treat a number of affected patients.[2] Regardless of limitations in this data, acute adrenal insufficiency appears to be associated with poor outcome in burn injury as has been suggested in other populations.

D. J. Dries, MSE, MD

References

1. Sheridan RL, Ryan CM, Tompkins RG. Acute adrenal insufficiency in the burn intensive care unit. *Burns.* 1993;19:63-66.
2. Rivers EP, Gaspari M, Saad GA, et al. Adrenal insufficiency in high-risk surgical ICU patients. *Chest.* 2001;119:889-896.

Esophageal Perforations: New Perspectives and Treatment Paradigms
Wu JT, Mattox KL, Wall MJ Jr (Baylor College of Medicine, Houston, TX)
J Trauma 63:1173-1184, 2007

Despite significant advances in modern surgery and intensive care medicine, esophageal perforation continues to present a diagnostic and therapeutic challenge. Controversies over the diagnosis and management of esophageal perforation remain, and debate still exists over the optimal therapeutic approach. Surgical therapy has been the traditional and preferred treatment; however, less invasive approaches to esophageal perforation continue to evolve. As the incidence of esophageal perforation increases with the advancement of invasive endoscopic procedures, early recognition of clinical features and implementation of effective treatment are essential for a favorable clinical outcome with minimal morbidity and mortality. This review will attempt to summarize the pathogenesis and diagnostic evaluation of esophageal injuries, and highlight the evolving therapeutic options for the management of esophageal perforation (Fig 1).

▶ Injury to the esophagus because of external trauma is relatively uncommon. Studies from major trauma centers report an incidence of injury to the cervical esophagus, which is more likely to be exposed to injury of approximately 5%. Injury in the thoracic esophagus is much less common to external trauma with reported incidence under 1%. Most of the penetrating esophageal injuries come from gunshot or shotgun wounds (approximately 80% of patients). Stab wounds are related to esophageal injury in approximately 20% of patients. Esophageal perforation from blunt trauma is rare and if seen, is related to high-speed motor

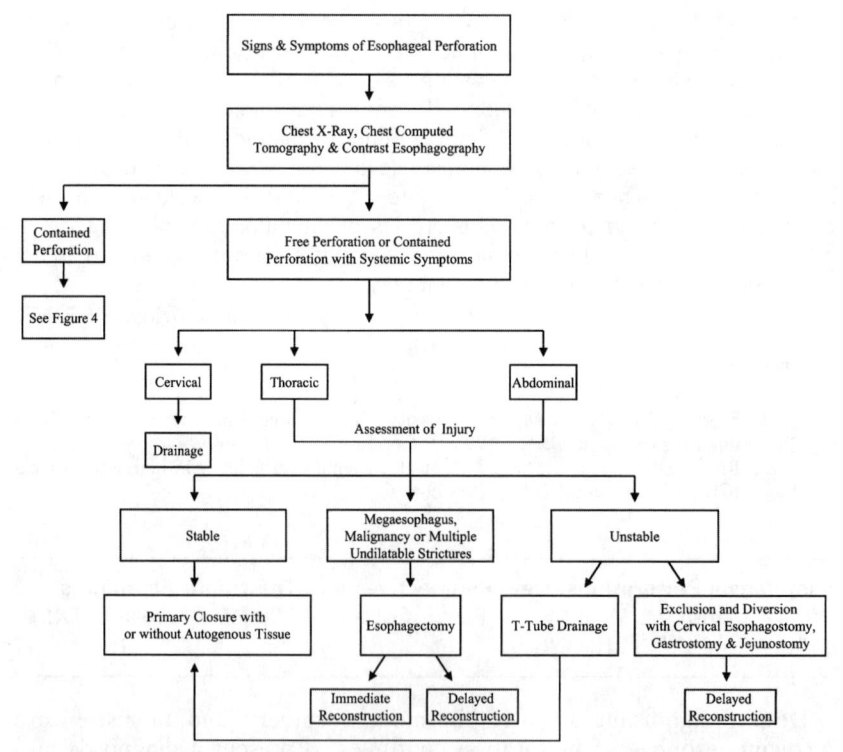

FIGURE 1.—Algorithm for surgical therapy of esophageal perforation. (Reprinted from Wu JT, Mattox KL, Wall MJ Jr. Esophageal perforations: new perspectives and treatment paradigms. *J Trauma*. 2007;63:1173-1184, with permission from Lippincott Williams & Wilkins.)

vehicle crashes. Blunt esophageal trauma occurs in the cervical and upper thoracic region in over 80% of victims. Most esophageal injuries overall, approximately 60%, are iatrogenic. Diagnosis of esophageal injury begins with plain radiographs, which reveal free air on cervical soft tissue films, or AP on lateral chest films. Plain chest films are suggestive of esophageal injury in 90% of patients with perforation. However, early chest radiographs may be normal. Contrast esophagography is the study of choice with an overall false negative rate of 10%. The initial material of choice is gastrograffin but because of higher density and better mucosal adherence, barium allows detection of smaller esophageal perforations. Chest computed tomography (CT) will show signs of mediastinal or extraluminal air, esophageal thickening, inflammation of surrounding structures, abscess cavities near the esophagus, and communication of an air-filled esophagus with an adjacent mediastinal air fluid collection. Esophagoscopy is not recommended as a primary diagnostic study but may provide visualization of perforation. A wide variety of approaches are not acceptable in the management of esophageal perforation. Patients with contained perforation and minimal systemic signs may be managed without surgical intervention as long as antibiotics and parenteral nutrition are provided. A contrast esophagram obtained after 7 to 10 days of therapy allows assessment of healing.[1] Exclusion and diversion techniques have been used in patients with extensive mediastinal contamination, devitalized esophagus, or hemodynamic instability unable to tolerate a definitive repair or esophageal resection. The contemporary approach to the contaminated mediastinum in severe esophageal injury includes preservation of esophageal continuity by placement of a staple line or removable ligature distally in conjunction with cervical esophagostomy. Another option for patients with major injuries, which cannot be repaired at the time of surgery or hemodynamic instability, is use of a large esophageal T-tube to create a controlled esophagocutaneous fistula. Placement of a T-tube allows drainage of the esophagus and time for surrounding tissues to heal. After patient stabilization, repair options for the esophagus managed with T-tube drainage can be considered.[2] Primary surgical repair with or without buttressing from adjacent tissues is the optimal modality in the surgical armamentarium with an average mortality of 12%. Esophagectomy has a mortality of 17%. Mortality rises to 24% with exclusion and diversion procedures and drainage of the esophagus alone is associated with a mortality of 37%. Success with primary is greatest if intervention occurs within hours of perforation. The likelihood of a failed repair increases as intervention is delayed.[3] It is essential that the surgeon be engaged in management of complex esophageal problems.

D. J. Dries, MSE, MD

References

1. Altorjay A, Kiss J, Vőrős A, Bohák A. Nonoperative management of esophageal perforations. Is it justified? *Ann Surg.* 1997;225:415-421.
2. Bufkin BL, Miller JI Jr, Mansour KA. Esophageal perforation: Emphasis on management. *Ann Thorac Surg.* 1996;61:1447-1452.
3. Wang N, Razzouk AJ, Safavi A, et al. Delayed primary repair of intrathoracic esophageal perforation: Is it safe? *J Thorac Cardiovasc Surg.* 1996;111:114-122.

9 Renal

Amino Acid Requirements in Critically Ill Patients with Acute Kidney Injury Treated with Continuous Renal Replacement Therapy
Btaiche IF, Mohammad RA, Alaniz C, et al (Univ of Michigan Hosps and Health Ctrs, Ann Arbor, MI; Long Island Univ, NY)
Pharmacotherapy 28:600-613, 2008

Acute kidney injury in critically ill patients is often a complication of an underlying condition such as organ failure, sepsis, or drug therapy. In these patients, stress-induced hypercatabolism results in loss of body cell mass. Unless nutrition support is provided, malnutrition and negative nitrogen balance may ensue. Because of metabolic, fluid, and electrolyte abnormalities, optimization of nutrition to patients with acute kidney injury presents a challenge to the clinician. In patients treated with conventional intermittent hemodialysis, achieving adequate amino acid intake can be limited by azotemia and fluid restriction. With the use of continuous renal replacement therapy (CRRT), however, better control of azotemia and liberalization of fluid intake allow amino acid intake to be maximized to support the patient's metabolic needs. High amino acid doses up to 2.5 g/kg/day in patients treated with CRRT improved nitrogen balance. However, to our knowledge, no studies have correlated increased amino acid intake with improved outcomes in critically ill patients with acute kidney injury. Data from large, prospective, randomized, controlled trials are needed to optimize the dosing of amino acids in critically ill patients with acute kidney injury who are treated with CRRT and to study the safety of high doses and their effects on patient morbidity and survival.

▶ In critically ill patients, there is often a negative nitrogen and protein balance that is the result of the high catabolic demands resulting from the underlying disease. Commonly, those patients also have acute kidney injury (AKI) that may require renal replacement therapy. In this article Btaiche et al presents the different ways to calculate nitrogen and protein balance and review the evidence for giving a higher amount of amino acids to patients of continuous renal replacement therapy (CRRT) because the latter can be responsible for clearing partly some of the given nutrients. On the other hand, the Surviving Sepsis guidelines[1] did not address the issue of amount of protein/amino acids to be given and if this dose needs to be modified in patients of CRRT. The reasons for this omission are probably the lack of major large prospective trials that studied this issue and the absence of evidence linking improved amino acid intake with outcomes. Btaich et al recommend giving higher doses of amino acids for patients on CRRT.

Some clinicians might be inclined to the opposite because of the fear of raising urea levels. However, as new evidence has been emerging over the years urea should no longer be considered as the only (if at all) uremic toxin.[2] The clinician treating critically ill patients on CRRT should prescribe higher doses of amino acids and keep close attention to the urine output because the high urea content can induce an osmotic diuresis resulting in hypernatremia, among other complications. Finally, in critically ill patients the clinician should institute early nutritional support within 24 to 48 hour of the ICU stay preferably using the enteral route with the addition of the parenteral route if needed.

J. S. Rachoin, MD
C. Bekes, MD

References

1. Vanholder R, Baurmeister U, Brunet P, Cohen G, Glorieux G, Jankowski J, European Uremic Toxin Work Group. A bench to bedside view of uremic toxins. *J Am Soc Nephrol.* 2008;19:863-870.
2. Scurlock C, Mechanick JI. Early nutrition support in the intensive care unit: a US perspective. *Curr Opin Clin Nutr Metab Care.* 2008;11:152-155.

Acute kidney injury criteria predict outcomes of critically ill patients
Barrantes F, Tian J, Vazquez R (Bridgeport Hosp and Yale Univ School of Medicine, CT)
Crit Care Med 36:1397-1403, 2008

Objective.—The Acute Kidney Injury Network's proposed definition for acute kidney injury (increment of serum creatinine ≥0.3 mg/dL or 50% from baseline within 48 hrs or urine output <0.5 mL/kg/hr for >6 hrs despite fluid resuscitation when applicable) predicts meaningful clinical outcomes.

Design.—Retrospective cohort study.

Setting.—A 350-bed community teaching hospital.

Patients.—The study population consisted of 471 patients with no recent history of renal replacement therapy who were admitted to the medical intensive care unit during 1 yr.

Interventions.—Medical records of all patients were reviewed using a data abstraction tool. Demographic information, diagnoses, risk factors for acute kidney disease, physiologic and laboratory data, and outcomes were recorded.

Measurements and Main Results.—Of 496 patients, 471 were not receiving renal replacement therapy in the weeks before medical intensive care unit admission; 213 had changes ≥.3 mg/dL in serum creatinine within 48 hrs and/or urine output of ≤.5 mL/kg/hr for >6 hrs. Detailed fluid challenge information was available for only 123 patients, who met acute kidney injury criteria, and three patients reversed after administration of ≥500 mL of intravenous fluid and/or blood products. All patients whose creatinine increased ≥50% also had increments ≥0.3 mg/dL. The

120 patients with acute kidney injury were older (mean ± SE: 69.3 ± 1.7 vs. 62.9 ± 1.3, $p < .01$), were more ill (Acute Physiology and Chronic Health Evaluation II score 18.7 ± .6 vs. 13.3 ± .4, $p < .01$), and had multiple comorbidities (two or more organs, 65% vs. 51.3%, $p < .01$) compared with those without acute kidney injury. The mortality rate of patients who met criteria for acute kidney injury was significantly higher than that of patients who did not have acute kidney injury (45.8 vs. 16.4%, $p < .01$). In multivariate logistic regression analyses, acute kidney injury was an independent predictor of mortality (adjusted odds ratio 3.7, 95% confidence interval 2.2–6.1). Acute kidney injury was a better predictor of in-hospital mortality than was Acute Physiology and Chronic Health Evaluation II score, advanced age, or presence of nonrenal organ failures. Median hospital stay was twice as long in patients with acute kidney injury (14 vs. 7 days, $p < .01$), and only patients with acute kidney injury required hemodialysis during hospitalization. The oliguria criterion of acute kidney injury did not affect the odds of in-hospital mortality.

Conclusions.—The Acute Kidney Injury Network definition of acute kidney injury predicts hospital mortality, need for renal replacement therapy, and prolonged hospital stay in critically ill patients. An increment of serum creatinine ≥0.3 mg/dL in 48 hrs alone predicts clinical outcomes as well as the full Acute Kidney Injury Network definition.

▶ Renal dysfunction or acute kidney injury (AKI) is a commonly encountered problem in critically ill patients that occurs in about 30% to 50% of cases. This study confirms others, which show that AKI is highly associated with increased mortality.[1,2] Prevention of AKI may improve mortality, so great effort has been devoted to devise strategies and treatments that would reduce the incidence of AKI; however, this effort has not led to significant advances in most cases. One major obstacle that researchers and clinicians faced when dealing with renal dysfunction was that until recently there was no consensual definition of this entity. In 2004, a panel of experts defined the risk, injury, failure, loss, and end-stage kidney disease (RIFLE) criteria,[3] followed by the Acute Kidney Injury Network (AKIN) criteria in 2005.[4] Those sets of criteria rely on the change of serum creatinine or urine output over a 1-week period (RIFLE) or 48-hour period (AKIN). Other differences include also the amount of rise in serum creatinine (> 0.5 mg/dL vs 0.3 mg/dL) .The 2 sets of criteria were compared in a recent large database query where the conclusion was that there was no superiority of one method over the other.[5] In this study, Barrantes et al examine the association between the AKIN criteria for renal failure (change of creatinine of more than 0.3 mg/dL over 48 hours) and outcomes in an effort to validate the AKIN definition of renal dysfunction. The authors found that when the criteria were met it was strongly associated with hospital lengths of stay (LOS), medical intensive care unit (MICU) LOS, and mortality, and after performing a multivariate analysis it was more strongly associated with the outcomes than Acute Physiology and Chronic Health Evaluation (APACHE) II score. This interesting study has, however, some limitations—its retrospective nature, the relatively small number and homogenous nature of patients, and the incomplete data collection. Moreover, the fact that it performed better than APACHE II may be due to the imperfect nature of the latter. In addition, even if it confirmed that AKIN criteria are associated with worse outcomes, several important issues remained unanswered such as the appropriate time period for change of serum creatinine or if sustained increases in serum creatinine over longer periods had worse outcomes. Clinicians should be aware that relatively small changes in serum creatinine over a short period of time can have a major negative impact on critically ill patients. In addition, this important step toward a validation of this definition of renal dysfunction should allow the researchers to adopt this consensual definition when performing studies. Such a step is crucial for global harmonization of research findings.

J.-S. Rachoin, MD
C. E. Bekes, MD, MHA

References

1. Uchino S, Kellum JA, Bellomo R, et al. Beginning and Ending Supportive Therapy for the Kidney (BEST Kidney) Investigators. Acute renal failure in critically ill patients: a multinational, multicenter Study. *JAMA.* 2005;294:813-818.
2. Lameire N, Van Biesen W, Vanholder R. Acute renal failure. *Lancet.* 2005;365: 417-430.
3. Bellomo R, Ronco C, Kellum JA, Mehta RL, Palevsky P, Acute Dialysis Quality Initiative workgroup. Acute renal failure - definition, outcome measures, animal models, fluid therapy and information technology needs: the Second International Consensus Conference of the Acute Dialysis Quality Initiative (ADQI) Group. *Crit Care.* 2004;8:R204-R212.
4. Mehta RL, Kellum JA, Shah SV, et al. Acute Kidney Injury Network: report of an initiative to improve outcomes in acute kidney injury. *Crit Care.* 2007;11:R31.
5. Bagshaw SM, George C, Bellomo RANZICS Database Management Committe. A comparison of the RIFLE and AKIN criteria for acute kidney injury in critically ill patients. *Nephrol Dial Transplant.* 2008;23:1569-1574.

Intra-abdominal hypertension and acute renal failure in critically ill patients
Dalfino L, Tullo L, Donadio I, et al (Univ of Bari, Italy)
Intensive Care Med 34:707-713, 2008

Objective.—To investigate the relationship between intra-abdominal hypertension (IAH) and acute renal failure (ARF) in critically ill patients.

Design and setting.—Prospective, observational study in a general intensive care unit.

Patients.—Patients consecutively admitted for > 24 h during a 6-month period.

Interventions.—None.

Measurements and Results.—Intra-abdominal pressure (IAP) was measured through the urinary bladder pressure measurement method. The IAH was defined as a IAP ≥12 mmHg in at least two consecutive measurements performed at 24-h intervals. The ARF was defined as the failure class of the RIFLE classification. Of 123 patients, 37 (30.1%)

developed IAH. Twenty-three patients developed ARF (with an overall incidence of 19%), 16 (43.2%) in IAH and 7 (8.1%) in non-IAH group ($p < 0.05$). Shock ($p < 0.001$), IAH ($p = 0.002$) and low abdominal perfusion pressure (APP; $p = 0.046$) resulted as the best predictive factors for ARF. The optimum cut-off point of IAP for ARF development was 12 mmHg, with a sensitivity of 91.3% and a specificity of 67%. The best cut-off values of APP and filtration gradient (FG) for ARF development were 52 and 38 mmHg, respectively. Age ($p = 0.002$), cumulative fluid balance ($p = 0.002$) and shock ($p = 0.006$) were independent predictive factors of IAH. Raw hospital mortality rate was significantly higher in patients with IAH; however, risk-adjusted and O/E ratio mortality rates were not different between groups.

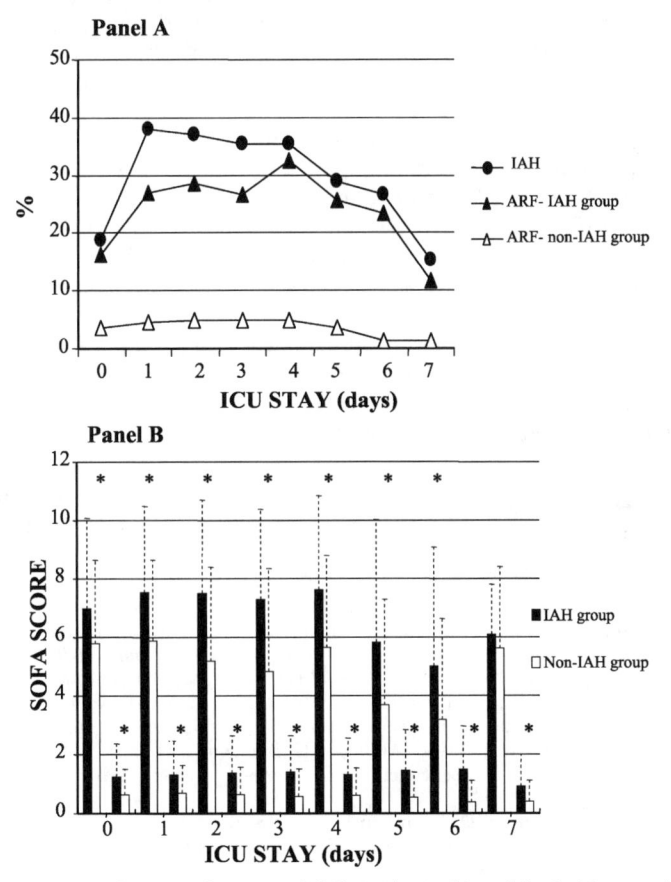

FIGURE 1.—a Prevalence on admission and daily incidence of intraabdominal hypertension (*IAH*) and acute renal failure (*ARF*) during the first week of ICU stay. b Mean extra-renal and renal sepsis-related organ failure assessment (*SOFA*) score during the first week of ICU stay in patients with and without IAH. For each day, extrarenal SOFA on the left and renal SOFA on the right. *$p<0.05$ vs. non-IAH group. (Reprinted from Dalfino L, Tullo L, Donadio I, et al. Intra-abdominal hypertension and acute renal failure in critically ill patients. *Intensive Care Med*. 2008;34:707-713, with kind permission from Springer Science+Business Media, Copyright, 2008.)

Conclusions.—In critically ill patients IAH is an independent predictive factor of ARF at IAP levels as low as 12 mmHg, although the contribution of impaired systemic haemodynamics should also be considered (Fig 1).

▶ More than a century ago, the occurrence of acute renal failure (ARF) in the setting of increased abdominal pressure (IAP) was reported.[1] More recently, however, there has been a resurgence of interest in this association that has generated a significant number of studies. Many hypotheses have been invoked as to how, when, and why an increase in the intra-abdominal pressure could impact renal function. Previous studies using higher cutoff values (eg, 18-25) estimated the incidence of IAP from 2% to more than 40%.[2-4] Current guidelines define IAP as being >12 mm Hg and a recent study showed that its occurrence may in fact be higher.[5] Abdominal trauma, higher acuity of illness, and massive fluid resuscitation have all been identified as reliable risk factors for IAP. Abdominal pressures >12 mm Hg affect hemodynamic status of patients by decreasing cardiac output and increasing vascular resistance.[6] Such processes are thought to underlie the associated renal dysfunction. Whether renal dysfunction is a true consequence or only merely associated with IAP is still unclear. In addition, the temporal relation is still undefined. In this study, Dalfino et al showed that, by using the newly approved consensual definition of IAP, there was an association with the presence of ARF occurring at 48 hours (Fig 1). It is tempting to link IAP and ARF in a cause-effect fashion; however, there has been no trial which demonstrated that improving or even reducing IAP impacts patient outcomes. Until such data become available, it would seem reasonable to measure abdominal pressure in patients with unexplained renal failure and at high risk of developing IAP. If found, noninvasive methods such as nasogastric (NG) tubes, sedation, and ultrafiltration should be attempted first and the use of surgical decompression should be carefully considered.

J. S. Rachoin, MD
C. Bekes, MD

References

1. Wendt E. Uber den einfluss des intraabdominalen Drukes auf die Absonderungsgeschwindigkeit des Harnes. *Arch Physiologische Heilkunde.* 1876;57:527-534.
2. Hong JJ, Cohn SM, Perez JM, Dolich MO, Brown M, McKenney MG. Prospective study of the incidence and outcome of intra-abdominal hypertension and the abdominal compartment syndrome. *Br J Surg.* 2002;89:591-596.
3. Sugrue M, Jones F, Deane SA, Bishop G, Bauman A, Hillman K. Intra-abdominal hypertensionis an independent cause of postoperative renal impairment. *Arch Surg.* 1999;134:1082-1085.
4. Sugrue M, Buist MD, Hourihan F, Deane S, Bauman A, Hillman K. Prospective study of intra-abdominal hypertension and renal function after laparotomy. *Br J Surg.* 1995;82:235-238.
5. Vidal MG, Ruiz Weisser J, Gonzalez F, et al. Incidence and clinical effects of intra-abdominal hypertension in critically ill patients. *Crit Care Med.* 2008;36:1823-1831.
6. Sugrue M. Abdominal compartment syndrome. *Curr Opin Crit Care.* 2005;11:333-338.

Five-year outcomes of severe acute kidney injury requiring renal replacement therapy
Schiffl H, Fischer R (Univ of Munich, Germany)
Nephrol Dial Transplant 23:2235-2241, 2008

Background.—Current research priorities in critical care medicine are focusing on long-term outcomes of survivors of critical illness. Severe acute kidney injury (AKI) is a common occurrence in intensive care. However, few studies have followed up these patients beyond 12 months after hospital discharge.

Methods.—Of a cohort of 425 patients, 226 survivors with severe AKI necessitating renal replacement therapy (RRT) were followed up for 60 months after hospital discharge. None of these patients had pre-existing kidney disease. Vital status and renal function were documented annually for 5 years.

Results.—None of the discharged or transferred patients was dependent on RRT; 57% had complete recovery and 43% had partial recovery of renal function. During the first year after hospital discharge, 18% of survivors died, during the second year 4% and during the third to fifth year 2% per year. At 5 years, 25% of the cohort were still alive. Further improvement in renal function (eGFR) was noted in 26 patients within the first year only. Deterioration of renal function occurred in eight patients. At 5 years, renal function was normal in 86% of the remaining survivors, it was impaired in 9% and 5% of the patients alive needed dialysis again. The proportional Cox regression analysis model showed that pre-existing extrarenal comorbidity, surgery and partial recovery of renal function were independent determinants of long-term survival.

Conclusions.—This prospective observational study indicates that severe AKI is not only a determinant of excess in-hospital case fatalities of critically ill patients, but it also carries significant implications for long-term mortality.

▶ Acute kidney injury (AKI) is commonly seen in critically ill patients and is significantly associated with increased morbidity and in-hospital mortality.[1,2] Most of the previous literature has focused on short-term end points such as in-hospital or 28-day mortality, but more recently, new data has emerged on long-term outcomes for critically ill patients with AKI.

In this study, Schiffl et al complete their previously published work[3] on critically ill patients with AKI who survive hospitalization.[4] They followed patients for 5 years and studied 2 main outcomes: survival and renal function.

The authors showed that the survival was only 25%, which contrasts with previous findings in a study by Liano[5] where survival was 69%. Survival was worsened by comorbidities, surgery, and chronic kidney disease (CKD). The difference in the 2 studies resides in that Schiffl only included patients that required renal replacement therapy (RRT), whereas in the study by Liano up to 70% did not. In addition, previous data had shown that RRT was required on discharge in up to one-third of critically ill patients with AKI.[6] In this study, no patient did, which is probably because they did not include any patient with previous CKD. Other interesting findings from this study are that the most renal function recovery was achieved within the first 12 months and that up to 14% had kidney dysfunction at the end of the study. Another recent study with longer follow-up (10 years) showed that the number of patients with deteriorating kidney function may be higher, and increased in patients with comorbidities and an older age.

Unfortunately, the conclusion that the authors make, namely that AKI is a determinant for long-term mortality, is not supported by their results. The patients in their study were old and had many comorbidities, which in and by itself decrease survival. Furthermore, the link between an episode of AKI and an increase in mortality a few years later is less plausible in the absence of such risk factors. What the conclusion of the study ought to be is that comorbidities (atherosclerosis burden, cardiovascular disease) increase the chance of RRT-requiring AKI, and negatively impact survival.

J. S. Rachoin, MD
C. Bekes, MD

References

1. Brivet FG, Kleinknecht DJ, Loirat P, Landais PJ. Acute renal failure in intensive care units: causes, outcome, and prognostic factors for hospital mortality–a prospective, multicenter study. *Crit Care Med*. 1996;24:192-198.
2. Levy MM, Macias WL, Vincent J-L, et al. Early changes in organ function predict eventual survival in severe sepsis. *Crit Care Med*. 2005;33:2194-2201.
3. Schiffl H. Renal recovery from acute tubular necrosis requiring renal replacement therapy: a prospective study in critically ill patients. *Nephrol Dial Transplant*. 2006;21:1248-1252.
4. Schiffl H, Fischer R. Five-year outcomes of severe acute kidney injury requiring renal replacement therapy. *Nephrol Dial Transplant*. 2008;23:2235-2241.
5. Liano F, Felipe C, Tenorio MT, et al. Long-term outcome of acute tubular necrosis: contribution to its natural history. *Kidney Int*. 2007;71:679-686.
6. Bagshaw SM, Laupland KB, Doig CJ, et al. Prognosis for long-term survival and renal recovery in critically ill patients with severe acute renal failure: a population-based study. *Crit Care*. 2005;9:R700-R709.

10 Trauma and Overdose

The Ratio of Blood Products Transfused Affects Mortality in Patients Receiving Massive Transfusions at a Combat Support Hospital
Borgman MA, Spinella PC, Perkins JG, et al (Brooke Army Med Ctr, Fort Sam Houston, TX)
J Trauma 63:805-813, 2007

Background.—Patients with severe traumatic injuries often present with coagulopathy and require massive transfusion. The risk of death from hemorrhagic shock increases in this population. To treat the coagulopathy of trauma, some have suggested early, aggressive correction using a 1:1 ratio of plasma to red blood cell (RBC) units.

Methods.—We performed a retrospective chart review of 246 patients at a US Army combat support hospital, each of who received a massive transfusion (≥10 units of RBCs in 24 hours). Three groups of patients were constructed according to the plasma to RBC ratio transfused during massive transfusion. Mortality rates and the cause of death were compared among groups.

Results.—For the low ratio group the plasma to RBC median ratio was 1:8 (interquartile range, 0:12–1:5), for the medium ratio group, 1:2.5 (interquartile range, 1:3.0–1:2.3), and for the high ratio group, 1:1.4 (interquartile range, 1:1.7–1:1.2) ($p < 0.001$). Median Injury Severity Score (ISS) was 18 for all groups (interquartile range, 14–25). For low, medium, and high plasma to RBC ratios, overall mortality rates were 65%, 34%, and 19%, ($p < 0.001$); and hemorrhage mortality rates were 92.5%, 78%, and 37%, respectively, ($p < 0.001$). Upon logistic regression, plasma to RBC ratio was independently associated with survival (odds ratio 8.6, 95% confidence interval 2.1–35.2).

Conclusions.—In patients with combat-related trauma requiring massive transfusion, a high 1:1.4 plasma to RBC ratio is independently associated with improved survival to hospital discharge, primarily by decreasing death from hemorrhage. For practical purposes, massive transfusion protocols should utilize a 1:1 ratio of plasma to RBCs for all patients who are hypocoagulable with traumatic injuries.

▶ Whole blood has been used in the military and historically for patients suffering significant trauma. Recent practice uses component therapy as opposed to whole blood therapy for patients with significant hemorrhage. Therapy for blood loss using individual stored components may not address patient needs when massive hemorrhage (>10 units lost per 24 h) occurs. This military report is intended to add additional data to the publications recommending a 1:1:1 ratio with equal parts of red blood cells (RBCs), fresh frozen plasma (FFP), and platelets that is more similar to the composition of whole blood in the patient facing major transfusion. Like civilian practice, most early deaths occurring in combat are related to uncontrolled hemorrhage.[1] Expeditious recognition and treatment of blood component deficits are critical because patients requiring a massive transfusion who succumb die within 6 to 12 hours of admission to hospital. This retrospective review evaluates the impact of varying ratios of plasma units to units of packed RBCs with respect to outcome from penetrating trauma at a combat hospital in Baghdad. I note that platelets are not available in this setting to the degree that they are found in civilian practice, and full platelet data from resuscitation is not provided in this article. Most remarkable in the data summarized in the attached figure is the collection of causes of death. Not surprisingly, increasing the use of FFP decreases the risk of hemorrhagic death. However, the risk of sepsis and multiple organ failure with later central nervous system complications is increased. Although this finding could simply reflect the shift of mortality to an interval after acute presentation, an ongoing concern in resuscitation research is modification of this practice to improve early survival while reducing late complications.

D. J. Dries, MSE, MD

Reference

1. Kauvar DS, Lefering R, Wade CE. Impact of hemorrhage on trauma outcome: An overview of epidemiology, clinical presentations, and therapeutic considerations. *J Trauma.* 2006;60:S3-S11.

Quality of life 2-7 years after major trauma
Ulvik A, Kvåle R, Wentzel-Larsen T, et al (Haukeland Univ Hosp, Bergen, Norway; et al)
Acta Anaesthesiol Scand 52:195-201, 2008

Background.—The aim of the present study was to assess potential long-term reduction in health-related quality of life (HRQOL) in adult trauma patients 2-7 years after discharge from an intensive care unit (ICU), and to study possible determinants of the HRQOL reduction.

Methods.—Follow-up study of a cohort of 341 trauma patients admitted to the ICU of a university hospital during 1998-2003. Of the 228 eligible patients, 210 (92%) completed the study. A telephone interview using the EuroQol 5-D (EQ-5D) was conducted. Patients reported their HRQOL both at present and before trauma.

Results.—Before trauma 88% reported in retrospect no problem in any EQ-5D dimension, compared with 20% at follow-up. After trauma (median 4.0 years) 58% suffered pain/discomfort, 44% reported alterations in usual activities, 40% reduced mobility, 35% anxiety/depression, and 15% limited autonomy. A total of 74% experienced reduction in

HRQOL. Severe problems were reported by 16%. Women experienced more anxiety/depression than men. Simplified Acute Physiology Score (SAPS) II and Injury Severity Score (ISS) were significantly associated with impaired HRQOL, while age was not. Patients with severe head injury reported better HRQOL than those without severe head injury.

Conclusion.—More than 2 years post-injury, 74% reported impaired HRQOL but only 16% had severe problems. The majority still suffered pain/discomfort, indicating that pain management is a key factor in improving long-term outcome after severe trauma.

▶ Although reports of outcomes associated with ICU stay and sepsis have been noted in various parts of the medical literature, long-term quality of life after injury receives less attention possibly because of the transient context of the victims of injury with the health care system. Ulvik and coworkers point out that a high number of patients with significant injury (injury severity score [ISS] > 25) have pain and discomfort up to 7 years after injury. These results are echoed by a recent study from the Netherlands that included approximately 300 patients having an ISS > 16. Mean ISS in both males and females in this study was 23. Although the Scandinavian report had a 92% response rate, this trial also reported an impressive response rate (85%). Twenty-six percent of patients in the Dutch trial were unable to work and dependent on social security. Thirty-three percent of survivors had to change their work or daily activity because of injuries. Problems with pain and cognitive ability were found in 58% and 57% of survivors. In addition to elevated ISS and number of body areas affected, female gender predicted worse long-term functional outcome.[1]

As I read these articles, I was concerned about underappreciation of post-traumatic stress disorder (PTSD). In a recent review, essential features of PTSD include reexperiencing of a traumatic event, avoidance of trauma-related situations, emotional withdrawal, and hyperarousal. Prevalence of PTSD in the United States is 8% with women affected more frequently compared with men.[2] Another characteristic of PTSD that rings true in these articles is hypervigilance to symptoms and poor pain coping mechanisms. Perhaps, PTSD requires greater consideration in patient populations such as those experiencing prominent, chronic pain. Unfortunately, identifying PTSD will not eliminate this component of post-traumatic disability. There are no widely successful pharmacotherapy or psychosocial treatment strategies in place. In addition, although I have not seen comparable data in the trauma patient population, I am confident that the use of formal rehabilitation resources has been reduced in the trauma population similar to reduction seen in medical patients.[3]

Fortunately, the news is not all bad. Another Dutch study compares 2 cohorts of injured patients (ISS > 15) the first treated from 1985-1990 and the second from September 2002 to January 2005.[4] Despite increased age in the Dutch population as a whole and the trauma population in particular, mortality was unchanged and the number of patients making a moderate or good recovery was 67% in the recent cohort compared with 40% 20 years ago. Unfortunately, the authors cannot pinpoint the source of improved functional outcome in this retrospective study.

D. J. Dries, MSE, MD

References

1. Vles WJ, Steyerberg EW, Essink-Bot ML, et al. Prevalence and determinants of disabilities and return to work after major trauma. *J Trauma.* 2005;58:126-135.
2. Davidson JR. Recognition and treatment of posttraumatic stress disorder. *JAMA.* 2001;286:584-588.
3. Ottenbacher KJ, Smith PM, Illig SB, Linn RT, Ostir GV, Granger CV. Trends in length of stay, living setting, functional outcome, and mortality following medical rehabilitation. *JAMA.* 2004;292:1687-1695.
4. Nijboer JM, van der Sluis CK, van der Naalt J, Nijsten MW, Ten Duis HJ. Two cohorts of severely injured trauma patients, nearly two decades apart: Unchanged mortality but improved quality of life despite higher age. *J Trauma.* 2007;63:670-675.

A comparison of central venous and arterial base deficit as a predictor of survival in acute trauma
Schmelzer TM, Perron AD, Thomason MH, et al (Maine Med Ctr, Portland, ME; Carolinas Med Ctr, Charlotte, NC)
Am J Emerg Med 26:119-123, 2008

Background.—The arterial base deficit has been demonstrated to be a marker of shock and predictive of survival in injured patients. The venous blood, however, may better reflect tissue perfusion. Its usefulness in trauma is unknown. We compared central venous with arterial blood gas analysis to determine which was a better predictor of survival in injured patients.

Methods.—A prospective, nonrandomized series of acutely injured patients was investigated. Patients who had an arterial blood gas analysis for acid-base determination had a simultaneous central venous blood gas analysis and routine blood tests. Patient demographics, Injury Severity Score, and survival past 24 hours were recorded. Arterial and venous blood samples were analyzed for pH, P_{CO_2}, P_{O_2}, HCO_3, hemoglobin-oxygen saturation, base deficit, and lactate.

Results.—One hundred patients were enrolled. There were 76 survivors and 24 nonsurvivors. Wilcoxon rank sum test and multivariate logistic regression were used for each recorded variable; only central venous base deficit was predictive of survival past 24 hours ($P = .0081$). Specifically, arterial base deficit was not predictive of survival past 24 hours.

Conclusion.—In a prospective series of acutely injured patients, central venous base deficit, not arterial base deficit, was predictive of survival past 24 hours.

▶ This study mirrors work with invasive central venous monitoring supporting the use of mixed venous saturation as a reflection of oxygen extraction through tissue beds.[1] In this study, 100 patients are evaluated for prognostic value of peripheral base deficit as opposed to arterial base deficit. Not surprisingly, venous base deficit offers more effective prognostic data. There are a number of practical observations to be made. First, most trauma centers do not obtain arterial blood specimens routinely in the emergency department. Thus, a venous sample could be quite valuable. However, the location of the venous sample point and the conditions under which the sample is obtained could affect the quality of data collected. A variety of factors also affect the quality of base deficit data. For example, patients receiving a large amount of chloride in resuscitation may have inappropriately depressed base deficit. If these patients received a large amount of normal saline or lactated Ringers in resuscitation, as we would expect nonsurvivors would, a depressed base deficit could be seen. In addition to hyperchloremic acidosis, chronic conditions such as renal failure and the presence of alcohol, a common problem among trauma patients, can affect the quality of base deficit data.[2] I am surprised at a 24% mortality in 100 patients with an Injury Severity Score (ISS) >15. This mortality rate seems quite high. There is abundant literature supporting the quality of lactate determination, either venous or arterial, in providing prognostic information in trauma resuscitation. Why didn't we see lactate data supporting the venous base deficit results reported? I suspect that this lack of correspondence reflects the relatively short duration of the study. Lactate is a stronger predictor of outcome as time passes after admission.[3]

D. J. Dries, MSE, MD

References

1. Scalea TM, Hartnett RW, Duncan AO, et al. Central venous oxygen saturation: a useful clinical tool in trauma patients. *J Trauma.* 1990;30:1539-1543.
2. Martin MJ, FitzSullivan E, Salim A, Brown CV, Demetriades D, Long W. Discordance between lactate and base deficit in the surgical intensive care unit: which one do you trust? *Am J Surg.* 2006;191:625-630.
3. Abramson D, Scalea TM, Hitchcock R, Trooskin SZ, Henry SM, Greenspan J. Lactate clearance and survival following injury. *J Trauma.* 1993;35:584-588.

Hypertonic Resuscitation of Hypovolemic Shock After Blunt Trauma: A Randomized Controlled Trial
Bulger EM, Jurkovich GJ, Nathens AB, et al (Harborview Med Ctr, Seattle, WA; et al)
Arch Surg 143:139-148, 2008

Background.—The leading cause of late mortality after trauma is multiple organ failure syndrome, due to a dysfunctional inflammatory response early after injury. Preclinical studies demonstrate that hypertonicity alters the activation of inflammatory cells, leading to reduction in organ injury. The purpose of this study was to evaluate the effect of hypertonicity on organ injury after blunt trauma.

Design.—Double-blind, randomized controlled trial from October 1, 2003, to August 31, 2005.

Setting.—Prehospital enrollment at a single level I trauma center.

Patients.—Patients older than 17 years with blunt trauma and prehospital hypotension (systolic blood pressure, ≤90 mm Hg).

Interventions.—Treatment with 250 mL of 7.5% hypertonic saline and 6% dextran 70 (HSD) vs lactated Ringer solution (LRS).

Main Outcome Measures.—The primary end point was survival without acute respiratory distress syndrome (ARDS) at 28 days. Cox proportional hazards regression was used to adjust for confounding factors. A preplanned subset analysis was performed for patients requiring 10 U or more of packed red blood cells in the first 24 hours.

Results.—A total of 209 patients were enrolled (110 in the HSD group and 99 in the LRS group). The study was stopped for futility after the second interim analysis. Intent-to-treat analysis demonstrated no significant difference in ARDS-free survival (hazard ratio, 1.01; 95% confidence interval, 0.63-1.60). There was improved ARDS-free survival in the subset (19% of the population) requiring 10 U or more of packed red blood cells (hazard ratio, 2.18; 95% confidence interval, 1.09-4.36).

Conclusions.—Although no significant difference in ARDS-free survival was demonstrated overall, there was benefit in the subgroup of patients requiring 10 U or more of packed red blood cells in the first 24 hours. Massive transfusion may be a better predictor of ARDS than prehospital hypotension. The use of HSD may offer maximum benefit in patients at highest risk of ARDS.

Trial Registration.—clinicaltrials.gov Identifier: NCT00113685.

▶ This is the latest in a series of trials investigating hemodynamic benefit with early administration of hypertonic saline after blunt trauma associated with hypotension.[1,2] Unfortunately, hypotension is a poor indicator of the need for this therapy and its potential value. The inaccuracy of prehospital blood pressure (BP) recording is also increased by the compromised circumstances in which these data are obtained. Consistent with data provided by the Los Angeles County group, these authors suggest, in retrospective analysis, that massive transfusion is a better marker for acute respiratory distress syndrome (ARDS), a key endpoint in this trial.[3] Although more than 4000 patients were assessed for eligibility, the number of individuals meeting inclusion criteria was 261. Only 209 patients were actually studied. Thus, the group of potential candidates for this trial was not consistent with most trauma patients seen at a well-known level I trauma center. Adverse events associated with massive transfusion are receiving increasing attention in the trauma population.[4] If a benefit to hypertonic saline administration is seen in these patients, it may come from enhancement of adaptive immune response as multiple authors have suggested.[5,6] Clinical studies translating attractive laboratory data into clinical benefit are pending. Finally, because we do not understand the clinical physiology of benefit associated with hypertonic saline administration (it is clearly not just BP changes), we struggle to design trials to evaluate clinical efficacy. In light of recent work on the adverse effects of massive transfusion, this may be a more appropriate target for hypertonic therapies as a part of trauma resuscitation.[7]

R. P. Dellinger, MD

References

1. Mattox KL, Maningas PA, Moore EE, et al. Prehospital hypertonic saline/dextran infusion for post-traumatic hypotension: The U.S.A. Multicenter Trial. *Ann Surg.* 1991;213:482-491.
2. Cooper DJ, Myles PS, McDermott FT, et al. Prehospital hypertonic saline resuscitation of patients with hypotension and severe traumatic brain injury: a randomized controlled trial. *JAMA.* 2004;291:1350-1357.
3. Plurad D, Martin M, Green D, et al. The decreasing incidence of late posttraumatic acute respiratory distress syndrome: the potential role of lung protective ventilation and conservative transfusion practice. *J Trauma.* 2007;63:1-7.
4. Sauaia A, Moore FA, Moore EE, Haenel JB, Read RA, Lezotte DC. Early predictors of postinjury multiple organ failure. *Arch Surg.* 1994;129:39-45.
5. Rizoli SB, Kapus A, Fan J, Li YH, Marshall JC, Rotstein OD. Immunomodulatory effects of hypertonic resuscitation on the development of lung inflammation following hemorrhagic shock. *J Immunol.* 1998;161:6288-6296.
6. Junger WG, Coimbra R, Liu FC, et al. Hypertonic saline resuscitation: a tool to modulate immune function in trauma patients? *Shock.* 1997;8:235-241.
7. Napolitano L. Cumulative risks of early red blood cell transfusion. *J Trauma.* 2006;60:S26-S34.

Blast Injury in a Civilian Trauma Setting is Associated with a Delay in Diagnosis of Traumatic Brain Injury

Bochicchio GV, Lumpkins K, O'Connor J, et al (Univ of Maryland School of Medicine, Baltimore, MD)
Am Surg 74:267-270, 2008

High-pressure waves (blast) account for the majority of combat injuries and are becoming increasingly common in terrorist attacks. To our knowledge, there are no data evaluating the epidemiology of blast injury in a domestic nonterrorist setting. Data were analyzed retrospectively on patients admitted with any type of blast injury over a 10-year period at a busy urban trauma center. Injuries were classified by etiology of explosion and anatomical location. Eighty-nine cases of blast injury were identified in 57,392 patients (0.2%) treated over the study period. The majority of patients were male (78%) with a mean age of 40 ± 17 years. The mean Injury Severity Score was 13 ± 11 with an admission Trauma and Injury Severity Score of 0.9 ± 0.2 and Revised Trauma Score of 7.5 ± 0.8. The mean intensive care unit and hospital length of stay was 2 ± 7 days and 4.6 ± 10 days, respectively, with an overall mortality rate of 4.5 per cent. Private dwelling explosion [n = 31 (35%)] was the most common etiology followed by industrial pressure blast [n = 20 (22%)], industrial gas explosion [n = 16 (18%)], military training-related explosion [n = 15 (17%)], home explosive device [n = 8 (9%)], and fireworks explosion [n = 1 (1%)]. Maxillofacial injuries were the most common injury (n = 78) followed by upper extremity orthopedic (n = 29), head injury (n = 32), abdominal (n = 30), lower extremity orthopedic (n = 29), and thoracic (n = 19). The majority of patients with head injury [28 of 32 (88%)] presented with a Glasgow Coma Scale score of

15. CT scans on admission were initially positive for brain injury in 14 of 28 patients (50%). Seven patients (25%) who did not have a CT scan on admission had a CT performed later in their hospital course as a result of mental status change and were positive for traumatic brain injury (TBI). Three patients (11%) had a negative admission CT with a subsequently positive CT for TBI over the next 48 hours. The remaining four patients (14%) were diagnosed with skull fractures. All patients (n = 4) with an admission Glasgow Coma Scale score of less than 8 died from diffuse axonal injury. Blast injury is a complicated disease process, which may evolve over time, particularly with TBI. The missed injury rate for TBI in patients with a Glasgow Coma Scale score of 15 was 36 per cent. More studies are needed in the area of blast injury to better understand this disease process.

▶ Blast injury with concomitant multisystem trauma is the most common form of terrorist insult to date.[1,2] Traumatic brain injury frequently is subtle with subacute hemorrhages and evolving axonal injury. Tympanic membrane perforation, a sensitive indicator of elevated atmospheric pressure, is among the markers of patients at increased risk for multisystem dysfunction in the setting of blast injury. Other markers include traumatic amputation, burns, and blast injury involving the lungs.[3] This report examines civilian blast injury noting the subtle nature of presentation. In itself, this is a valuable observation and reflects the lack of sensitivity for the Glasgow Coma Score, particularly if obtained only on admission, to assess evolution of brain injury in these patients. Unfortunately, there are many limitations in this data. Coexisting injuries suggestive of increasing severity of brain trauma are not reported.[4] Did these patients have a transient loss of consciousness? In our trauma center, transient loss of consciousness in the setting of blast injury would trigger computed tomography (CT) scan and inpatient (formal) cognitive and motor assessment by trauma center staff. We need more data such as this to better identify markers of patients at risk for evolution of brain injury and to develop criteria for more aggressive screening of blast injury victims.

D. J. Dries, MSE, MD

References

1. Frykberg ER. Principles of mass casualty management following terrorist disasters. *Ann Surg*. 2004;239:319-321.
2. Frykberg ER. Medical management of disasters and mass casualties from terrorist bombings: how can we cope? *J Trauma*. 2002;53:201-212.
3. Ciraulo DL, Frykberg ER. The surgeon and acts of civilian terrorism: blast injuries. *J Am Coll Surg*. 2006;203:942-950.

Pain in the aftermath of trauma is a risk factor for post-traumatic stress disorder
Norman SB, Stein MB, Dimsdale JE, et al (Univ of California, San Diego, CA)
Psychol Med 38:533-542, 2008

Background.—Identifying risk factors for the development of post-traumatic stress disorder (PTSD) is important for understanding and ultimately preventing the disorder. This study assessed pain shortly after traumatic injury (i.e. peritraumatic pain) as a risk factor for PTSD.

Method.—Participants ($n = 115$) were patients admitted to a Level 1 Surgical Trauma Center. Admission to this service reflected a severe physical injury requiring specialized, emergent trauma care. Participants completed a pain questionnaire within 48 h of traumatic injury and a PTSD diagnostic module 4 and 8 months later.

Results.—Peritraumatic pain was associated with an increased risk of PTSD, even after controlling for a number of other significant risk factors other than acute stress disorder symptoms. An increase of 0.5 s.D. from the mean in a 0–10 pain rating scale 24–48 h after injury was associated with an increased odds of PTSD at 4 months by more than fivefold, and at 8 months by almost sevenfold. A single item regarding amount of pain at the time of hospital admission correctly classified 65% of participants.

Conclusions.—If these findings are replicated in other samples, high levels of peritraumatic pain could be used to identify individuals at elevated risk for PTSD following traumatic injury (Table 3).

▶ There was a time when about all we could worry about in the ICU was improving mortality. Now that mortality from many disorders continues to fall and safety programs are helping to reduce morbidities, there is a greater focus on the intermediate and long-term outcomes of critical illness. One potentially devastating disorder is PTSD. This study demonstrates that a measure as simple as the initial pain score may be highly predictive of a patient developing PTSD (Table 3). If this is subsequently verified, there may not be a simpler, cost-effective approach to early identification of these patients. The study has some important limitations: all patients were < 65 years old, there is no control group, there was a fairly high (up to 20%) drop out rate, and there was a simultaneous competing study evaluating pharmacoprevention of PTSD. In addition, most (94%) of the patients had previously suffered a traumatic event, and it is unclear what role that may have played in their evaluation of pain at a subsequent traumatic event.

T. Dorman, MD

TABLE 3.—Stepwise Logistic Regression Model to Predict PTSD Status at 4 and 8 Months Post-Trauma

	Block 1	Block 2	Block 3	Block 4
4-month PTSD status				
Peritraumatic MPQ-SF VAS	1.39 (1.13–1.71)**	1.34 (1.07–1.67)**	1.23 (0.98–1.54)	1.10 (0.85–1.41)
Opiate use at 4 months		0.72 (0.20–2.58)	0.60 (0.14–2.61)	0.43 (0.08–2.34)
MPQ-SF VAS at 4 months		1.13 (0.94–1.35)	1.18 (0.96–1.45)	1.13 (0.91–1.41)
Female gender			6.38 (2.25–18.11)*	3.74 (1.20–11.63)*
Prior psychiatric history			2.55 (0.90–7.25)	3.56 (1.11–11.42)*
Prior sexual trauma			1.18 (0.31–4.43)	0.84 (0.20–3.52)
Total ASD score				1.26 (1.10–1.45)**
Model r^2	0.15	0.17	0.37	0.50
8-month PTSD status				
Peritraumatic MPQ-SF VAS	1.47 (1.13–1.92)	1.41 (1.97–1.85)*	1.34 (1.02–1.76)*	1.22 (0.90–1.66)
Opiate use at 8 months		0.56 (0.10–3.17)	0.44 (0.06–2.87)	0.47 (0.07–3.08)
MPQ-SF VAS at 8 months		1.22 (0.99–1.52)	1.34 (1.06–1.70)*	1.27 (0.99–1.62)
Female gender			4.65 (1.37–15.78)*	2.67 (0.70–10.24)
Total ASD symptoms				1.16 (1.01–1.33)*
Model r^2	0.16	0.21	0.30	0.37
Peritraumatic MPQ-SF total score	1.04 (1.00–1.09)*	1.03 (0.98–1.08)	1.03 (0.98–1.09)	1.00 (0.95–1.06)
Opiate use at 8 months		0.74 (0.13–3.98)	0.62 (0.09–4.16)	0.51 (0.07–3.41)
MPQ-SF total score at 8 months		1.12 (0.98–1.29)	1.17 (1.01–1.37)*	1.15 (0.98–1.36)
Female gender			5.21 (1.59–17.04)**	2.79 (0.78–0.99)
Total ASD score				1.23 (1.06–1.42)**
Model r^2	0.06	0.12	0.25	0.38
Peritraumatic affective pain score	1.20 (1.04–1.38)**	1.19 (1.02–1.38)*	1.18 (1.01–1.38)	1.06 (0.89–1.25)
Opiate use at 8 months		1.23 (0.22–6.61)	1.30 (0.20–8.36)	0.90 (0.14–5.78)
Affective pain at 8 months		1.31 (0.87–1.97)	1.44 (0.92–2.26)	1.39 (0.85–2.27)
Female gender			4.28 (1.35–13.55)*	2.35 (0.67–8.19)
Total ASD score				1.23 (1.06–1.42)**
Model r^2	0.11	0.15	0.25	0.37

OR, Odds ratio; CI, confidence interval; ASD, Acute stress disorder; MPQ-SF VAS, McGill Pain Questionnaire visual analog scale.
*p<0.05.
**p<0.01.
(Reprinted from Norman SB, Stein MB, Dimsdale JE, et al. Pain in the aftermath of trauma is a risk factor for post-traumatic stress disorder. *Psychol Med.* 2008;38:533-542, with permission from Cambridge University Press.)

A Trauma Mortality Prediction Model Based on the Anatomic Injury Scale

Osler T, Glance L, Buzas JS, et al (Univ of Vermont, Burlington; Univ of Rochester, NY; et al)
Ann Surg 247:1041-1048, 2008

Objective.—To develop a statistically rigorous trauma mortality prediction model based on empiric estimates of severity for each injury in the abbreviated injury scale (AIS) and compare the performance of this new model with the injury severity score (ISS).

Summary Background Data.—Mortality rates at trauma centers should only be compared after adjusting for differences in injury severity, but no reliable measure of injury severity currently exists. The ISS has served as the standard measure of anatomic injury for 30 years. However, it relies on the individual injury severities assigned by experts in the AIS, is nonmonotonic with respect to mortality, and fails to perform even as well as a far simpler model based on the single worst injury a patient has sustained.

Methods.—This study is based on data from 702,229 injured patients in the National Trauma Data Bank (NTDB 6.1) hospitalized between 2001 and 2005. Sixty percent of the data was used to derive an empiric measure of severity of each of the 1322 injuries in the AIS lexicon by taking the weighted average of coefficients estimated using 2 separate regression models. The remaining 40% of the data was used to create 3 exploratory mortality prediction models and compare their performance with the ISS using measures of discrimination (C statistic), calibration (Hosmer Lemeshow statistic and calibration curves), and the Akaike information criterion.

Results.—Three new models based on empiric AIS injury severities were developed. All of these new models discriminated survivors from nonsurvivors better than the ISS, but one, the trauma mortality prediction model (TMPM), had both better discrimination [$ROC_{TMPM} = 0.901$ (0.898–0.905), $ROC_{ISS} = 0.871$ (0.866–0.877)] and better calibration [$HL_{TMPM} = 58$ (35–91), $HL_{ISS} = 296$ (228–357)] than the ISS. The addition of age, gender, and mechanism of injury improved all models, but the augmented TMPM dominated ISS by every measure [$ROC_{TMPM} = 0.925 (0.921–0.928)$, $ROC_{ISS} = 0.904 (0.901–0.909)$, $HL_{TMPM} = 18$ (12–31), $HL_{ISS} = 54$ (30–64)].

Conclusions.—Trauma mortality models based on empirical estimates of individual injury severity better discriminate between survivors and nonsurvivors than does the current standard, ISS. One such model, the TMPM, has both superior discrimination and calibration when compared with the ISS. The TMPM should replace the ISS as the standard measure of overall injury severity.

▶ Osler and coworkers are among the most important writers currently describing outcome measures in the setting of injury. They appropriately point out limitations of the time-honored injury severity score (ISS) and using the massive retrospective database of the National Trauma Data Bank

(NTDB), propose a more sophisticated, broadly applicable comparative measure for dose of trauma.[1,2] Perhaps, the greatest limitation of the widely used ISS relates to head injury.[3] Massive orthopedic and abdominal trauma may score identically with traumatic brain injury although the latter has a far greater impact on patient outcome. Nonetheless, ISS can be calculated at the bedside unlike the present, more sophisticated parameters that require a laptop computer at least. There is also the issue of history. The trauma literature has used the ISS as a grading criterion for general severity of injury for decades. A ready translation of ISS into trauma mortality prediction model (TMPM) is not possible. Finally, as the authors point out, simple addition of age, gender, and mechanism of injury improves predictive value of all indices. These parameters could readily be added to improve ISS. Neither ISS nor TMPM includes physiologic data.[4] This could also be easily added. Although TMPM may be an appropriate tool for administrative comparisons among trauma centers, ISS, preferably modified by age, gender, physiologic data, and mechanism of injury remains a valuable bedside tool.

D. J. Dries, MSE, MD

References

1. Baker SP, O'Neill B, Haddon W, et al. The injury severity score: a method for describing patients with multiple injuries and evaluating emergency care. *J Trauma*. 1974;14:187-196.
2. Champion HR, Copes WS, Sacco WJ, et al. A new characterization of injury severity. *J Trauma*. 1990;30:539-546.
3. Kilgo PD, Meredith JW, Hensberry R, Osler TM. A note on the disjointed nature of the injury severity score. *J Trauma*. 2004;57:479-485.
4. Boyd CR, Tolson MA, Copes WS. Evaluating trauma care: the TRISS method. *J Trauma*. 1987;27:370-378.

The use of leukoreduced red blood cell products is associated with fewer infectious complications in trauma patients
Friese RS, Sperry JL, Phelan HA, et al (Univ of Texas Southwestern Med Ctr at Dallas; Univ of Pittsburgh Med Ctr, PA)
Am J Surg 196:56-61, 2008

Background.—Clinical studies suggest that leukocytes in banked blood may increase infectious complications after transfusion. However, these investigations included few injured patients. Therefore, the effect of the use of leukoreduced red blood cell (RBC) products in this patient population is unknown. In addition, large numbers of RBC transfusions are frequently required in the treatment of patients with hemorrhagic shock, which may have a more profound effect on infectious risk. The purpose of this study was to determine the effect of prestorage leukoreduction on infectious complications in injured patients.

Methods.—A retrospective before-and-after cohort study was conducted at an urban level 1 trauma center. A policy of using leukoreduced RBC products commenced in January 2002. Patients treated from March

2002 through December 2003 received leukoreduced RBC products. Those transfused from March 2000 through December 2001 served as controls. Inclusion criteria were age ≥18 years, survival ≥2 days after admission, and transfusion of ≥2 U RBCs within 24 hours of admission. There were 240 patients in the leukoreduction group, and 438 patients in the control group. Multivariate logistic regression controlling for age, sex, injury severity, and number of transfusions was used to determine if leukoreduction status was an independent predictor of infectious complications. Subset analysis was performed on patients receiving massive transfusion (ie, >6 units in 24 hours; n = 168).

Results.—Patient demographics and injury severity characteristics were similar during both treatment periods. Overall, those patients receiving leukoreduced RBC products had a 45% reduction in nosocomial pneumonia (odds ratio [OR] .55; 95% confidence interval [CI] .33–.91) and a significant reduction in the development of any type of infection (OR .48; 95% CI .31–.73). In the massive-transfusion subset, the OR for development of any infection was .33 (95% CI, .15–.73), and the OR for the development of pneumonia was .29 (95% CI, .11–.76) in those patients receiving leukoreduced RBC products. There were no differences in mortality within the overall- or massive-transfusion subset analyses.

Conclusion.—Prestorage leukoreduction is associated with a reduction of infectious complications in injured patients. Furthermore, this protective effect appears more pronounced in patients receiving massive transfusion (>6 U packed RBCs).

▶ The incidental presence of white blood cells (WBCs) in packed red blood cells (PRBC) intended for transfusion as a cause of immunologically mediated adverse events such as transfusion reactions has been well-known for decades. More recently, WBCs have also been implicated as factors in a variety of other adverse effects of PRBC transfusion, including, but not limited to, transfusion-associated lung injury, infection, and cardiac dysrhythmias. In this study, the investigators used a retrospective, before and after methodology to assess the impact of leukoreduction (LR) of PRBC transfused to trauma patients in the first 24 hours on the incidence of infection and mortality. They found that LR was associated with a significant reduction in the rates of overall infection and nosocomial pneumonia, both in the entire study population and in the subset of patients classified as receiving massive transfusion. No impact on mortality was identified. Overall, the data regarding the benefits of universal LR of PRBC remain to be determined, although the preponderance of literature evaluating the impact of leukoreduced blood in an acutely ill patient population appears to be a beneficial one, and none demonstrates a harmful effect. Interestingly, the beneficial effects vary from study to study, with some showing a lower infection rate and some a mortality benefit. The literature in the elective surgical population is more variable. This variability in outcomes in studies may be not only related to differences in methodologies and study population characteristics, but also due in large part to the fact that WBC may not be the entire story for why PRBC have adverse effects on the recipient. Even in the era of universal LR, patients receiving PRBC appear to have significantly more infectious complications and other adverse events compared with their nontransfused counterparts, even when adjusted for comorbidities, acuity, and other confounding factors. The morphological and biochemical degradation that PRBC undergo during storage are well documented, which may impair their ability to deliver oxygen at the cellular level after transfusion. In addition, the increased fragility of stored PRBC may result in release of a host of toxic substances that may impair microcirculatory flow and cellular and immune function, independent of the presence or absence of WBC in the stored blood. Although LR of PRBC is likely to be a significant step in improving the safety of the blood supply, it does not appear to be the ultimate solution to the problem.

D. R. Gerber, DO

Perceived value of trauma autopsy among trauma medical directors and coroners
Santanello S, Dean D, Hayes JR, et al (Grant Med Ctr, Columbus, OH; Central Ohio Trauma System, Columbus, OH; et al)
Injury 39:1075-1081, 2008

Introduction.—Although autopsy is acknowledged as essential for improving quality of medical care of trauma patients and accuracy of injury surveillance systems, the autopsy rate has remained well below 100% for certain categories of trauma. We obtained recent documentation of the frequency of autopsy among trauma-related deaths in Ohio, and surveyed coroners and trauma program medical directors (TMDs) about the perceived benefits and challenges of performing autopsy.

Materials and Methods.—Copies of death certificates were obtained for the years 1996–2001. Death and autopsy rates were calculated and examined for trends over time. Surveys covering the topics of mechanisms of injury prompting autopsy, uses and users of autopsy data, and barriers to performing autopsy were sent to Ohio's coroners, coroners from nearby states, and Ohio TMDs. The χ^2-test for trend analysed autopsy rates over time, while responses among groups were compared using the χ^2-test.

Results.—The autopsy rate for injury related deaths increased from 50% in 1996 to 66.5% in 2001 ($p = .0018$). During the study period the volume of autopsies rose by 18%, from 2990 to 3546. There was no review by the coroner in almost 10% of trauma deaths. TMDs more often indicated that autopsies advance medical knowledge than did Ohio and non-Ohio coroners (62.9% versus 33.4% and 47.6%, respectively, $p = .016$). TMDs more frequently reported themselves as users of autopsy information than did Ohio and non-Ohio coroners (91.4% versus 14.6% and 20%, respectively, $p < .0001$). All groups reported inadequate funds and personnel as the two most common barriers to performing autopsies, although TMDs were more likely to identify these as barriers than coroners ($p < .0001$). Almost 27% of Ohio coroners agreed with the statement, "I do not feel that trauma-related autopsies are necessary".

Conclusion.—Significant barriers exist to improving autopsy rates among trauma patients who die. These include not only more well-recognised impediments such as inadequate funds and personnel, but less commonly reported issues concerning differing points of view on the role of trauma-related autopsy among coroners and TMDs. To improve trauma-related autopsy rates, each of these issues requires attention and cooperation among all parties.

▶ This survey research highlights improving use of autopsy data in Ohio, particularly as related to trauma-related mortality. Not surprisingly, injury associated with legal investigation received significant attention from the coroner, whereas cases less likely to be associated with litigation seemed to receive less attention. I was not surprised to see the discordant views of the value of autopsy between coroners and trauma administrators. Trauma centers rely heavily on autopsy data as a part of the quality assurance process. When the pattern of mortality after trauma is assessed, events in the ICU, for example, become very important after initial trauma mortality related to hemorrhage is identified.[1]

As a medical student, I was taught that the best medical education included the combined input of primary clinicians, focused consultants and, where appropriate, the pathologist. The departure of gross pathology and its disconnect from physiology in medical education and practice today is obvious. As a trauma surgeon, I rarely see the pathologists in my hospital and have little contact with medical examiners despite the presence of our county coroner's office on the hospital campus. As we attempt to further document the quality and process of care in trauma systems, consistent input of autopsy data grow in importance.

Perhaps, clinicians in the United States should not be too upset about a relative lack of autopsy data. A recent review from the Netherlands, discloses a 23% autopsy rate based on medical examiner advice.[2] Autopsies were more commonly used for prehospital deaths. In medical/legal circumstances, the autopsy rate was 46%. Authors deny the low rate of medical/legal and clinically desirable autopsies noting that the limited activity of the Amsterdam system focuses resources mainly on medical/legal cases and educational opportunities are largely ignored. Other recent work from the United Kingdom questions the quality of autopsy material where autopsy was performed. In this review from the Victorian Institute of Forensic Medicine, a review of autopsies revealed that only 52% of reports were considered satisfactory and only 4% of autopsy reports were marked as excellent. Over 25% of autopsies were felt to be poor.[3]

D. J. Dries, MSE, MD

References

1. Kauvar DS, Lefering R, Wade CE. Impact of hemorrhage on trauma outcome: an overview of epidemiology, clinical presentations, and therapeutic considerations. *J Trauma.* 2006;60:S3-S11.

2. Fung Kon Jin PH, Klaver JF, Maes A, Ponsen KJ, Das C, Goslings JC. Autopsies following death due to traumatic injuries in The Netherlands: an evaluation of current practice. *Injury.* 2008;39:83-89.
3. Ranson D. Coroners' autopsies: quality concerns in the United Kingdom. *J Law Med.* 2007;14:315-318.

Acute Coagulopthy of Trauma: Hypoperfusion Induces Systemic Anticoagulation and Hyperfibrinolysis

Brohi K, Cohen MJ, Ganter MT, et al (The Royal London Hosp, London, UK; Univ of California San Francisco, CA; et al)
J Trauma 64:1211-1217, 2008

Background.—Coagulopathy is present at admission in 25% of trauma patients, is associated with shock and a 5-fold increase in mortality. The coagulopathy has recently been associated with systemic activation of the protein C pathway. This study was designed to characterize the thrombotic, coagulant and fibrinolytic derangements of trauma-induced shock.

Methods.—This was a prospective cohort study of major trauma patients admitted to a single trauma center. Blood was drawn within 10 minutes of arrival for analysis of partial thromboplastin and prothrombin times, prothrombin fragments 1 + 2 (PF1 + 2), fibrinogen, factor VII, thrombomodulin, protein C, plasminogen activator inhibitor-1 (PAI-1), thrombin activatable fibrinolysis inhibitor (TAFI), tissue plasminogen activator (tPA), and D-dimers. Base deficit was used as a measure of tissue hypoperfusion.

Results.—Two hundred eight patients were studied. Systemic hypoperfusion was associated with anticoagulation and hyperfibrinolysis. Coagulation was activated and thrombin generation was related to injury severity, but acidosis did not affect Factor VII or PF1 + 2 levels. Hypoperfusion-induced increase in soluble thrombomodulin levels was associated with reduced fibrinogen utilization, reduction in protein C and an increase in TAFI. Hypoperfusion also resulted in hyperfibrinolysis, with raised tPA and D-Dimers, associated with the observed reduction in PAI-1 and not alterations in TAFI.

Conclusions.—Acute coagulopathy of trauma is associated with systemic hypoperfusion and is characterized by anticoagulation and hyperfibrinolysis. There was no evidence of coagulation factor loss or dysfunction at this time point. Soluble thrombomodulin levels correlate with thrombomodulin activity. Thrombin binding to thrombomodulin contributes to hyperfibrinolysis via activated protein C consumption of PAI-1.

▶ Common causes of coagulopathy after trauma include clotting factor consumption associated with vascular injury, acidosis, and hypothermia associated with reduced enzymatic activity as well as hemodilution from massive administration of crystalloids and administration of packed cells without adequate clotting factors. This has led to recognition of the importance of aggressive administration of fresh frozen plasma (FFP) along with packed red cells in the initial minutes of transfusion therapy in patients with clinical signs of massive blood loss.[1] Another group of patients has coagulopathy after injury before these changes can occur. These patients are frequently normothermic and not severely acidotic. In a previous study, these workers demonstrated coagulopathy associated with post-traumatic shock that could be identified on admission to hospital. Modification in thrombomodulin and reduction in protein C levels were observed.[2] Thrombomodulin is a local anticoagulant present in the endothelium working to prevent thrombosis through generation of activated protein C (APC). Exaggerated release of thrombomodulin with subsequent complex formation with thrombin and activation of protein C in global low flow conditions appears to contribute to the anticoagulant environment seen with post-traumatic shock. Reduced plasminogen activator inhibitor, consumed by APC, in association with increased release of plasminogen activators from small vessel walls contribute to hyperfibrinolysis. Contemporary efforts to address traumatic coagulopathy use administration of FFP or recombinant factor VIIa.[3,4] These strategies may not be sufficiently specific or successful to address the early coagulopathy after trauma described by these authors.

D. J. Dries, MSE, MD

References

1. Malone DL, Hess JR, Fingerhut A. Massive transfusion practices around the globe and a suggestion for a common massive transfusion protocol. *J Trauma.* 2006;60: S91-S96.
2. Brohi K, Singh J, Heron M, Coats T. Acute traumatic coagulopathy. *J Trauma.* 2003;54:1127-1130.
3. Boffard KD, Riou B, Warren B, et al. Recombinant factor VIIa as adjunctive therapy for bleeding control in severely injured trauma patients: two parallel randomized, placebo-controlled, double-blind clinical trials. *J Trauma.* 2005;59: 8-15.
4. Cotton BA, Gunter OL, Isbell J, et al. Damage control hematology: the impact of a trauma exsanguination protocol on survival and blood product utilization. *J Trauma.* 2008;64:1177-1182.

The Evolution of Blunt Splenic Injury: Resolution and Progression
Savage SA, Zarzaur BL, Magnotti LJ, et al (Wilford Hall Med Ctr, Lackland AFB, TX; Univ of Tennessee Health Science Ctr, Memphis, Tennessee; et al)
J Trauma 64:1085-1092, 2008

Background.—Nonoperative management of blunt splenic injury (BSI) has become the standard of care for hemodynamically stable patients. Successful nonoperative management raises two related questions: (1) what is the time course for splenic healing and (2) when may patients safely return to usual activities? There is little evidence to guide surgeon recommendations regarding return to full activities. Our hypothesis was that time to healing is related to severity of BSI.

Methods.—The trauma registry at a level I trauma center was queried for patients diagnosed with a BSI managed nonoperatively between 2002 and 2007. Follow-up abdominal computed tomography scans were reviewed with attention to progression to healing of BSI. Kaplan-Meier curves were compared for mild (American Association for the Surgery of Trauma grades I–II) and severe (grades III–V) BSI.

Results.—Six hundred thirty-seven patients (63.9% mild spleen injury and 36.1% severe injury) with a BSI were eligible for analysis. Fifty-one patients had documented healing as inpatients. Ninety-seven patients discharged with BSI had outpatient computed tomography scans. Nine had worsening of BSI as outpatients and two (1 mild and 1 severe) required intervention (2 splenectomies). Thirty-three outpatients were followed to complete healing. Mild injuries had faster mean time to healing compared with severe (12.5 vs. 37.2 days, $p < 0.001$). Most healing occurred within 2 months but approximately 20% of each group had not healed after 3 months.

Conclusion.—Although mild BSIs heal faster than severe BSIs, nearly 10% of all the BSIs followed as outpatients worsened. Close observation of patients with BSI should continue until healing can be confirmed.

▶ Nonoperative management with selective embolization has become the standard-of-care in the management of blunt splenic injury.[1] Patients are frequently discharged with damaged spleens where late rupture is a risk. The general trend in the trauma community is moving away from follow-up imaging in these individuals unless a high acuity or high complexity constellation of injuries exists. This is born out in the recent survey of the Eastern Association for the Surgery of Trauma regarding practices in blunt splenic injury.[1] There is little recent data, however, on the natural history of this injury. Savage and coworkers fill in some of this gap. Practices at the Presley Trauma Center are similar to those in other major centers. Initial screening CT is performed with embolization of patients with complex injuries, obvious pseudoaneurysm detection, or contrast blush in the injured splenic parenchyma.[2] Patients are discharged with activity limitations typically measured in months. These investigators provide a limited long horizon dataset with outcome parameters for blunt splenic injury. The likelihood of healing with either blunt or mild injury is good at 90 days. Two patients in this series underwent late splenectomy. The first patient had concomitant injuries that should have been repaired at initial hospitalization. The second had what was described as an American Association for the Surgery of Trauma (AAST) grade II spleen injury.[3] This patient presented to the emergency department with abdominal pain and hypotension, and ultimately underwent splenectomy. Using the Social Security Death Index, the authors were unable to identify any patient discharged alive with a splenic injury who died within 90 days of hospitalization.[4] These authors suggest that this data represent a starting point for "organized out-patient care." I believe that the authors have added to our understanding of outcomes for blunt splenic injury. Clearly, discharge of patients with damaged spleens can be safely done if appropriate precautions are instituted and follow-up is available. This data is not sufficient to convince me of the need for additional CT scanning. Splenectomy is a clinical decision. Clearly, activity limitation for patients with blunt splenic injury should extend for at least 90 days.

D. J. Dries, MSE, MD

References

1. Fata P, Robinson L, Fakhry SM. A survey of EAST member practices in blunt splenic injury: a description of current trends and opportunities for improvement. *J Trauma.* 2005;59:836-842.
2. Davis KA, Fabian TC, Croce MA, et al. Improved success in nonoperative management of blunt splenic injuries: embolization of splenic artery pseudoaneurysms. *J Trauma.* 1998;44:1008-1013.
3. Social Security Death Index. http://ssa-custhelp.ssa.gov/cgi-bin/ssa.cfg/php/enduser/std_alp.php?p_faqid=149. Accessed February 13, 2009.
4. Moore EE, Shackford SR, Pachta HL, et al. Organ injury scaling: spleen, liver, and kidney. *J Trauma.* 1989;29:1664-1666.

Impact of the Method of Initial Stabilization for Femoral Shaft Fractures in Patients With Multiple Injuries at Risk for Complications (Borderline Patients)

Pape H-C, Rixen D, Morley J, et al (Univ of Pittsburgh Med Ctr, PA; Univ of Witten, Herdecke, Germany; St. James Univ Hosp, Leeds, UK; et al)
Ann Surg 246:491-499, 2007

Objectives.—The timing of definitive fixation for major fractures in patients with multiple injuries is controversial. To address this gap, we randomized patients with blunt multiple injuries to either initial definitive stabilization of the femur shaft with an intramedullary nail or an external fixateur with later conversion to an intermedullary nail and documented the postoperative clinical condition.

Methods.—Multiply injured patients with femoral shaft fractures were randomized to either initial (<24 hours) intramedullary femoral nailing or external fixation and later conversion to an intramedullary nail. Inclusion: New Injury Severity Score >16 points, or 3 fractures and Abbreviated Injury Scale score ≥ 2 points and another injury (Abbreviated Injury Scale score ≥ 2 points), and age 18 to 65 years. Exclusion: patients in unstable or critical condition. Patients were graded as stable or borderline (increased risk of systemic complications).

Outcomes.—Incidence of acute lung injuries.

Results.—Ten European Centers, 165 patients, mean age 32.7 ± 11.9 years. Group intramedullary nailing, n = 94; group external fixation, n = 71. Preoperatively, 121 patients were stable and 44 patients were in borderline condition. After adjusting for differences in initial injury severity between the 2 treatment groups, the odds of developing acute lung injury were 6.69 times greater in borderline patients who underwent intramedullary nailing in comparison with those who underwent external fixation, $P < 0.05$.

Conclusion.—Intramedullary stabilization of the femur fracture can affect the outcome in patients with multiple injuries. In stable patients, primary femoral nailing is associated with shorter ventilation time. In borderline patients, it is associated with a higher incidence of lung dysfunctions when compared with those who underwent external fixation and later conversion to intramedullary nail. Therefore, the preoperative condition should be when deciding on the type of initial fixation to perform in patients with multiple blunt injuries.

▶ It is generally accepted that definitive stabilization of major fractures in patients with multiple blunt injuries is advantageous for mortality, pulmonary morbidity, and resource consumption. Controversy arises in the patient with severe head injury, which has recently been associated with pulmonary complications, and in patients with significant multisystem trauma who are then subjected to a shower of fat microemboli-associated with intramedullary stabilization of long bone fractures. For the patient with multiple injuries, which preclude standard orthopedic repairs, external fixator application, which can be done in the emergency room, intensive care unit, or during a brief stay in the operating room, has gained popularity.[1] However, the role of standard intramedullary fixation as opposed to placement of the external fixator has never been clearly defined. Here, the authors examine early definitive fixation as opposed to placement of external fixators with later definitive stabilization in patients broken into 2 groups based on emergency department assessment. Previous orthopedic trauma studies describe 4 clinical categories for patients evaluated in this work—stable, borderline, unstable, or in extremis.[2,3] Here, treatment group differences were examined separately in stable and borderline patient groups. Patients who were unstable or in extremis were eliminated from the study. Outcome variables such as acute lung injury (ALI) and systemic inflammatory response syndrome were defined using standard criteria. Of approximately 165 evaluable patients, three-quarters were in stable and one-quarter (44 patients) were in borderline condition. Among borderline patients, pneumonia, ALI, acute respiratory distress syndrome (ARDS), sepsis, and multiple organ failure were more common in patients who underwent primary intramedullary nailing, but the only outcome that was statistically significant was that for ALI. I believe that this reflects the relatively small number of patients in borderline condition who were evaluated. The authors make 3 observations: (1) When treatments groups were compared, patients undergoing external fixation were more severely injured and had a higher degree of head trauma. When data was corrected for injury severity, the incidence of complications was comparable across treatment groups. Thus, early intramedullary nailing and external fixation, if used in appropriate patients, is associated with a comparable incidence of complications. (2) In stable patients, there was a longer duration of mechanical ventilation with external fixation in comparison with intramedullary nailing. As I review the data, this is not surprising as clinicians may hold patients on the ventilator longer waiting for the transition from damage control orthopedics to definitive stabilization. Investigators admit that ventilator management strategy was not standardized between sites. (3) In patients defined as borderline, a higher incidence of ALI occurred in individuals who underwent initial intramedullary fixation as opposed to external fixation. The authors admit to a higher incidence of head injury in borderline patients. Head injury and adverse pulmonary outcomes have been linked in blunt trauma.[4,5] Thus, an operation alone may not explain all the differences seen. In part, because of small sample size in the borderline group and lack of control over some clinical practices, I do not believe that this data offers definitive evidence that one type of orthopedic approach is better than another in the more severely injured patient. The authors do provide new insight into the potential for pulmonary dysfunction associated with early intramedullary nailing in high risk patients and offer a way to think about the propriety of nailing as opposed to external fixator placement based on injury severity.

D. J. Dries, MSE, MD

References

1. Scalea TM, Boswell SA, Scott JD, Mitchell KA, Kramer ME, Pollak AN. External fixation as a bridge to intramedullary nailing for patients with multiple injuries and with femur fractures: damage control orthopedics. *J Trauma*. 2000;48: 613-621.
2. Pape HC, Giannoudis P, Krettek C. The timing of fracture treatment in polytrauma patients: relevance of damage control orthopedic surgery. *Am J Surg*. 2002;183: 622-629.
3. Pape HC, Giannoudis PV, Krettek C, Trentz O. Timing of fixation of major fractures in blunt polytrauma: role of conventional indicators in clinical decision making. *J Orthop Trauma*. 2005;19:551-562.
4. Giannoudis PV, Veysi VT, Pape HC, Krettek C, Smith MR. When should we operate on major fractures in patients with severe head injuries? *Am J Surg*. 2002;183: 261-267.
5. Jaicks RR, Cohn SM, Moller BA. Early fracture fixation may be deleterious after head injury. *J Trauma*. 1997;42:1-7.

11 Neurologic: Traumatic and Non-traumatic

Posttraumatic Cerebral Infarction: Incidence, Outcome, and Risk Factors
Tawil I, Stein DM, Mirvis SE, et al (Univ of New Mexico, Albuquerque)
J Trauma 64:849-853, 2008

Background.—Outcome in patients with traumatic brain injury (TBI) is often affected by secondary insults including posttraumatic cerebral infarction (PTCI). The incidence of PTCI after TBI was previously reported to be 2% with no mortality impact. We suspected that recent advances in imaging modalities and treatment might affect incidence and outcome. We sought to define the incidence and mortality impact of PTCI. We also identified risk factors associated with PTCI.

Methods.—We retrospectively reviewed all patients admitted between 2004 and 2006 with severe TBI (brain Abbreviated Injury Scale [AIS] score >2, Glasgow Coma Scale score [GCS] <9). Demographics, injury specifics, and clinical data were abstracted. All brain imaging studies were reviewed with an attending trauma radiologist. Statistical analysis of outcome data were performed using χ^2 and Student's t test and multivariate analysis was performed using logistic regression to identify independent risk factors.

Results.—Of the 384 patients identified with severe TBI; 93% sustained a blunt injury, 75% were men. Mortality was 21%, and 48% had a brain AIS score of 5. Mean age was 36 years (11–90 years), admission GCS score was 5 (3–8), and Injury Severity Score was 32 (9–75). Thirty-one (8%) had a confirmed PTCI. The PTCI group had a significantly increased mortality (45% vs. 19%, $p < 0.002$), hospital length of stay (LOS) (25 days vs. 18 days, $p < 0.02$), and intensive care unit LOS (21 days vs. 15 days, $p < 0.03$). In multivariate analysis, sex, age, Injury Severity Score, Revised Trauma Score, admission GCS, and brain AIS were not associated with PTCI; whereas the presence of blunt cerebral vascular injury [odds ratio (OR) 4.0, 95% confidence interval (CI) 1.9-8.7], the need for craniotomy (OR 3.0, 95% CI 1.2–6.9), or treatment with recombinant factor VIIa (OR 3.1, 95% CI 1.1–8.0) were each independently associated with an increased risk of PTCI.

Conclusions.—The incidence of PTCI in patients with severe TBI is higher after severe brain injury than previously thought. PTCI has a significant impact on mortality and LOS. The presence of a blunt cerebral vascular injury, the need for craniotomy, or treatment with factor VIIa are risk factors for PTCI. Recognition of this secondary brain insult and the associated risk factors may help identify the group at risk and tailor management of patients with severe TBI.

▶ Secondary cerebral insults such as hypoxia or hypoperfusion have been noted to increase morbidity and mortality for a number of years.[1] This article focuses on a frequently recognized but little discussed complication of traumatic brain injury (TBI), regional cerebral infarction, and identifies risk factors including craniotomy and treatment with recombinant factor VIIa (rFVIIa). Although neither of these observations is surprising, a detailed study such as this has been unavailable up to now. The senior author is particularly noted for extensive experience with rFVIIa in a variety of settings associated with injury. The authors offer a variety of mechanisms for post-traumatic cerebral infarction (PTCI) including embolic events from carotid and other extracranial arteries and local vascular injury associated with direct trauma, regional hemorrhage with compression, or cerebral edema.[2] Craniotomy, as a marker for injury severity, is also associated with cerebral infarction. The important observations in this article are the incidence of blunt cerebrovascular injury (8%) and the increased potential of microvascular and embolic injury to create this phenomenon. RFVIIa, although important in acute control of bleeding, may not improve outcome to the degree originally imagined if microvascular injury and cerebral infarction result. In fact, Mayer and coworkers found in the Factor Seven for Acute Hemorrhagic Stroke (FAST) trial recently published in the *New England Journal of Medicine* that use of rFVIIa controlled hematoma expansion in hemorrhagic stroke but did not improve survival or functional outcome.[3] There are several important lessons here. First, rFVIIa may control bleeding but is not a panacea in the patient with severe TBI, even if associated with significant hemorrhage.[4] Second, risks associated with craniotomy must be expanded to include a small but realistic risk of associated infarction. As strategies for craniotomy and craniectomy are explored, additional criteria for evaluating effectiveness of these interventions should include the incidence and volume of postoperative PTCI. Modern cerebral imaging allows reliable evaluation of this complication. Finally, as interventions are designed to treat the next order of secondary insults with TBI, cerebral infarction must be considered.

D. J. Dries, MSE, MD

References

1. Chestnut RM, Marshall LF, Klauber MR, et al. The role of secondary brain injury in determining outcome from severe head injury. *J Trauma.* 1993;34:216-222.
2. Miller PR, Fabian TC, Croce MA, et al. Prospective screening for blunt cerebrovascular injuries: Analysis of diagnostic modalities and outcomes. *Ann Surg.* 2002;236:386-395.
3. Mayer SA, Brun NC, Begtrup K, et al. Efficacy and safety of recombinant activated factor VII for acute intracerebral hemorrhage. *N Engl J Med.* 2008;358: 2127-2137.
4. Connell KA, Wood JJ, Wise RP, et al. Thromboembolic adverse events after use of recombinant human coagulation factor VIIa. *JAMA.* 2006;295:293-298.

Monitoring brain tissue oxygen tension in brain-injured patients reveals hypoxic episodes in normal-appearing and in peri-focal tissue

Longhi L, Pagan F, Valeriani V, et al (Univ of Milano, Italy)
Intensive Care Med 33:2136-2142, 2007

Objective.—We compared brain tissue oxygen tension (PtiO$_2$) measured in peri-focal and in normal-appearing brain parenchyma on computerized tomography (CT) in patients following traumatic brain injury (TBI).

Design.—Prospective observational study.

Setting.—Neurointensive care unit.

Patients and Participants.—Thirty-two consecutive TBI patients were subjected to PtiO$_2$ monitoring.

Interventions.—Peri-focal tissue was identified by the presence of a hypodense area of the contusion and/or within 1 cm from the core of the contusion. The position of the tip of the PtiO$_2$ probe was assessed at follow-up CT scan.

Measurements and Results.—Mean PtiO$_2$ in the peri-contusional tissue was 19.7 ± 2.1 mmHg and was lower than PtiO$_2$ in normal-appearing tissue (25.5 ± 1.5 mmHg, $p < 0.05$), despite a greater cerebral perfusion pressure (CPP) (73.7 ± 2.3 mmHg vs. 67.4 ± 1.4 mmHg, $p < 0.05$). We observed both in peri-focal tissue and in normal-appearing tissue episodes of brain hypoxia (PtiO$_2$ < 20 mmHg for at least 10 min), whose median duration was longer in peri-focal tissue than in normal-appearing tissue (51% vs. 34% of monitoring time, $p < 0.01$). In peri-focal tissue, we observed a progressive PtiO$_2$ increase from pathologic to normal values ($p < 0.01$).

Conclusions.—Multiple episodes of brain hypoxia occurred over the first 5 days following severe TBI. PtiO$_2$ was lower in peri-contusional tissue than in normal-appearing tissue. In peri-contusional tissue, a progressive increase of PtiO$_2$ from pathologic to normal values was observed over time, suggestive of an improvement at microcirculatory level.

▶ It is becoming increasingly clear that what goes on in the rest of the body doesn't particularly correlate with what is happening in the brain. This seems to be most pertinent in traumatic brain injury. There was an example of this phenomenon with brain hypoglycemia without systemic hypoglycemia that was reported recently.[1] Now we have an example of brain oxygen depletion that doesn't correlate with cerebral perfusion pressure or systemic oxygenation. Moreover, the abnormalities were noted not only in areas of obvious damage (pericontusional white matter with cerebral edema) but also in normal-appearing brain by imaging.

The ramifications of these findings are that invasive brain monitoring may become the norm for patients with brain injury. Although invasive monitoring has its obvious disadvantages, there are increasingly recognized advantages. Particularly when it comes to substrate delivery and use, it is apparent that measuring in the periphery may lead clinicians to undertreat potentially outcome worsening abnormalities. Monitoring techniques in the brain beyond pressure are still in their infancy. As the techniques become validated in multiple settings, intensive care physicians outside the realm of neurology/neurosurgery will have to learn how to use them and evaluate the data. This will be a new horizon for medically- and surgically-focused practitioners who still consider the brain a black box.

J. J. Provencio, MD

Reference

1. Vespa P, Boonyaputthikul R, McArthur DL, et al. Intensive insulin therapy reduces microdialysis glucose values without altering glucose utilization or improving the lactate/pyruvate ratio after traumatic brain injury. *Crit Care Med.* 2006;34: 850-856.

Goal-Directed Fluid Management by Bedside Transpulmonary Hemodynamic Monitoring After Subarachnoid Hemorrhage
Mutoh T, Kazumata K, Ajiki M, et al (Teine Keijinkai Med Ctr, Sapporo, Japan)
Stroke 38:3218-3224, 2007

Background and Purpose.—Optimal monitoring of cardiac output and intravascular volume is of paramount importance for good fluid management of patients with subarachnoid hemorrhage (SAH). The aim of this study was to demonstrate the feasibility of advanced hemodynamic monitoring with transpulmonary thermodilution and to provide descriptive data early after SAH.

Methods.—Forty-six patients with SAH treated within 24 hours of the ictus were investigated. Specific targets for cardiac index (≥ 3.0 L·min^{-1}·m^{-2}), global end-diastolic volume index (700 to 900 mL/m^2), and extravascular lung water index (≤ 14 mL/kg) were established by the single-indicator transpulmonary thermodilution technique, and a fluid management protocol emphasizing supplemental colloid administration was used to attain these targets. Plasma hormones related to stress and fluid regulation were also measured.

Results.—A higher cardiac index (mean value of 5.3 L·min^{-1}·m^{-2}) and a lower global end-diastolic volume index (555 mL/m^2) were observed on initial measurement, for which elevations of plasma adrenaline, noradrenaline, and cortisol were also detected. Cardiac index was progressively decreased (3.5 L·min^{-1}·m^{-2}) and global end-diastolic volume index was normalized by fluid administration aimed at normovolemia. The extent of the initial hemodynamic and hormonal profile was greater in patients with a poor clinical status ($P<0.05$). The extravascular lung water index was mildly elevated but within the target range throughout the study period. No patients developed pulmonary edema or congestive heart failure.

Conclusions.—The impact of sympathetic hyperactivity after SAH predisposes patients to a hyperdynamic and hypovolemic state, especially

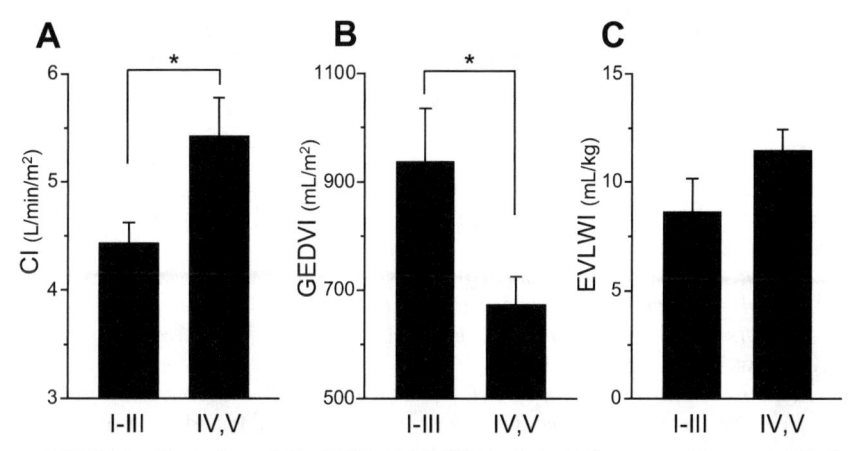

FIGURE 3.—Comparison of CI, GEDVI, and EVLWI between SAH patients with a good (WFNS grades I–III; n = 23) and a poor (grades IV and V; n = 23) clinical grade. These hemodynamic variables were obtained immediately after application of the transpulmonary thermodilution system. *$P<0.05$ vs grades I–III. (Reprinted from Mutoh T, Kazumata K, Ajiki M, et al. Goal-directed fluid management by bedside transpulmonary hemodynamic monitoring after subarachnoid hemorrhage. *Stroke.* 2007;38:3218-3224.)

in those whose clinical status is poor. Bedside monitoring with the transpulmonary thermodilution system may be a powerful tool for the systemic management of such patients (Fig 3).

▶ This study demonstrates that when we try to implement hyperdynamic, hypertensive, and hypervolemic therapy we may accomplish only components of all 3, especially if one of the goals is to prevent the accumulation of extravascular lung water (EVLWI). Furthermore, these authors were indeed able to induce hyperdynamic and hypertensive therapy at lower EVLWI indices, but when they failed to achieve all targets it was because they could not maximize intravascular volume as determined by global end-diastolic volume index (GEDVI). Of concern is whether or not these measures of EVLWI and GEDVI are indeed accurately measuring what they are purported to measure in this population of patients. Furthermore, the most important aspect of these management strategies is their potential association with improvements in outcomes, a factor sorely missing from this article and clearly needed to understand whether this paradigm of monitoring and management is truly a useful paradigm. A peak into these associations can be found in Fig 3 where patients with a worse grade of subarachnoid hemorrhage (SAH) initially demonstrated lower GEDVI; yet, a higher cardiac index (CI) as a marker of the hyperadrenergic state they were in. Importantly, if one had placed a pulmonary artery catheter and used it staticly to determine CI one may have drawn the wrong conclusion as to the adequacy of hyperdynamic, hypertensive, and hypervolemic therapy.

T. Dorman, MD

Nonconvulsive electrographic seizures after traumatic brain injury result in a delayed, prolonged increase in intracranial pressure and metabolic crisis
Vespa PM, Miller C, McArthur D, et al (Univ of California Los Angeles, CA)
Crit Care Med 35:2830-2836, 2007

Objective.—To determine whether nonconvulsive electrographic post-traumatic seizures result in increases in intracranial pressure and microdialysis lactate/pyruvate ratio.
Design.—Prospective monitoring with retrospective data analysis.
Setting.—Single center academic neurologic intensive care unit.
Patients.—Twenty moderate to severe traumatic brain injury patients (Glasgow Coma Score 3–13).
Measurements and Main Results.—Continuous electroencephalography and cerebral microdialysis were performed for 7 days after injury. Ten patients had seizures and were compared with a matched cohort of traumatic brain injury patients without seizures. The seizures were repetitive and constituted status epilepticus in seven of ten patients. Using a within-subject design, post-traumatic seizures resulted in episodic increases in intracranial pressure (22.4 ± 7 vs. 12.8 ± 4.3 mm Hg; $p < .001$) and an episodic increase in lactate/pyruvate ratio (49.4 ± 16 vs. 23.8 ± 7.6; $p < .001$) in the seizure group. Using a between-subjects comparison, the seizure group demonstrated a higher mean intracranial pressure (17.6 ± 6.5 vs. 12.2 ± 4.2 mm Hg; $p < .001$), a higher mean lactate/pyruvate ratio (38.6 ± 18 vs. 27 ± 9; $p < .001$) compared with nonseizure patients. The intracranial pressure and lactate/pyruvate ratio remained elevated beyond postinjury hour 100 in the seizure group but not the nonseizure group ($p < .02$).
Conclusion.—Post-traumatic seizures result in episodic as well as long-lasting increases in intracranial pressure and microdialysis lactate/pyruvate ratio. These data suggest that post-traumatic seizures represent a therapeutic target for patients with traumatic brain injury.

▶ This meticulously prepared and important report sheds light on a common, but nearly invisible, complication of traumatic brain injury–nonconvulsive (NC) seizures. These investigators with painstaking precision document the metabolic and intracranial pressure implications of an underappreciated phenomenon.[1,2,3] Perhaps most concerning are the 2 peaks of seizure activity. The first peak of seizure activity occurred in just over 1 day after injury, whereas the second occurred toward the end of the standard week of anticonvulsive therapy received by these patients.[4] Thus, NC seizures are not eliminated by standard postinjury seizure prophylaxis. It is possible that this prophylaxis reduces the incidence of convulsive seizures while blinding us to NC central nervous system (CNS) insults.

Because of the small number of patients enrolled, there are several critical questions that require answers. First, is there a pattern of injury that increases the likelihood of NC seizures? What is the effect of secondary brain injury (hypotension and hypoxia) on the predisposition to NC seizures? What is the optimal prophylactic strategy? These patients received phenytoin for 7 days, but 7 individuals had silent status epilepticus. Clearly, better drug therapy is needed. It is possible that other nonmedication care strategies could predispose to seizures. It is not clear that other medication use was standardized in these patients. Most important, the impact of seizure activity on outcome awaits evaluation in multiple centers with larger groups of patients. Finally, the importance of electroencephalogram (EEG) monitoring, which I have heard neurointensivists alluding to for several years, seems clear if only to improve the epidemiologic database for a potentially significant problem.

D. J. Dries, MSE, MD

References

1. Vespa PM, Nuwer MR, Nenov V, et al. Increased incidence and impact of nonconclusive and conclusive seizures after traumatic brain injury as detected by continuous electroencephalographic monitoring. *J Neurosurg.* 1999;91:750-760.
2. Claassen J, Mayer SA, Kowalski RG, Emerson RG, Hirsch LJ. Detection of electrographic seizures with continuous EEG monitoring in critically ill patients. *Neurology.* 2004;62:1743-1748.
3. Vespa PM, O'Phelan K, Shah M, et al. Acute seizures after intracerebral hemorrhage: a factor in progressive midline shift and outcome. *Neurology.* 2003;60: 1441-1446.
4. Brain Trauma Foundation, American Association of Neurological Surgeons, Congress of Neurological Surgeons, et al. Guidelines for the management of severe traumatic brain injury. XIII. Antiseizure prophylaxis. *J Neurotrauma.* 2007;24: S83-S86.

Effect of Sedation With Dexmedetomidine vs Lorazepam on Acute Brain Dysfunction in Mechanically Ventilated Patients: The MENDS Randomized Controlled Trial
Pandharipande PP, Pun BT, Herr DL, et al (Vanderbilt Univ Schools of Med and Nursing, Nashville, TN; et al)
JAMA 298:2644-2653, 2007

Context.—Lorazepam is currently recommended for sustained sedation of mechanically ventilated intensive care unit (ICU) patients, but this and other benzodiazepine drugs may contribute to acute brain dysfunction, ie, delirium and coma, associated with prolonged hospital stays, costs, and increased mortality. Dexmedetomidine induces sedation via different central nervous system receptors than the benzodiazepine drugs and may lower the risk of acute brain dysfunction.

Objective.—To determine whether dexmedetomidine reduces the duration of delirium and coma in mechanically ventilated ICU patients while providing adequate sedation as compared with lorazepam.

Design, Setting, Patients, and Intervention.—Double-blind, randomized controlled trial of 106 adult mechanically ventilated medical and surgical ICU patients at 2 tertiary care centers between August 2004 and April 2006. Patients were sedated with dexmedetomidine or lorazepam for as many as 120 hours. Study drugs were titrated to achieve the desired level of sedation, measured using the Richmond Agitation-Sedation Scale (RASS). Patients were monitored twice daily for delirium using the Confusion Assessment Method for the ICU (CAM-ICU).

Main Outcome Measures.—Days alive without delirium or coma and percentage of days spent within 1 RASS point of the sedation goal.

Results.—Sedation with dexmedetomidine resulted in more days alive without delirium or coma (median days, 7.0 vs 3.0; $P = .01$) and a lower prevalence of coma (63% vs 92%; $P < .001$) than sedation with lorazepam. Patients sedated with dexmedetomidine spent more time within 1 RASS point of their sedation goal compared with patients sedated with lorazepam (median percentage of days, 80% vs 67%; $P = .04$). The 28-day mortality in the dexmedetomidine group was 17% vs 27% in the lorazepam group ($P = .18$) and cost of care was similar between groups. More patients in the dexmedetomidine group (42% vs 31%; $P = .61$) were able to complete post-ICU neuropsychological testing, with similar scores in the tests evaluating global cognitive, motor speed, and attention functions. The 12-month time to death was 363 days in the dexmedetomidine group vs 188 days in the lorazepam group ($P = .48$).

Conclusion.—In mechanically ventilated ICU patients managed with individualized targeted sedation, use of a dexmedetomidine infusion resulted in more days alive without delirium or coma and more time at the targeted level of sedation than with a lorazepam infusion.

TABLE 2.—Outcomes in Mechanically Ventilated Patients Sedated With Dexmedetomidine vs Lorazepam[a]

Outcome Variable	Dexmedetomidine (n = 52)	Lorazepam (n = 51)	P Value
Duration of brain organ dysfunction, d			
Delirium-free and coma-free[b]	7 (1-10)	3 (1-6)	.01
Delirium-free[b]	9 (5-11)	7 (5-10)	.09
Coma-free[b]	10 (9-12)	8 (5-10)	<.001
Delirium	2.5 (1-5)	4 (1-5)	.71
Coma	2 (0-3)	3 (2-5)	.003
Prevalence of brain organ dysfunction, No. (%)[c]			
Delirium or coma	45 (87)	50 (98)	.03
Delirium	41 (79)	42 (82)	.65
Coma	33 (63)	47 (92)	<.001
Other clinical outcomes			
Mechanical ventilator-free, d[d]	22 (0-24)	18 (0-23)	.22
Intensive care unit length of stay, d	7.5 (5-19)	9 (6-15)	.92
28-Day mortality, No. (%)	9 (17)	14 (27)	.18

[a]Median (interquartile range) unless otherwise noted.
[b]Indicates the number of days alive without stated dysfunction from study days 1 to 12.
[c]Prevalence is used to describe the rates of brain organ dysfunction instead of incidence because preintensive care unit delirium or coma status could not be determined. Prevalence represents the occurrence of brain organ dysfunction at any time during the 12-day assessment period.
[d]Indicates the number of days alive, breathing without mechanical ventilator assistance, from study day 1 to 28.
(Reprinted from Pandharipande PP, Pun BT, Herr DL, et al. Effect of sedation with dexmedetomidine vs lorazepam on acute brain dysfunction in mechanically ventilated patients: the MENDS randomized controlled trial. *JAMA.* 2007;298:2644-2653, with permission from the American Medical Association.)

TABLE 3.—Efficacy of Sedation With Dexmedetomidine vs Lorazepam[a]

Variable	Dexmedetomidine (n = 52)	Lorazepam (n = 51)	P Value
Outcome			
Received study drug, d	5 (2-6)	4 (2-6)	.52
RASS score within 1 point of nurse goal, % (IQR)[b]	80 (58-100)	67 (48-83)	.04
RASS score within 1 point of physician goal, % (IQR)[b]	67 (50-85)	55 (8-67)	.008
Sedated deeper than nurse goal RASS score, % (IQR)[c]	15 (0-33)	33 (11-48)	.01
Oversedated on study drug, d	1 (0-2.2)	2 (1-3.5)	.01
Other drugs received during study			
Median fentanyl, μg/d	575 (140-2206)	150 (0-922)	.006
Any antipsychotics, No. (%)	24 (46)	18 (35)	.26
Any propofol, No. (%)	7 (13)	4 (8)	.36
Received antipsychotics, d	0 (0-5)	0 (0-3)	.32

Abbreviations: IQR, interquartile range; RASS, Richmond Agitation-Sedation Scale.
[a]Median (IQR) unless otherwise noted.
[b]The nurse and physician goal RASS score outcomes indicate the percentage of days while on study drug when patients were either at goal or within 1 RASS point of the stated goal.
[c]Percentage of days the RASS scores were 2 or more points deeper than the nurse goal for RASS score.
(Reprinted from Pandharipande PP, Pun BT, Herr DL, et al. Effect of sedation with dexmedetomidine vs lorazepam on acute brain dysfunction in mechanically ventilated patients: the MENDS randomized controlled trial. *JAMA*. 2007;298:2644-2653, with permission from the American Medical Association.)

Trial Registration.—clinicaltrials.gov Identifier: NCT00095251 (Tables 2 and 3).

▶ Sedating critically ill patients and avoiding unwanted side effects is an important clinical goal. This well-popularized study seems to support the use of dexmedetomidine (DEX) for ICU sedation as compared with lorazepam if one desires to limit the combined outcome of delirium and coma in critically ill patients. These results are best seen in Table 2. It should, however, be noted that there was no difference in the rate of delirium, and the primary outcome benefit was driven solely by a difference in coma rate. Given the nurses were to target a specific sedation level that presumably did not include coma, it is hard to tease out whether the benefits accrued were attributable to DEX as a drug effect or whether these outcomes were attributable to the provider. Obviously if the providers can't effectively use a particular agent this is of great concern and should lead us away from such an agent. However, this study was not designed to evaluate the impact of focused training on provider performance. This is especially important given the therapy with DEX cost about twice as much as lorazepam. Table 3 seems to show that the nurses and physicians had different sedation goals for these patients, which in and of itself is possibly the most fascinating finding in this study.

T. Dorman, MD

Hyponatremia in neurological patients: cerebral salt wasting versus inappropriate antidiuretic hormone secretion

Brimioulle S, Orellana-Jimenez C, Aminian A, et al (Free Univ of Brussels, Belgium)
Intensive Care Med 34:125-131, 2008

Objective.—To assess whether hyponatremia in acute neurological patients is associated with the syndrome of inappropriate antidiuretic hormone secretion (SIADH) or with the cerebral salt-wasting syndrome (CSWS).

Design.—Clinical, controlled, prospective study.

Setting.—Department of intensive care of a tertiary care academic hospital.

Patients.—Forty acute neurological patients with hyponatremia suggesting SIADH or CSWS (20) or with normonatremia (20).

Interventions.—None.

Measurements and Main Results.—Measurement of clinical and biological variables. Measurement of blood, plasma, and red blood cell volumes to discriminate SIADH and CSWS. Renal, adrenal and thyroid functions were normal in all patients. Average blood, plasma, and red blood cell volumes were 54, 37 and 17 ml/kg in control patients and 54, 37 and 18 ml/kg in hyponatremic patients, respectively.

Conclusions.—The adequate blood volumes in hyponatremic patients confirm the diagnosis of SIADH and do not support the concept of CSWS.

▶ The debate over the syndrome of inappropriate antidiuretic hormone secretion (SIADH) versus cerebral salt-wasting syndrome (CSWS) in patients with neurologic injury has been hotly contested since Wijdicks published the first report of worsening neurologic outcome with volume restriction in patients with low sodium and subarachnoid hemorrhage (SAH) in 1985.[1] Now Brimioulle and colleagues have opened the debate again. In their study, they tested 20 patients with neurologic disease who had hyponatremia and no clinical evidence of volume depletion. In this group, they found that they did indeed have volume depletion compared with normal subjects. They also tested a group of neurologic patients with normonatremia and found the same volume depletion. Finally, CSWS has been best described in SAH patients. It is unclear if this is an entity seen in most of the patients with traumatic brain injury in this study.

They conclude that the volume depletion is an inherent property of neurologic critical care and that it is normal for this population, therefore supporting the diagnosis of SIADH in all the patients.

This finding is short-sighted and in many ways misses the point. First, a more appropriate control would have been patients in a critical care setting with no brain injury and hyponatremia thought to be because of SIADH. Because there is no inherent reason why brain-injured patients should develop low volume in the intensive care unit (ICU), comparing these patients with true SIADH critically ill patients would have been more appropriate. Second, choosing patients who are clinically not volume depleted favors the result of SIADH. It is likely that these flaws in the study made the findings a forgone conclusion. To summarize the findings, one could make the statement that "The major theoretic distinction between SIADH and CSWS is the presence of hypovolemia in CSWS. This study shows that all patients in the study were hypovolemic and therefore must have CSWS." The authors came to the opposite conclusion that because all patients were hypovolemic, hypovolemia must be normovolemia in neurologic patients and, therefore, the diagnosis of SIADH is more appropriate.

Although it is true that neurologic intensivists have become enamored with the diagnosis of CSWS, administering hypertonic salt solutions to patients who clearly have SIADH, there is 1 population in which, regardless of how the hyponatremia is defined, treatment decision can make a great difference. In SAH, Wijdicks showed that treatment of hyponatremia with volume restriction led to increase in stroke during vasospasm and worse outcome. This then becomes a concern. If the authors are right, in that all hyponatremia in neurologic patients is because of SIADH, then there is a population in which the treatment for SIADH is contraindicated. This may be too nuanced an argument for the bedside. Better to just call it CSWS so that the patient gets appropriate treatment.

J. J. Provencio, MD

Reference

1. Wijdicks EF, Vermeulen M, Hijdra A, et al. Hyponatremia and cerebral infarction in patients with ruptured intracranial aneurysms: is fluid restriction harmful? *Ann Neurol.* 1985;17:137-140.

Emergency Administration of Abciximab for Treatment of Patients With Acute Ischemic Stroke: Results of an International Phase III Trial: Abciximab in Emergency Treatment of Stroke Trial (AbESTT-II)
Adams HP Jr, Effron MB, Torner J, et al (Univ of Iowa, Iowa City)
Stroke 39:87-99, 2008

Background and Purpose.—A previous randomized, placebo-controlled, double-blind study suggested that abciximab may be safe and effective in treatment of acute ischemic stroke. The current phase 3 study was planned to test the relative efficacy and safety of abciximab in patients with acute ischemic stroke with planned treatment within 5 hours since symptoms onset.

Methods.—An international, randomized, placebo-controlled, double-blind phase 3 trial tested intravenous administration of abciximab in 2 study cohorts using stratification variables of time since onset and stroke severity. The planned enrollment was 1800 patients. The primary cohort enrolled those patients who could be treated within 5 hours of onset of stroke. A companion cohort enrolled patients that were treated 5 to 6 hours after stroke as well as a smaller cohort of patients who could be treated within 3 hours of stroke present on awakening. The primary efficacy measure was the dichotomous modified Rankin Scale score at 3 months as adjusted to the baseline severity of stroke among subjects in the primary cohort. The primary safety outcome was the rate of symptomatic or fatal intracranial hemorrhage that occurred within 5 days of stroke.

Results.—The trial was terminated prematurely after 808 patients in all cohorts were enrolled by recommendation of an independent safety and efficacy monitoring board due to an unfavorable benefit-risk profile. At 3 months, approximately 33% of patients assigned placebo (72/218) and 32% of patients assigned abciximab (71/221; $P = 0.944$) in the primary cohort were judged to have a favorable response to treatment. The distributions of outcomes on the modified Rankin Scale were similar between the treated and control groups. Within 5 days of enrollment, $\approx 5.5\%$ of abciximab-treated and 0.5% of placebo-treated patients in the primary cohort had symptomatic or fatal intracranial hemorrhage ($P = 0.002$). The trial also did not demonstrate an improvement in outcomes with abciximab among patients in the companion and wake-up cohorts. Although the number of patients was small, an increased rate of hemorrhage was noted within 5 days among patients in the wake-up population who received abciximab (13.6% versus 5% for placebo).

Conclusions.—This trial did not demonstrate either safety or efficacy of intravenous administration of abciximab for the treatment of patients with acute ischemic stroke regardless of end point or population studied. There was an increased rate of symptomatic or fatal intracranial hemorrhage in the primary and wake-up cohorts.

▶ Treatment for acute stroke has been relegated to the intravenous (IV) administration of tissue plasminogen activator (tPA) for the last 13 years. The realization that many patients do not qualify for, or if they do qualify they do not respond to, tPA has put pressure on the medical establishment to develop complementary or parallel therapies to offer patients. The research has moved in 2 directions—intra-arterial therapies to disrupt clot, and new IV thrombolytics. Trials with modified plasminogen activators have failed despite promising early results.[1,2] The Abciximab in Emergency Stroke Treatment Trial-II (AbESTT-II) trial was an attempt to use a therapy that was not a plasminogen activator. In this case, they tried the glycoprotein IIa/IIIb receptor antagonist, abciximab within 5 hours of the onset of stroke.

The most daunting challenge for the treatment of acute stroke with thrombolytic therapies is the interplay between efficacy of the therapy and the risk of bleeding. This trial was stopped early because of an excessive bleeding risk and mortality in patients who received abciximab compared with placebo.

It is becoming apparent that bleeding risk in thrombolysis is what separates therapies in stroke from the relatively successful treatments for acute myocardial infarction. Overcoming this hurdle is going to be a challenge.

J. J. Provencio, MD

References

1. Haley EC Jr, Lyden PD, Johnston KC, Hemmen TM, et al. TNK in Stroke Investigators. A pilot dose-escalation safety study of tenecteplase in acute ischemic stroke. *Stroke*. 2005;36:607-612.
2. Hacke W Preliminary results of the Desmoteplase In Acute Ischemic Stroke 2 (DIAS-2) trial. Presented at the 16th European Stroke Conference. May 29-June 1, 2007.

Dose–response relationship of mannitol and intracranial pressure: a metaanalysis
Sorani MD, Manley GT (Univ of California, San Francisco)
J Neurosurg 108:80-87, 2008

Object.—Brain edema can increase intracranial pressure (ICP), potentially leading to ischemia, herniation, and death. Edema and elevated ICP are often treated with osmotic agents to remove water from brain tissue. Mannitol is the osmotic diuretic most commonly used in the intensive care unit; however, despite its clinical importance, treatment protocols vary from center to center, and the dose–response relationship is not understood. The goal of this metaanalysis was to aggregate and analyze data from studies in which authors have described the dose–response relationship between mannitol and ICP.

Methods.—The authors identified 18 studies that quantitatively characterized the dose–response relationship of mannitol and ICP. We also examined study designs and mannitol administration protocols.

Results.—Meta-regression found a weak linear relationship between change in ICP (ΔICP) and dose (ΔICP = 6.6 × dose − 1.1; p = 0.27, R^2 = 0.05). The lack of statistical significance could reflect the variation in protocols among studies and the variation in patients both within and among studies. However, the authors found a highly significant difference (p < 0.001) in decrease in ICP when the initial ICP was higher or lower than 30 mm Hg. Nonlinear regression suggested that ICP decrease is greatest shortly after mannitol is given (R^2 = 0.63). Finally, the authors found that recent studies tend to include fewer patients and set a lower ICP threshold for mannitol administration but report more parameters of interest; the duration of mannitol's effect was the most frequently unreported parameter.

Conclusions.—Despite its clinical importance, the determination of the mannitol dose–response curve continues to be challenging for many reasons. This metaanalysis highlights the need for a consensus of methods and results required to determine this important relationship.

▶ Mannitol has been a mainstay of treatment for increased intracranial pressure (ICP) in the 1970s. Despite this, little is known about the mechanism of mannitol's action and the efficacy of treatment. This is most obvious in the Brain Trauma Foundation Guidelines for ICP management where the recommendation is to administer a weight-adjusted dose of mannitol between 0.25 g/kg to 1.00 g/kg.[1] This wide range of dose is indicative of an absence of evidence.

This work by Sorani and Manley attempts to address this issue using previous studies of mannitol therapy in ICP management. Unfortunately, the variability of the previous studies precludes a definitive understanding of the dose kinetics of mannitol. It does confirm that mannitol is an effective therapy for the treatment of ICP. It, for the first time, makes the correlation between the initial ICP and efficacy of mannitol. The authors recommend a larger rigorous study to settle this issue.

There is an interesting finding hidden in this study to which the authors allude but is often overlooked by clinicians. The most common understanding of the mechanism of mannitol therapy is that the osmotic pressure generated by the administration creates an osmotic gradient that takes water out of the brain. Fig 3 in the original article shows that the magnitude of ICP decline is greatest in the first 10 minutes. This is likely too fast to be attributed to an osmotic gradient. The authors propose a rheostatic theory that has been presented in the past. It is likely that mannitol works by multiple mechanisms to lower ICP. This bears further study.

J. J. Provencio, MD

Reference

1. Sorani MD, Manley GT. Dose-response relationship of mannitol and intracranial pressure: a metaanalysis. *J Neurosurg.* 2008;108:80-87.

Noninvasive Ventilation in Myasthenic Crisis
Seneviratne J, Mandrekar J, Wijdicks EFM, et al (Mayo Clinic, Rochester, MN)
Arch Neurol 65:54-58, 2008

Background.—Myasthenic crisis (MC) is often associated with prolonged intubation and with respiratory complications.

Objectives.—To assess predictors of ventilation duration and to compare the effectiveness of endotracheal intubation and mechanical ventilation (ET-MV) with bilevel positive airway pressure (BiPAP) noninvasive ventilation in MC.

Design.—Retrospective cohort study.

Setting.—Academic research.

Patients.—We reviewed consecutive episodes of MC treated at the Mayo Clinic, Rochester, Minnesota.

Main Outcome Measures.—Collected information included patients' demographic data, immunotherapy, medical complications, mechanical ventilation duration, and hospital lengths of stay, as well as baseline and preventilation measurements of forced vital capacity, maximal inspiratory and expiratory pressures, and arterial blood gases.

Results.—We identified 60 episodes of MC in 52 patients. BiPAP was the initial method of ventilatory support in 24 episodes and ET-MV was performed in 36 episodes. There were no differences in patient demographics or in baseline respiratory variables and arterial gases between the groups of episodes initially treated using BiPAP vs ET-MV. In 14 episodes treated using BiPAP, intubation was avoided. The mean duration of BiPAP in these patients was 4.3 days. The only predictor of BiPAP failure (ie, requirement for intubation) was a P_{CO_2} level exceeding 45 mm Hg on BiPAP initiation ($P = .04$). The mean ventilation duration was 10.4 days. Longer ventilation duration was associated with intubation ($P = .02$), atelectasis ($P < .005$), and lower maximal expiratory pressure on arrival ($P = .02$). The intensive care unit and hospital lengths of stay statistically significantly increased with ventilation duration ($P < .001$ for both). The only variable associated with decreased ventilation duration was initial BiPAP treatment ($P < .007$).

Conclusions.—BiPAP is effective for the treatment of acute respiratory failure in patients with myasthenia gravis. A BiPAP trial before the development of hypercapnia can prevent intubation and prolonged ventilation, reducing pulmonary complications and lengths of intensive care unit and hospital stay.

▶ This retrospective study spans almost 20 years of experience caring for patients with myasthenic crisis (MC). One can argue that over 20 years there were many changes in our approach to management of MC and our ability to skillfully use noninvasive ventilatory support. Nonetheless, the conclusion that those patients with MS who can be managed with noninvasive ventilatory support and avoid endotracheal intubation will have a shorter hospital course and better outcome. Another interesting finding was the failure of the traditional bedside tools used to evaluate respiratory muscle function to predict the success or failure of ventilatory support.

R. A. Balk, MD

Arterial gas embolism: a review of cases at Prince of Wales Hospital, Sydney, 1996 to 2006
Trytko BE, Bennett MH (Prince of Wales Hosp, Sydney, NSW, Australia)
Anaesth Intensive Care 36:60-64, 2008

Arterial gas embolism may occur as a complication of diving or certain medical procedures. Although relatively rare, the consequences may be disastrous. Recent articles in the critical care literature suggest the non-hyperbaric medical community may not be aware of the role for hyperbaric oxygen therapy in non-diving related gas embolism. This review is part of an Australian appraisal of experience in the management of arterial gas embolism over the last 10 years.

We identified all patients referred to Prince of Wales Hospital Department of Diving and Hyperbaric Medicine with a diagnosis of arterial gas embolism from 1996 to 2006. Twenty-six patient records met our selection criteria, eight iatrogenic and 18 diving related. All patients were treated initially with a 280 kPa compression schedule. At discharge six patients were left with residual symptoms. Four were left with minor symptoms that did not significantly impact quality of life. Two remained severely affected with major neurological injury. Both had non-diving-related arterial gas embolism.

There was a good outcome in the majority of patients who presented with arterial gas embolism and were treated with compression.

▶ The authors state that hyperbaric therapy is underused for nondiving-related arterial gas embolism (AGE) in critically ill patients principally because practitioners fail to think of it. Thus they present a case series of patients seen at their center. Unfortunately, the limitations of the article potentially compromise its ability to draw attention to an efficacious therapy. As a case series it is subject to significant referral bias. Most importantly although is the fact that the authors want to stress nondiving-related episodes of gas embolism but present a series in which 18 of the 26 patients have had diving-related accidents. This significantly limits any potential lessons learned from this case series. In addition, the 8 patients who had nondiving-related events undergo a variety of treatment regimens, some of which also included treatment with Heliox. I would hope that despite these limitations that these authors have indeed reminded the critical care community that hyperbaric therapy should at least be considered for AGE patients not because it's a perioperative evidence-based therapy but because through pathophysiologic reasoning it makes sense that it should have efficacy in these syndromes. Of note, however, is that a formal study would be beneficial because it is possible that despite the potential clinical efficacy of the treatment itself, that the difficulty in providing full critical care services to the critically ill during the therapy could, in theory counterbalance any benefit.

T. Dorman, MD

Beta-Blockers in Isolated Blunt Head Injury
Inaba K, Teixeira PGR, David J-S, et al (Univ of Southern California, Los Angeles, CA; Claude Bernard Univ, Lyons, France; et al)
J Am Coll Surg 206:432-438, 2008

Background.—The purpose of this study was to evaluate the effect of β-blockers on patients sustaining acute traumatic brain injury. Our hypothesis was that β-blocker exposure is associated with improved survival.

Study Design.—The trauma registry and the surgical ICU databases of an academic Level I trauma center were used to identify all patients sustaining blunt head injury requiring ICU admission from July 1998 to

December 2005. Patients sustaining major associated injuries (Abbreviated Injury Score ≥ 4 in any body region other than the head) were excluded. Patient demographics, injury profile, Injury Severity Score, and β-blocker exposure were abstracted. The primary outcomes measure evaluated was in-hospital mortality.

Results.—During the 90-month study period, 1,156 patients with isolated head injury were admitted to the ICU. Of these, 203 (18%) received β-blockers and 953 (82%) did not. Patients receiving β-blockers were older (50 ± 21 years versus 38 ± 20 years, p < 0.001), had more frequent severe (Abbreviated Injury Score ≥ 4) head injury (54% versus 43%, p < 0.01), Glasgow Coma Scale ≤ 8 less often (37% versus 47%, p = 0.01), more skull fractures (20% versus 12%, p < 0.01), and underwent craniectomy more frequently (23% versus 4%, p < 0.001). Stepwise logistic regression identified β-blocker use as an independent protective factor for mortality (adjusted odds ratio: 0.54; 95% CI, 0.33 to 0.91; p = 0.01). On subgroup analysis, elderly patients (55 years or older) with severe head injury (Abbreviated Injury Score ≥ 4) had a mortality of 28% on β-blockers as compared with 60% when they did not receive them (odds ratio: 0.3; 96% CI, 0.1 to 0.6; p = 0.001).

Conclusions.—Beta-blockade in patients with traumatic brain injury was independently associated with improved survival. Older patients with severe head injuries demonstrated the largest reduction in mortality with β-blockade.

▶ This is the largest retrospective trial to date examining the impact of β-blockade on outcome in patients sustaining traumatic brain injury (TBI).[1,2] As noted in the abstract, there were multiple differences between patients who received β-blockade and those who did not receive this therapy. In addition, there was no consistent β-blocker regimen provided. Nonetheless, head-injured patients, particularly the elderly appeared to sustain benefit with use of β-blockade during the course of hospitalization. The authors admit that the reason for this outcome is unknown. An attractive hypothesis, however, is suppression of inappropriate catecholamine output that has been identified in both clinical and preclinical settings after various forms of TBI.[3,4] In patients with TBI undergoing plasma norepinephrine (NE) sampling, for example, abnormal NE levels were inversely proportional to the patient's Glasgow Coma Score. Where NE levels normalized, injury outcome appeared to be improved. Unfortunately, there are no data to demonstrate the impact of any form of β-blocker administration on NE levels. Elevated catecholamines may contribute to cerebral vasospasm and administration of β-blockers may help deflect this process and protect remote organs, particularly the cardiopulmonary system from adverse effects of excessive catecholamine release.[5]

D. J. Dries, MSE, MD

References

1. Arbabi S, Campion EM, Hemmila MR, et al. Beta-blocker use is associated with improved outcomes in adult trauma patients. *J Trauma.* 2007;62:56-62.

2. Cotton BA, Snodgrass KB, Fleming SB, et al. Beta-blocker exposure is associated with improved survival after severe traumatic brain injury. *J Trauma*. 2007;62: 26-33.
3. Cruickshank JM, Neil-Dwyer G, Degaute JP, et al. Reduction of stress-catecholamine-induced cardiac necrosis by beta 1-selective blockade. *Lancet*. 1987;2: 585-589.
4. Colgan FJ, Sawa T, Teneyck LG, Izzo JL Jr. Protective effects of beta blockade on pulmonary function when intracranial pressure is elevated. *Crit Care Med*. 1983; 11:368-372.
5. Chai CL, Tu YK, Huang SJ. Can cerebral hypoperfusion after sympathetic storm be used to diagnose brain death? A retrospective survey in traumatic brain injury patients. *J Trauma*. 2008;64:688-697.

Effect of Equiosmolar Solutions of Mannitol versus Hypertonic Saline on Intraoperative Brain Relaxation and Electrolyte Balance

Rozet I, Tontisirin N, Muangman S, et al (Univ of Washington, Seattle, WA)
Anesthesiology 107:697-704, 2007

Background.—The purpose of the study was to compare the effect of equiosmolar solutions of mannitol and hypertonic saline (HS) on brain relaxation and electrolyte balance.

Methods.—After institutional review board approval and informed consent, patients with American Society of Anesthesiologists physical status II–IV, scheduled to undergo craniotomy for various brain pathologies, were enrolled into this prospective, randomized, double-blind study. Patients received 5 ml/kg 20% mannitol (n = 20) or 3% HS (n = 20). Partial pressure of carbon dioxide in arterial blood was maintained at 35–40 mmHg, and central venous pressure was maintained at 5 mmHg or greater. Hemodynamic variables, fluid balance, blood gases, electrolytes, lactate, and osmolality (blood, cerebrospinal fluid, urine) were measured at 0, 15, 30, and 60 min and 6 h after infusion; arteriovenous difference of oxygen, glucose, and lactate were calculated. The surgeon assessed brain relaxation on a four-point scale (1 = relaxed, 2 = satisfactory, 3 = firm, 4 = bulging). Appropriate statistical tests were used for comparison; $P < 0.05$ was considered significant.

Results.—There was no difference in brain relaxation (mannitol = 2, HS = 2 points; $P = 0.8$) or cerebral arteriovenous oxygen and lactate difference between HS and mannitol groups. Urine output with mannitol was higher than with HS ($P < 0.03$) and was associated with higher blood lactate over time ($P < 0.001$, compared with HS). Cerebrospinal fluid osmolality increased at 6 h in both groups ($P < 0.05$, compared with baseline). HS caused an increase in sodium in cerebrospinal fluid over time ($P < 0.001$, compared with mannitol).

Conclusion.—Mannitol and HS cause an increase in cerebrospinal fluid osmolality, and are associated with similar brain relaxation scores and arteriovenous oxygen and lactate difference during craniotomy.

▶ Previous attempts to evaluate the effects of these 2 agents did not control for osmolarity. This study is the first to provide equimolar solutions but, unfortunately, the measure of brain relaxation was subjective and not objective. Furthermore, this measure was not previously validated by intraobserver or interobserver analysis. Not withstanding those limitations, the study is well done and offers a few insights. In Fig 1, in the original article, it can be seen that the osmolality of blood and cerebrospinal fluid (CSF) were equally affected by the administered fluids. Importantly, the impact of the fluid could be seen as early as 15 minutes after administration and the effect persisted for the 6 hours that were studied. It should also be noted that the 15-minute time point was the first studied and so, in fact, the impact may have been even faster. The similarity in osmolar response seemed to parallel the similarity in subjective relaxation. An important difference, however, can be seen in Fig 3 in the original article where arterial lactate was not elevated early during the study period but was elevated in the mannitol group implying some differences in systemic perfusion or flow.

T. Dorman, MD

Recognition and labeling of delirium symptoms by intensivists: Does it matter?
Cheung CZ, Alibhai SMH, Robinson M, et al (Univ of Toronto, Toronto, ON; Queen's Univ, Kingston, ON; et al)
Intensive Care Med 34:437-446, 2008

Objective.—The approach to acute cognitive dysfunction varies among physicians, including intensivists. Physicians may differ in their labeling of cognitive abnormalities in critically ill patients. We aimed to survey: (a) what Canadian intensive care unit (ICU) physicians identify as "delirium"; (b) choices of non-pharmacological and pharmacological management; and (c) consultation patterns among ICU patients with cognitive abnormalities.

Design.—A mail-in self-administered survey was sent to Canadian intensivists registered with the Canadian Critical Care Society. The survey contained three clinical scenarios which described cognitively abnormal patients with: (a) hepatic encephalopathy; (b) multiple drug overdose; and (c) post-operative aortic aneurysm repair. Symptoms, which included fluctuating level of consciousness, inattention, disorientation, hallucinations, sleep/wake cycle disturbance, and paranoia, all fulfilled DSM-IV criteria for delirium. We asked for diagnoses in short-answer format for each scenario, and offered multiple selections of non-pharmacological and pharmacological therapies and consultation options.

Participants.—All intensivists registered with the Canadian Critical Care Society.

Measurements and Results.—One-hundred thirty surveys were returned, for a response rate of 58.3%. When an etiological cognitive dysfunction diagnosis was obvious, 83–85% responded with the medical diagnosis to explain the cognitive abnormalities; only 43–55% used the term "delirium". In contrast, where an underlying medical problem was lacking, 74% of respondents diagnosed "delirium" ($p = 0.002$). Non-pharmacological and pharmacological management varied considerably by physician and scenario but independently from whether the term "delirium" was selected. Commonly selected pharmacological agents were antipsychotics and benzodiazepines, followed by narcotics, non-narcotic analgesics, and other sedatives. Whether and when intensivists chose to consult other services varied.

Conclusions.—Canadian intensivists diagnose delirium based upon the presence or absence of an obvious medical etiology. Wide variation exists in approach to management, as well as patterns of consultation (Figs 1 and 2).

▶ Delirium appears to be a frequent occurrence in ICU patients, and a growing body of literature implies an association with higher rates of morbidity and mortality. Thus a better understanding of delirium, its risk factors, assessment tools, and therapeutic options is required. This study evaluates how care providers think about the diagnosis of delirium by use of 3 case vignettes.

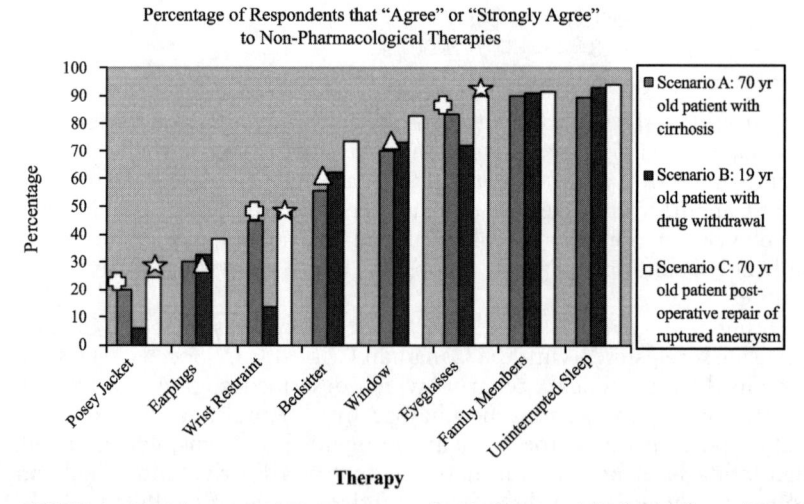

FIGURE 1.—Non-pharmacological management. *Star* indicates statistically significant difference between scenarios B and C ($p < 0.05$); *cross* indicates statistically significant difference between scenarios A and B ($p < 0.05$); *triangle* indicates statistically significant difference between scenarios A and C ($p < 0.05$). (Reprinted from Cheung CZ, Alibhai SMH, Robinson M, et al. Recognition and labeling of delirium symptoms by intensivists: does it matter? *Intensive Care Med.* 2008;34:437-446, with kind permission from Springer Science+Business Media. Copyright 2008.)

Chapter 11–Neurologic: Traumatic and Non-traumatic / 231

Drug Therapies by Scenario

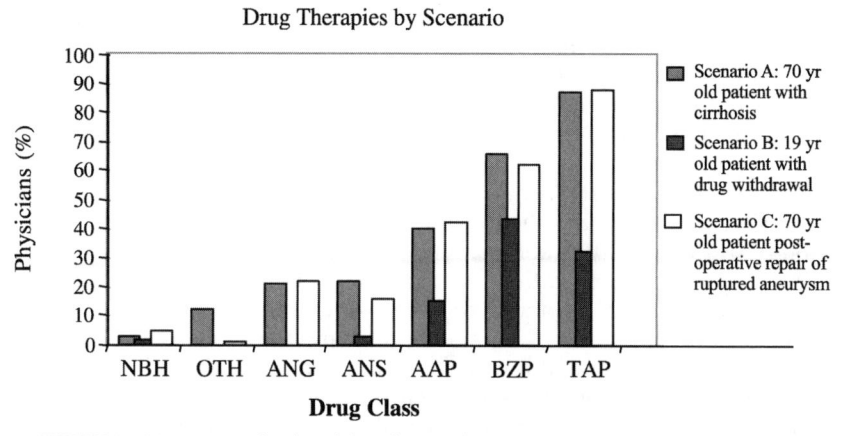

FIGURE 2.—Most commonly selected drug therapies by scenario ($n = 130$). Drug Class: *AAP*, atypical antipsychotic; *ANG*, analgesic; *ANS*, anesthetic; *BZP*, benzodiazepine; *NBH*, nonbenzodiazepine hypnotic; *OTH*, other; *TAP*, typical antipsychotic. (Reprinted from Cheung CZ, Alibhai SMH, Robinson M, et al. Recognition and labeling of delirium symptoms by intensivists: does it matter? *Intensive Care Med.* 2008;34:437-446, with kind permission from Springer Science+Business Media. Copyright, 2008.)

Importantly, the study found a high degree of variability in the recognition of delirium, labeling the patient as delirious and for the intended pharmacologic and nonpharmacologic interventions (Figs 1 and 2). Clearly, this variability will compromise future research attempts, and this study helps to establish the fact that the variability itself needs to be an early target for improvement. Unfortunately, the study did not evaluate whether or not participants used objectives scales for delirium. Additionally, if a participant identified a medical cause of altered consciousness like encephalopathy, it is not clear if they clearly understood that they also needed to mark the patient as delirious; thus, the finding regarding diagnosis frequency may be in question. Finally, most intensivists are from a medical background, and it is not clear how this may have impacted the results.

T. Dorman, MD

IMPACT OF NOSOCOMIAL INFECTIOUS COMPLICATIONS AFTER SUBARACHNOID HEMORRHAGE
Frontera JA, Fernandez A, Schmidt JM, et al (Mount Sinai School of Medicine, New York, NY; Columbia Univ College of Physicians and Surgeons, New York, NY)
Neurosurgery 62:80-87, 2008

Objective.—Critically ill neurological patients are susceptible to infections that may be distinct from other intensive care patients. The aim of this study is to quantify the prevalence, risk factors, and effect on the outcome of nosocomial infectious complications in patients with subarachnoid hemorrhage (SAH).

Methods.—We studied 573 consecutive patients with SAH, identified the most prevalent infectious complications, and performed univariate analyses to determine risk factors for each complication. Multiple logistic regression models were constructed to calculate adjusted odds ratios for associated risk factors and to assess the impact of infectious complications on 3-month outcome as evaluated with the modified Rankin Scale.

Results.—The most prevalent nosocomial infections were pneumonia (n = 114, 20%), urinary tract infection (n = 77, 13%), bloodstream infection (BSI) (n = 48, 8%), and meningitis/ventriculitis (n = 28, 5%). Significant independent associations with pneumonia included older age, poor Hunt and Hess grade, intubation/mechanical ventilation, and loss of consciousness at ictus. Urinary tract infection was associated with female sex and central line use. BSI was also associated with central line use, and meningitis/ventriculitis was associated with the presence of intraventricular hemorrhage and external ventricular drainage (all $P < 0.05$). After adjustment for Hunt and Hess grade, aneurysm size, and age, pneumonia (adjusted odds ratio, 2.04; 95% confidence interval, 1.12–3.71; $P = 0.020$) and BSI (adjusted odds ratio, 2.51; 95% confidence interval, 1.14–5.56; $P = 0.023$) independently predicted death or severe disability at 3 months. Prolonged length of stay was significantly associated with all infection types ($P < 0.001$).

Conclusion.—Pneumonia and BSI are common infectious complications of SAH and independently predict poor outcome. The implementation of infection-control measures may be needed to improve outcome after SAH.

▶ Neurologic intensive care has grown from the need to manage patients whose complex medical problems demand an understanding of both neurology/neurosurgery and more general critical care. This study by Frontera and colleagues is another example of how non-neurological complications in subarachnoid hemorrhage (SAH) importantly impact the prognosis of our patients.

In this retrospective study, the authors evaluate the impact of the 4 most common infections in patients with aneurysmal SAH: pneumonia, urinary tract infections, bloodstream infections, and meningitis/ventriculitis. There are concerns about the way that particularly meningitis/ventriculitis are diagnosed both in this study and in general clinical practice, but the authors chose a reasonable definition.

The findings are quite striking. Pneumonia has an independent risk of death or poor outcome of more than 2 times. Similarly, the risk of death or poor outcome in blood stream infections was 2.5 times. Fig 1, in the original article, shows the actual mortality of patients with and without these infections. The sobering truth remains that most interventions we are investigating for brain injury will have far lower benefit in mortality than reducing the incidence of nosocomial pneumonia. Yet little research in the neurological and neurosurgical intensive care unit fields is devoted to nosocomial infection prevention.

J. J. Provencio, MD

Serum inflammatory adhesion molecules and high-sensitivity C-reactive protein correlates with delayed ischemic neurologic deficits after subarachnoid hemorrhage
Kubo Y, Ogasawara K, Kakino S, et al (Iwate Med Univ, Morioka, Japan)
Surg Neurol 69:592-596, 2008

Background.—The purpose of the present study was to investigate the relationship between serum concentrations of the immunoglobulin-like superfamily, selectins, hsCRP, and the development of DIND in patients with aneurysmal SAH.

Methods.—Serum ICAM-1, VCAM-1, E-selectin, P-selectin, L-selectin, and hsCRP were measured in 33 patients with SAH who underwent aneurysmal clipping within 48 hours of the onset of symptoms. Serum samples were obtained during the early period (day 0) and the late period (day 7).

Results.—The serum concentrations of ICAM-1 ($P = .009$), VCAM-1 ($P = .0383$) and hsCRP ($P = .0014$) during the early period were significantly higher in patients with SAH than in control patients. Further, serum hsCRP concentration during the late period was significantly higher in patients with SAH than in control patients ($P = 0033$). Finally, serum concentrations of ICAM-1, VCAM-1, and hsCRP during the early ($P = .0055$, $P = .0266$, and $P = .0266$) and late ($P = .0423$, $P = .0041$, and $P = .0004$) period were significantly higher in patients with DIND than in patients without DIND.

Conclusions.—Serum levels of ICAM-1, VCAM-1 and hsCRP during the early and late period following SAH correlate with DIND.

▶ The cause of delayed cerebral injury (DCI) after subarachnoid hemorrhage has been vexingly difficult to pin down. The syndrome, commonly called vasospasm, usually becomes clinically manifest between 5 days and 2 weeks after the original hemorrhage. It is associated with angiographic vasculopathy and stroke in some patients. There has been a great deal of research focusing on the vasculopathy and how mediators of vasoconstriction and dilation can be modulated to improve outcome. Interestingly, we have had 2 major trials of vasoactive agents with conflicting results. A trial of a cerebroselective calcium channel blocker showed no improvement in angiographic vasculopathy but improved patient outcome.[1] A second trial of an endothelin-1 antagonist successfully vasodilated the cerebral vasculature but did not improve patient outcome.[2] These confusing results have lead to a resurgence of study into other possible causes of DCI.

This work is part of a growing body of work that is investigating inflammation as the cause. Unlike other studies that have looked closely at the time when vasospasm was diagnosed, this study looked immediately after the hemorrhage. The authors found an elevation in intracellular adhesion molecule-1 (ICAM-1), vascular cell adhesion molecule-1 (VCAM-1), and the high-sensitivity C-reactive protein (hsCRP) on the day of the hemorrhage in patients who later developed DCI. This suggests that the process leading to DCI begins at the time of the hemorrhage and takes days to manifest. This is promising because it allows time for possible treatments to interact with this process.

I think this study also makes a strong case that DCI is an inflammatory condition. It is likely that the damage from inflammation is responsible for the vascular damage but may also have ramifications directly in the brain that may account for part of the morbidity of the disease.

J. J. Provencio, MD

References

1. Pickard JD, Murray GD, Illingworth R, et al. Effect of oral nimodipine on cerebral infarction and outcome after subarachnoid haemorrhage: British aneurysm nimodipine trial. *BMJ.* 1989;298:636-642.
2. Vajkoczy P, Meyer B, Weidauer S, et al. Clazosentan (AXV-034343), a selective endothelin A receptor antagonist, in the prevention of cerebral vasospasm following severe aneurysmal subarachnoid hemorrhage: results of a randomized, double-blind, placebo-controlled, multicenter phase IIa study. *J Neurosurg.* 2005;103:9-17.

Focal motor seizures induced by alerting stimuli in critically ill patients
Hirsch LJ, Pang T, Claassen J, et al (Columbia Univ, NY)
Epilepsia 49:968-973, 2008

Purpose.—We have previously demonstrated that it is common for alerting stimuli to induce electrographic seizures and other periodic or rhythmic patterns in the critically ill; however, only 1 of the first 33 patients we reported with this phenomenon had a detectable clinical correlate.

Methods.—Review of charts and video EEG findings in critically ill patients in a neurological ICU at a tertiary care medical center in Manhattan.

Results.—We identified nine patients who had focal motor seizures repeatedly induced by alerting stimuli. All patients were comatose, and 8/9 had nonconvulsive status epilepticus at some point during their acute illness. Imaging abnormalities involved bilateral thalami in three patients, upper brainstem in one, and the perirolandic region in five.

Discussion.—We hypothesize that in encephalopathic patients, alerting stimuli activate the arousal circuitry, and, when combined with hyperexcitable cortex, result in epileptiform activity or seizures. This activity can be focal or generalized, and is usually nonconvulsive, as is true of seizures in general in the critically ill. However, when the cortex is hyperexcitable in a specific region only, focal EEG findings arise. If the electrographic seizure activity is adequately synchronized and involves motor pathways, this can present as focal motor seizures, as seen in these nine patients.

Alerting can induce seizures in encephalopathic/comatose patients. The observation of clear focal clinical seizures removes the last remaining doubt that these stimulus-induced patterns are indeed seizures by any definition, not simply abnormal arousal patterns.

▶ As the field of neurocritical care has evolved, the use of continuous electroencephalogram (CEEG) in the comatose patient has become more prevalent. Work by Hirsh and colleagues has led the way in determining which patients are at risk for subtle or nonconvulsive seizures. This report is a slight variation on this theme. Instead of determining what existing seizure syndromes are found in ICU patients, the authors have found a novel type of seizure in patients in the ICU.

This phenomenon is more familiar to nurses in the ICU compared with that of physicians. It is not uncommon to hear nurses say that every time a patient gets a bath, their arm or leg begins to twitch. This can last anywhere from seconds to minutes. The classical teaching (addressed by the authors) is that stimulus-invoked seizures in the ICU do not exist. This flies in contrast to reports that stimuli such as flashing lights and even some foods can precipitate seizures.

This report is the first that systematically evaluates EEG with stereotyped movements in the ICU. What Hirsh and coinvestigators have found is that there is such thing as stimulus-invoked seizures in ICU patients. He also found that this phenomenon is largely limited to patients who had other evidence of seizure (either convulsive or nonconvulsive). It is still to be seen if there are a significant number of patients without neurologic injury who experience this type of seizure.

J. J. Provencio, MD

An Acute Ischemic Stroke Classification Instrument That Includes CT or MR Angiography: The Boston Acute Stroke Imaging Scale
Torres-Mozqueda F, He J, Yeh IB, et al (Harvard Med School, Boston, MA)
AJNR Am J Neuroradiol 29:1111-1117, 2008

Background and Purpose.—A simple classification instrument based on imaging that predicts outcomes in patients with actute ischemic stroke is lacking. We tested the hypotheses that the Boston Acute Stroke Imaging Scale (BASIS) classification instrument effectively predicts patient outcomes and is superior to the Alberta Stroke Program Early CT Score (ASPECTS) in predicting outcomes in acute ischemic stroke.

Materials and Methods.—Of 230 prospectively screened, consecutive patients with acute ischemic stroke, 87 had noncontrast CT (NCCT)/CT angiography (CTA), and 118 had MR imaging/MR angiography (MRA) at admission and were classified as having major stroke by BASIS criteria if they had a proximal cerebral artery occlusion or, if no occlusion, imaging evidence of significant parenchymal ischemia; all of the others were classified as minor strokes. Outcomes included death, length of hospitalization, and discharge disposition. BASIS was compared with ASPECTS (dichotomized > or ≤7) in 87 patients who had NCCT/CTA.

Results.—BASIS classification by NCCT/CTA was equivalent to MR imaging/MRA. Fifty-six of 205 patients were classified as having major strokes including all 6 of the deaths. A total of 71.4% and 15.4% of major and minor stroke survivors, respectively, were discharged to a rehabilitation facility, whereas 14.3% and 79.2% of patients with major and minor strokes were discharged to home. The mean length of hospitalization was 12.3 and 3.3 days for the major and minor stroke groups, respectively (all outcomes, $P < .0001$). In 87 NCCT/CTA patients, BASIS and ASPECTS agreed in 22 major and 44 minor strokes. BASIS classified 21 patients as having major strokes who were classified as having minor strokes by ASPECTS. The BASIS major/ASPECTS minor stroke group had outcomes similar to those classified as major strokes by both instruments.

Conclusions.—The BASIS classification instrument is effective and appears superior to ASPECTS in predicting outcomes in acute ischemic stroke.

▶ With the growing aggressiveness of treatment in stroke, there is increasing need to categorize stroke as major or minor. Specifically, interventional procedures to remove and lyse clots or angioplasty stenotic blood vessels are riskier compared with intravenous tissue plasminogen activator. Better prediction of which patients will have significant disease burden without intervention can justify riskier therapy to try to improve their outcome. Conversely, an understanding of who will do well can temper enthusiasm for risky procedures.

This study by Torres-Mozqueda and colleagues has a number of advantages. First, they developed the Boston Acute Stroke Imaging Scale based on studies that are now increasingly available in emergency departments (EDs). Second, they based the first step of the algorithm on an easily diagnosed finding, major artery occlusion. The algorithm is easy to follow and can be implemented in most EDs that have radiology support. This classification may have important ramifications for how we evaluate treatments for stroke in the future.

J. J. Provencio, MD

Aggressive Blood Pressure–Lowering Treatment Before Intravenous Tissue Plasminogen Activator Therapy in Acute Ischemic Stroke
Martin-Schild S, Hallevi H, Albright KC, et al (Univ of Texas Health Science Ctr, Houston; Univ of California, San Diego, et al)
Arch Neurol 65:1174-1178, 2008

Background.—Patients with acute ischemic stroke (AIS) commonly have elevated blood pressure (BP). Guidelines have recommended against treatment with intravenous tissue plasminogen activator (tPA) when aggressive measures such as continuous infusion with nicardipine hydrochloride are required to maintain BP lower than 185/110 mm Hg. We evaluated the effect of elevated BP and its management on clinical outcomes after tPA therapy in AIS.

Objectives.—To evaluate safety and outcome in patients with AIS who require treatment to lower BP before tPA therapy and to compare safety and outcome in patients who received aggressive treatment with nicardipine with those who received labetalol hydrochloride before tPA.

Design.—Retrospective review of medical records for all patients who received intravenous tPA within 3 hours of AIS onset.

Setting.—Emergency department.

Patients.—One hundred seventy-eight patients with AIS treated with tPA.

Main Outcome Measures.—Occurrence of symptomatic intracerebral hemorrhage and neurologic deterioration.

Results.—Fifty patients required BP lowering before tPA therapy. Twenty-four of these patients (48%) received nicardipine either after labetalol or as first-line therapy. Patients requiring antihypertensive agents had higher baseline blood glucose concentrations, incidence of hypertension, and National Institutes of Health Stroke Scale scores. The rate of adverse events and of modified Rankin score at discharge were not significantly different in patients without BP-lowering treatment compared with patients given either labetalol or nicardipine before intravenous tPA therapy.

Conclusions.—Blood pressure lowering before intravenous tPA therapy, even using aggressive measures, may not be associated with a higher rate of hemorrhage or poor outcome. Data suggest that patients with AIS requiring aggressive treatment to lower BP should not be excluded from receiving tPA therapy. A prospective study is needed to support these conclusions.

▶ An important problem that clinicians face in the emergency department and ICU setting is whether to treat patients who have an acute stroke and accelerated hypertension with intravenous tissue plasminogen activator (tPA). The National Institute of Neurological Disorders and Stroke Trial (NINDS) which initially evaluated the efficacy of tPA excluded patients with systolic blood pressures (BPs) > 180 mm Hg after a number of doses of bolus intravenous antihypertensives.[1] The rationale for this exclusion was previous data using both tPA and streptokinase that showed that after administration of the drug, hypertension is associated with increased bleeding.

The difficult question is whether elevated BP is a true risk for hemorrhage or is accelerated hypertension a sign of blood vessel damage that, in turn, leads to hemorrhage. If the former is true, BP management alone should suffice to mitigate the risk. If the latter is true, BP control would essentially do nothing.

This work by Martin-Schild and colleagues attempts to answer this question. Although this study is limited by its retrospective nature and the lack of outcome data, it suggests that there is little early danger to aggressively controlling BP in patients who are eligible for tPA. This study needs to be repeated in a randomized trial because of the finding that neurologic deterioration was increased in patients receiving aggressive lowering of BP. This study does not have the power to address whether this increase is a statistical variant or real.

J. J. Provencio, MD

Reference

1. The National Institute of Neurological Disorders and Stroke rt-PA Stroke Study Group. Tissue plasminogen activator for acute ischemic stroke. *N Engl J Med.* 1995;333:1581-1587.

Outcome After Decompressive Craniectomy for the Treatment of Severe Traumatic Brain Injury

Howard JL, Cipolle MD, Anderson M, et al (Lehigh Valley Hosp, Allentown, PA)
J Trauma 65:380-386, 2008

Background.—Using decompressive craniectomy as part of the treatment regimen for severe traumatic brain injury (STBI) has become more common at our Level I trauma center. This study was designed to examine this practice with particular attention to long-term functional outcome.

Methods.—A retrospective review of prospectively collected data was performed for patients with STBI admitted from January 1, 2003 to December 31, 2005. Our institution manages patients using the Brain Trauma Foundation Guidelines. Data collected from patients undergoing decompressive craniectomy included: age, Injury Severity Score, admission and follow-up Glasgow Coma Score, timing of, and indication for decompressive craniectomy, and procedure-related complications. The Extended Glasgow Outcome Scale (GOSE) was performed by an experienced trauma clinical research coordinator using a structured phone interview to assess long-term outcome in the survivors. Student's t test and χ^2 were used to examine differences between groups.

Results.—Forty STBI patients were treated with decompressive craniectomy; 24 were performed primarily in conjunction with urgent evacuation of extra-axial hemorrhage and 16 were performed primarily in response to increased intracranial pressure with 4 of these after an initial craniotomy. Decompressive craniectomy was very effective at lowering intracranial pressure in these 16 patients (35.0 mm Hg ± 13.5 mm Hg to 14.6 mm Hg ± 8.7 mm Hg, $p = 0.005$). Twenty-two decompressive craniectomy patients did not survive to hospital discharge, whereas admission Glasgow Coma Score and admission pupil size and reactivity correlated with outcome, age, and Injury Severity Score did not. At a mean of 11 months (range, 3–26 months) after decompressive craniectomy, 6 survivors had a poor functional outcome (GOSE 1–4), whereas 12 survivors had a good outcome (GOSE 5–8). Therefore, 70% of these patients had an unfavorable outcome (death or severe disability), and 30% had a favorable long-term functional outcome. Fifteen of 18 survivors went on to cranioplasty, whereas 4 of 18 had cerebrospinal infection.

Conclusion.—The majority of survivors after decompressive craniectomy have a good functional outcome as analyzed by GOSE. Overall, 30% of patients with STBI who underwent decompressive craniectomy had a favorable long-term outcome. Improving patient selection and optimizing timing of this procedure may further improve outcome in these very severely brain injured patients.

▶ Traumatic brain injury continues to dictate outcomes in patients with multisystem blunt trauma.[1] Thus, any intervention that may improve adverse outcomes seen in head injury is important. The Brain Trauma Foundation, citing a wealth of historic data notes that intracranial pressure (ICP) control, is one of the pillars of head trauma management.[2] It is not uncommon, however, that medical management of ICP is inadequate. Decompressive craniectomy is not a new intervention, but has seen increasing application in the setting of improved critical care support for patients with severe brain injury. This study provides contemporary outcome data.

There are several issues that cannot be addressed in this series. The first issue is surgical technique. A larger craniectomy appears to be superior to a very small opening in the cranial vault if aggressive decompression is required. There is no evidence of standardization of craniectomy technique in this article. Second, timing of intervention is probably important. For decompressive craniectomy to be most effective, early intervention seems appropriate. This data set is too small to address the timing issue. A significant number of patients in this series underwent decompressive craniectomy after the failure of medical management. Third, it is likely that some patients are unlikely to improve regardless of decompressive craniectomy. We need a larger data set to identify patients who are likely to do poorly or to better predict the likelihood of poor outcomes with aggressive surgical intervention. For example, the trauma community is widely aware of the poor outcomes associated with cardiac arrest in the setting of blunt trauma (1.6% survival).[3] Frequently, blunt trauma patients in cardiac arrest are not aggressively resuscitated. Finally, management of patients after decompressive craniectomy must be standardized. Recent neurosurgical data suggests that patients undergoing cranioplasty have improved outcomes after decompressive craniectomy.[4] Although many explanations are possible, improved venous drainage has been proposed as one explanation as venous return is enhanced when the skull is intact.

These authors effectively review the state-of-the-art in craniectomy care. A mortality rate over 50% overall in these patients indicates that we still have a long way to go.

D. J. Dries, MSE, MD

References

1. Sarrafzadeh AS, Peltonen EE, Kaisers U, et al. Secondary insults in severe head injury? Do multiply injured patients do worse? *Crit Care Med.* 2001;29:1116-1123.
2. Brain Trauma Foundation, American Association of Neurological Surgeons, Congress of Neurological Surgeons. Guidelines for the management of severe traumatic brain injury. *J Neurotrauma.* 2007;24:S1-S106.
3. Working Group, Ad Hoc Subcommittee on Outcomes, American College of Surgeons Committee on Trauma. Practice management guidelines for emergency department thoracotomy. *J Am Coll Surg.* 2001;193:303-309.
4. Stiver SI, Wintermark M, Manley GT. Reversible monoparesis following decompressive hemicraniectomy for traumatic brain injury. *J Neurosurg.* 2008;109:245-254.

Outcomes in 140 critically ill patients with status epilepticus

Legriel S, Mourvillier B, Bele N, et al (Hôpital Saint-Louis, Paris, France; Hôpital Robert Ballanger, France)
Intensive Care Med 34:476-480, 2008

Objective.—Despite recent management guidelines, no recent study has evaluated outcomes in ICU patients with status epilepticus (SE).

Design and Setting.—An 8-year retrospective study.

Subjects and Intervention.—Observational study in 140 ICU patients with SE, including 81 (58%) with continuous SE and 59 (42%) with intermittent SE (repeated seizures without interictal recovery).

Measurements and Results.—The 95 men and 45 women had a median age of 49 years (IQR 24–71). Median seizure time was 60 min (IQR 20–180), and 58 patients had seizures longer than 30 min. The SE was nonconvulsive in 16 (11%) patients and convulsive in 124 (89%), including 89 (64%) with tonic-clonic generalized seizures, 27 (19%) with partial seizures, 7 (5%) with myoclonic seizures, and 1 with tonic seizures. The most common causes of SE were cerebral insult in 53% and anticonvulsant drug withdrawal in 20% of patients. No cause was identified in 35% of patients. Median time from SE to treatment was 5 min (IQR 0–71). The SE was refractory in 35 (25%) patients. Mechanical ventilation was needed in 106 patients. Hospital mortality was 21%. By multivariate analysis, independent predictors of 30-day mortality were age (OR 1.03/year; 95% CI 1.00–1.06), GCS at scene (OR 0.84/point; 95% CI 0.72–0.98), continuous SE (OR 3.17; 95% CI 1.15–8.77), symptomatic SE (OR 4.08; 95% CI 1.49–11.10), and refractory SE (OR 2.83; 95% CI 1.06–7.54).

Conclusion.—Mortality in SE patients remains high and chiefly determined by seizure severity. Further studies are needed to evaluate the possible impact of early maximal anticonvulsant treatment on outcomes.

▶ Management of patients with status epilepticus (SE) in the ICU may be a struggle because of various causes and associated pathologies. However, the incidence of SE is on the rise and mortality remains high. Will early recognition, diagnosis, and treatment improve outcome and decrease mortality in SE as in septic shock and early antibiotics? Legriel and colleagues set out to identify factors associated with death and identify areas for improvement of ICU patients with SE. This single center study of a university-affiliated ICU in Paris, France, retrospectively evaluated SE patients over an 8-year period. Findings of this study are similar to other studies showing high mortality in patients with continuous seizures versus intermittent seizures. However, the authors found that outcomes for patients with refractory SE may be affected most by earlier management or diverse treatment methods. The authors were unsuccessful in meeting their second objective of identifying factors for improvement. Efforts to identify area for improvement may be more appropriately identified in a prospective study and concurrent data collection using the more recent standardized operational definitions of SE. The results of this study point to the importance of varying predictors of death based on the operational definition that may be identified early in the ICU stay. Further analysis on earlier maximal and combination therapies may provide additional information to improving management in patients with SE.

C. A. Schorr, RN, MSN

The Effect of Anemia and Blood Transfusions on Mortality in Closed Head Injury Patients
Duane TM, Mayglothling J, Grandhi R, et al (Virginia Commonwealth Univ Med Ctr, Richmond, VA)
J Surg Res 147:163-167, 2008

Background.—The purpose of this study was to determine if anemia in isolated head trauma patients results in a higher mortality rate that would justify a more liberal use of blood transfusions.

Methods.—A retrospective review of isolated blunt head trauma patients was performed between January 2001 and December 2006. Comparisons were made between survivors and nonsurvivors regarding demographics, laboratory values, transfusions received, and lengths of stay.

Results.—There were 788 patients with 735 survivors who were significantly younger (46.3 y ± 21.5 survivors versus 68.9 y ± 18.8 nonsurvivors, $P < 0.0001$) and less injured [(ISS: 14.7 ± 5.2 survivors versus 23.2 ± 4.7 nonsurvivors, $P < 0.0001$), (head abbreviated injury severity: 3.7 ± 0.7 survivors versus 4.7 ± 0.5 nonsurvivors, $P < 0.0001$)] than those who died ($n = 53$). The survivors also had shorter lengths of stay (days) [(ICU: 2.4 ± 4.2 versus 5.6 ± 11.7, $P = 0.03$), (hospital: 6.3 ± 9.8 versus 7.8 ± 14.8, $P = 0.02$)]. Multivariate logistic regression showed age (OR 1.063, CI 1.042–1.084), ISS (OR 1.376, CI 1.270–1.491), minimum hemoglobin (OR 0.855, CI 0.732–1.000), and total blood products transfused (OR 1.073, CI 1.008–1.142) to be independent predictors of mortality with an ROC of 0.942. Outcome was independent of the operative procedures, hematocrit and packed red blood cells transfused at 24, 48, and 72 h. Hemoglobin levels of <8 mg/dL were more predictive of death than >8 mg/dL ($P = 0.01$).

Conclusions.—This study supports the need to balance mild anemia with judicious blood product use in the head trauma patient. Given the risk with blood product use, each transfusion should be carefully considered and the patient re-evaluated regularly to determine the need for further intervention.

▶ It has been traditionally accepted that maintenance of a hematocrit of > 30% is necessary for better outcomes in the neurosurgical patient population to maintain adequate cerebral perfusion and oxygen delivery. However, there is no reason to presume that the problems that have been identified in the ability of stored packed red blood cells (PRBC) to traverse the microcirculation and to ultimately deliver oxygen at the cellular level in other clinical situations are not present in the neurosurgical patient also. In this study, these authors report the first significant evaluation of the impact of transfusion on outcomes in patients with closed head injuries (CHIs). As with other patient populations, in this study significant anemia was indeed identified as a poor prognostic indicator. However, as with many of its predecessor studies, transfusion as a means of increasing hematocrit (or hemoglobin) was not found to be beneficial in yet another patient population that had long been assumed to benefit from this intervention. Indeed, as with many previous studies, infectious complications were correlated with the amount of PRBC transfused, although in this study mortality was not. As the authors point out, numerous factors other than anemia are responsible for morbidity and mortality in cases of significant CHI. They conclude that a balance between mild anemia and a judicious use of blood transfusion is appropriate in this patient population, and call for prospective studies for more detailed and formal evaluation of this question, all of which seem appropriate.

D. R. Gerber, DO

Early complications of high-dose methylprednisolone in acute spinal cord injury patients

Suberviola B, González-Castro A, Llorca J, et al (Hospital Universitario Marqués de Valdecilla, Santander, Spain; Univ of Cantabria, Santander, Spain)
Injury 39:748-752, 2008

Background.—To evaluate the early complications and effect on neurological outcome of methylprednisolone (MP) treatment in spinal cord injury (SCI) patients during the acute phase.

Methods.—We retrospectively reviewed the whole cohort of patients admitted to our ICU between January 1994 and December 2005 due to acute SCI. Patients were grouped according to the medical treatment received (MP group versus no-MP group). Patient data as age, gender, Glasgow coma score (GCS), APACHE II, injury severity score (ISS) and

ICU stay were recorded. Outcome at ICU discharge and neurological function based on Frankel grade was recorded at ICU admission and at ICU discharge. Early complications were also noted.

Results.—There were no differences between both groups in ICU mortality (OR = 0.48; 95% CI: 0.08–3.64) nor neurological function at ICU discharge. (OR = 1.09; 95% CI: 0.35–3.66). MP group presented an increase in respiratory tract infections (OR = 8.19; 95% CI: 1.10–358.6) and in total infections (OR = 4.90; 95% CI: 1.46–18.83) compared to no-MP group during the ICU stay. There was a significant increase in the incidence of hyperglycaemia in the MP group (OR = 17.0; 95% CI: 4.52–66.3).

Conclusions.—The use of MP in patients with acute SCI is not associated with an improvement in outcome or neurological function at ICU discharge. Moreover, the use of MP is associated with an increased risk of infectious and metabolic complications during ICU stay.

▶ Since the original report in the New England Journal of Medicine in 1990,[1] there has been considerable debate about the merits of high-dose methylprednisolone. Despite the conclusion that there is little evidence of efficacy for high-dose steroids, the risks in this patient population have not been categorized. This study by Suberviola and colleagues is an attempt to quantify the risks of high-dose steroids in this specific patient population.

This review of 1 hospital's experience shows that there is an increase in pneumonia and total infections. There was also routinely an increase in hyperglycemia that likely contributes to the infection risk.

Despite the recommendation from the American Association of Neurological Surgeons that high-dose steroids are only an option, use of steroids in patients with spinal cord injury is still practiced.[2] Evidence of increased risk with the therapy will likely diminish further enthusiasm for high-dose steroids.

It is very likely that the enthusiasm for steroids was in part because of the lack of other effective therapies. Unfortunately, it is also likely that the embrace of high-dose steroids may have set back work on other promising therapies. This may serve as a lesson for other diseases that are likewise searching for first treatments.

J. J. Provencio, MD

References

1. Bracken MB, Shepard MJ, Collins WF, et al. A randomized, controlled trial of methylprednisolone or naloxone in the treatment of acute spinal cord injury: results of the Second National Acute Spinal Cord Injury Study. N Engl J Med. 1990;322:1405-1411.
2. Pharmacotherapy after acute cervical spinal cord injury. Neurosurgery. 2002; 50(suppl):63-72.

12 Ethics/Socioeconomic/Administrative Issues

Quality of Life/End of Life/Outcome Prediction

Simulation-Based Education Improves Quality of Care During Cardiac Arrest Team Responses at an Academic Teaching Hospital: A Case-Control Study
Wayne DB, Didwania A, Feinglass J, et al (Northwestern Univ Feinberg School of Med, Chicago, IL)
Chest 133:56-61, 2008

Background.—Simulation technology is widely used in medical education. Linking educational outcomes achieved in a controlled environment to patient care improvement is a constant challenge.

Methods.—This was a retrospective case-control study of cardiac arrest team responses from January to June 2004 at a university-affiliated internal medicine residency program. Medical records of advanced cardiac life support (ACLS) events were reviewed to assess adherence to ACLS response quality indicators based on American Heart Association (AHA) guidelines. All residents received traditional ACLS education. Second-year residents (simulator-trained group) also attended an educational program featuring the deliberate practice of ACLS scenarios using a human patient simulator. Third-year residents (traditionally trained group) were not trained on the simulator. During the study period, both simulator-trained and traditionally trained residents responded to ACLS events. We evaluated the effects of simulation training on the quality of the ACLS care provided.

Results.—Simulator-trained residents showed significantly higher adherence to AHA standards (mean correct responses, 68%; SD, 20%) vs traditionally trained residents (mean correct responses, 44%; SD, 20%; $p = 0.001$). The odds ratio for an adherent ACLS response was 7.1 (95% confidence interval, 1.8 to 28.6) for simulator-trained residents compared to traditionally trained residents after controlling for patient age, ventilator, and telemetry status.

Conclusions.—A simulation-based educational program significantly improved the quality of care provided by residents during actual ACLS events. There is a growing body of evidence indicating that simulation can be a useful adjunct to traditional methods of procedural training.

▶ As the use of medical simulation has grown significantly during the past decade, there is considerable interest in using simulation-based medical education for teaching and assessment of medical students and residents. Recent attention to medical errors, the need to improve patient safety, and a shift to outcomes-based education has led both the public and medical educators to champion this new method of medical education. Medical simulators allow educators to reproduce a wide variety of high risk, low frequency clinical conditions on demand, and allow the novice learner to use deliberate repetitive practice to improve his management of these clinical situations.

As the use of medical simulators increases, so does the need to provide evidence of the effectiveness of this method of education and to link the quality of patient care delivered to simulation education. This retrospective case-control study on the adherence of a cardiac arrest team to American Heart Association (AHA) guidelines on advanced cardiac life support (ACLS) response is an important evaluation of whether patient care improved because of deliberate practice using a human patient simulator. Their research demonstrates the ability of a simulation-based education program to improve adherence to AHA ACLS guidelines, among students who took part in a simulation-based ACLS program 6 months before the study period, even though they had less clinical experience and less traditional ACLS courses, but is not able to show improved outcomes among these patients. Most of the patients died regardless of the treatment they received. Although this patient outcome reflects the high morbidity of this patient population, it is therefore difficult to evaluate the competence of the team caring for these patients.

The study has several limitations, as it represents a small sample of events at a single institution, uses a case-control retrospective design, and relies on charts and records kept during a cardiac event. Even with these limitations, the skill improvements of the students who attended the simulation program, and their adherence to accepted algorithms is clearly improved.

A. Burden, MD
C. Bekes, MD

Survival From In-Hospital Cardiac Arrest During Nights and Weekends
Peberdy MA, Ornato JP, Larkin GL, et al (Virginia Commonwealth Univ, Richmond, VA; Yale School of Med, New Haven, CT; et al)
JAMA 299:785-792, 2008

Context.—Occurrence of in-hospital cardiac arrest and survival patterns have not been characterized by time of day or day of week. Patient physiology and process of care for in-hospital cardiac arrest may be different at night and on weekends because of hospital factors unrelated to patient, event, or location variables.

Objective.—To determine whether outcomes after in-hospital cardiac arrest differ during nights and weekends compared with days/evenings and weekdays.

Design and Setting.—We examined survival from cardiac arrest in hourly time segments, defining day/evening as 7:00 AM to 10:59 PM, night as 11:00 PM to 6:59 AM, and weekend as 11:00 PM on Friday to 6:59 AM on Monday, in 86 748 adult, consecutive in-hospital cardiac arrest events in the National Registry of Cardiopulmonary Resuscitation obtained from 507 medical/surgical participating hospitals from January 1, 2000, through February 1, 2007.

Main Outcome Measures.—The primary outcome of survival to discharge and secondary outcomes of survival of the event, 24-hour survival, and favorable neurological outcome were compared using odds ratios and multivariable logistic regression analysis. Point estimates of survival outcomes are reported as percentages with 95% confidence intervals (95% CIs).

Results.—A total of 58 593 cases of in-hospital cardiac arrest occurred during day/evening hours (including 43 483 on weekdays and 15 110 on weekends), and 28 155 cases occurred during night hours (including 20 365 on weekdays and 7790 on weekends). Rates of survival to discharge (14.7% [95% CI, 14.3%-15.1%] vs 19.8% [95% CI, 19.5%-20.1%], return of spontaneous circulation for longer than 20 minutes (44.7% [95% CI, 44.1%-45.3%] vs 51.1% [95% CI, 50.7%-51.5%]), survival at 24 hours (28.9% [95% CI, 28.4%-29.4%] vs 35.4% [95% CI, 35.0%-35.8%]), and favorable neurological outcomes (11.0% [95% CI, 10.6%-11.4%] vs 15.2% [95% CI, 14.9%-15.5%]) were substantially lower during the night compared with day/evening (all P values <.001). The first documented rhythm at night was more frequently asystole (39.6% [95% CI, 39.0%-40.2%] vs 33.5% [95% CI, 33.2%-33.9%], $P < .001$) and less frequently ventricular fibrillation (19.8% [95% CI, 19.3%-20.2%] vs 22.9% [95% CI, 22.6%-23.2%], $P < .001$). Among in-hospital cardiac arrests occurring during day/evening hours, survival was higher on weekdays (20.6% [95% CI, 20.3%-21%]) than on weekends (17.4% [95% CI, 16.8%-18%]; odds ratio, 1.15 [95% CI, 1.09-1.22]), whereas among in-hospital cardiac arrests occurring during night hours, survival to discharge was similar on weekdays (14.6% [95% CI, 14.1%-15.2%]) and on weekends (14.8% [95% CI, 14.1%-15.2%]; odds ratio, 1.02 [95% CI, 0.94-1.11]).

Conclusion.—Survival rates from in-hospital cardiac arrest are lower during nights and weekends, even when adjusted for potentially confounding patient, event, and hospital characteristics (Table 3).

▶ In-hospital cardiac arrest is a major public health problem. Several small studies have shown worse outcomes with in-hospital cardiac arrest in the night compared with daytime.[1,2]

This large study looked at differences in outcome for in-hospital cardiac arrest during nights and weekends compared with days/evenings and

TABLE 3.—Cardiac Arrest Outcomes by Day/Evening vs Night[a]

	No. (%) [95% Confidence Interval]			Odds Ratio (95% Confidence Interval)	
	Day/Evening (n = 58 593)[b]	Night (n = 28 155)[b]	Total (N = 86 748)	Unadjusted Odds Ratio (Day/Evening vs Night) (N = 86 748)	Adjusted Odds Ratio[c] (Day/Evening vs Night) (N = 86 748)
Survived to discharge	11 604 (19.8) [19.5-20.1]	4139 (14.7) [14.3-15.1]	15 743 (18.1) [17.9-18.4]	1.43 (1.38-1.49)	1.18 (1.12-1.23)
Return of spontaneous circulation longer than 20 min	29 920 (51.1) [50.7-51.5]	12 581 (44.7) [44.1-45.3]	42 501 (49) [48.7-49.3]	1.29 (1.26-1.33)	1.15 (1.12-1.19)
Survival at 24 h	20 236 (35.4) [35.0-35.8]	7931 (28.9) [28.4-29.4]	28 167 (32.5) [32.2-32.8]	1.35 (1.31-1.39)	1.19 (1.15-1.23)
Favorable neurological outcome[d]	8918 (15.2) [14.9-15.5]	3097 (11) [10.6-11.4]	12 015 (13.9) [13.6-14.1]	1.45 (1.39-1.52)	1.17 (1.11-1.23)

[a]$P < .001$ for day/evening vs night for all 4 outcomes.
[b]Day/evening was defined as 7:00 AM to 10:59 PM, night as 11:00 PM to 6:59 AM.
[c]Regression adjusted for sex, age, race, illness category, discovery status at time of event, witnessed event, first documented pulseless rhythm, duration of cardiopulmonary resuscitation, preexisting conditions, immediate factors related to event, defibrillation, delay in cardiopulmonary resuscitation, delay in vasopressor use, weekend, hospital bed size, time from admission to event, interventions in place at time of event, and pharmacologic interventions.
[d]Either a cerebral performance category score of 1 or 2 (range, 1-5) or no change from baseline cerebral performance category score.
(Reprinted from Peberdy MA, Ornato JP, Larkin GL, et al. Survival from in-hospital cardiac arrest during nights and weekends. *JAMA*. 2008;299:785-792, with permission from the American Medical Association.)

weekdays. Fewer patients survived to hospital discharge during nights and weekends compared with day/evening times on weekdays, even after accounting for potentially confounding variables like patient, arrest event, and hospital factors (see Table 3).

Operational processes of care could partly explain the difference in outcome. These include hospital staffing patterns and lower nurse-patient ratio at night. Physician staffing also differs during night, with cross coverage being provided for most patients by attending physicians and residents. Consequently, fewer healthcare professionals are available at night to respond to a resuscitation event. Interestingly enough, emergency department and trauma services were the only locations that had the same survival outcomes at night compared with day/evening. In addition to physiologic differences in these patient populations, availability of attending and resident physicians at all times along with similar staffing ratios may have positively impacted survival.

This study does have several limitations. Although this was a large multicenter registry of patients, the sample may not be representative of all United States hospitals. The data is self-reported and there may be issues related to integrity.

Findings of this study emphasize the need to focus on operational factors at night and during weekends to potentially improve patient survival after cardiac arrest. Further studies are needed to determine whether there is a physiologic basis for poorer survival from in-hospital cardiac arrests during nights and weekends.

M. K. Athar, MD
C. Bekes, MD

References

1. Marcu CB, Juhasz D, Donahue TJ. Circadian variation and outcome of in-hospital cardiopulmonary resuscitation. *Conn Med.* 2005;69:389-393.
2. Peng TC, Sum TC. Evaluation of in hospital cardiopulmonary resuscitation. *Ma Zui Xue Za Zhi.* 1989;27:137-142.

Family Member Satisfaction With End-of-Life Decision Making in the ICU
Gries CJ, Curtis JR, Wall RJ, et al (Univ of Washington, Seattle, WA)
Chest 133:704-712, 2008

Rationale.—Families of ICU patients may be at risk for increased psychological morbidity due to end-of-life decision making. The identification of chart-based quality indicators of palliative care that predict family satisfaction with decision making may help to guide interventions to improve decision making and family outcomes.

Objective.—To determine patient and family characteristics and chart the documentation of processes of care that are associated with increased family satisfaction with end-of-life decision making for ICU patients.

Methods.—We conducted a cohort study of ICU patients dying in 10 medical centers in the Seattle-Tacoma area.

Measurement.—Outcomes from family surveys included summary scores for family satisfaction with decision making and a single-item score that indicated feeling supported during decision making. Predictor variables were obtained from surveys and chart abstraction.

Main Results.—The survey response rate was 41% (442 of 1,074 families responded). Analyses were conducted of 356 families with questionnaire and chart abstraction data. Family satisfaction with decision making was associated with the withdrawal of life support, and chart documentation of physician recommendations to withdraw life support, discussions of patients' wishes, and discussions of families' spiritual needs. Feeling supported during decision making was associated with the withdrawal of life support, spiritual care involvement, and chart documentation of physician recommendations to withdraw life support, expressions of families' wishes to withdraw life support, and discussions of families' spiritual needs.

Conclusions.—Increased family satisfaction with decision making is associated with withdrawing life support and the documentation of palliative care indicators including the following: physician recommendations to withdraw life support; expressions of patients' wishes; and discussions of families' spiritual needs. These findings provide direction for future studies to investigate approaches to improving family satisfaction in end-of-life decision making. In addition, because there were few nonwhites in this study, these results may not be generalizable to more diverse populations. Future studies should target diverse populations in order to test whether similar factors are similarly important for end-of-life decision making.

▶ Twenty percent of all deaths in the United States occur in the intensive care unit (ICU). Most of them involve decisions to withdraw life support. The Study to Understand Prognoses and Preferences for Outcomes and Risks of Treatments (SUPPORT) showed that many physicians were unaware of their patients' preferences for end-of-life treatment.[1] Because of the inability of patients to express their wishes, a surrogate decision maker, usually a family member is often involved. Other studies have shown that surrogate decision makers remain dissatisfied with physician-family communication in the ICU.[2,3] There is a wide gulf between the family's understanding of the diagnosis and physician's explanation of their loved one's condition. A significant number of family members experience symptoms of anxiety, depression, and post-traumatic stress disorder (PTSD) if they are involved in end-of-life decision-making. A recent randomized trial has suggested that standardizing end-of-life family conferences decreased family symptoms of anxiety, depression, and PTSD. This exploratory study looked into predictors of family satisfaction with decision making and feeling supported in the ICU when a loved one died. Although the decision to withdraw life-sustaining treatment was associated with greater family satisfaction, the decision itself remains a complex one. The family members may take their time to come to terms with their loved one's impending death. Secondly, the nature of the illness may make it difficult to predict the outcome with any degree of certainty and make clear-cut recommendations. Therefore, supporting family members through a decision to withdraw life support when survival is unlikely could be an important area for future research. Additionally, addressing the spiritual needs of family members and discussing patients' wishes are important interventions that increase family satisfaction with end-of-life decision making. This study does have several limitations. These include the low response rates (41%) and response bias (responders were more likely to be white). This may limit application to a more diverse patient population. At the same time it opens avenues for further research to look into predictors of family satisfaction regarding end-of-life decision-making among minorities.

M. K. Athar, MD
C. Bekes, MD

References

1. A controlled trial to improve care for seriously ill hospitalized patients. The study to understand prognoses and preferences for outcomes and rise of treatments (SUPPORT). The SUPPORT Principal Investigators. *JAMA.* 1995;274:1591-1598.
2. Malaerida R, Bettelini CM, Degrate A, et al. Reasons for dissatisfaction: a survey of relatives of intensive care unit patients who died. *Crit Care Med.* 1998;26: 1187-1193.
3. Azoulay E, Pochard F, Chevret S, et al. Half the family members of intensive care unit patients do not want to share in decision-making process: a study in 78 French intensive care units. *Crit Care Med.* 2004;32:1832-1838.

A simple device to increase rates of compliance in maintaining 30-degree head-of-bed elevation in ventilated patients
Williams Z, Chan R, Kelly E (Brigham and Women's Hospital, Boston, MA)
Critical Care Medicine 36:1155-1157, 2008

Objective.—To determine whether a highly visible device that clearly indicates whether the head-of-bed is adequately elevated would increase rates of compliance with head-of-bed elevation guidelines.

Design.—A prospective, single-center, multi-unit, two-phase study.

Setting.—Surgical, thoracic, trauma, and medical intensive care units.

Patients.—Cohort of intubated patients.

Interventions.—A 4-wk trial was performed. At the onset of the trial, nurses were reminded to maintain head-of-bed elevation >30 degrees. Over the subsequent 2 wks, head-of-bed elevations of intubated patient beds were measured. An Angle Indicator, designed to clearly display whether the head-of-bed was adequately elevated, was then placed on side rails of beds of ventilated patients, and head-of-bed elevation measurements were taken for an additional 2 wks. A survey was then handed out to nursing staff to assess satisfaction with the device.

Measurements and Main Results.—A total of 268 bed measurements were made. The average head-of-bed elevation was 21.8 degrees on beds without the device (n = 166) and 30.9 degrees on beds with the device (n = 102; $p < .005$). When compliance is defined as a bed angle of ≥28 degrees, 23% of beds without the device were compliant while 71.5% of the beds with the device were compliant. The relative risk and odds ratio of having the device on a compliant bed were 2.2 and 9.25, respectively ($p < .005$). Seventy-two percent of nurses surveyed (n = 32) found it to be an improvement over existing methods, 88% found it helpful, and 84% would like it routinely used.

Conclusions.—The Angle Indicator improved rates of adherence to bed-elevation guidelines, and hospital staff found it helpful.

▶ Employing a bundle approach to prevent ventilator-associated pneumonia (VAP) results in better outcomes and decreased cost. One of the bundle elements, maintaining the head-of-bed (HOB) elevation > 30 degrees for intubated patients, seems so simple, yet continues to be an obstacle in many intensive care units (ICUs). Despite multiple studies and agencies supporting the HOB elevation, compliance remains low in many ICUs with reports that clinicians overestimate the angle of the HOB. The lack of a built-in device in many beds and inability to easily view the degree measurement may also impact compliance. Williams and colleagues evaluated the use of a simple angle indicator device to improve compliance with HOB elevation.

Before the use of the angle indicator, Williams and colleagues conducted a survey. The survey found that 94% of nurses were aware of the guidelines and that education was not a factor in maintaining the HOB elevation. The authors describe a simple device with minimal expense to assist the nurse in clearly recognizing adequate HOB elevation. Making the device visible using red/green indicators rather than degrees and the ability to accurately view from a distance were the key elements to ensuring success of the device.

The study clearly allowed for successful improvement based on the increased awareness of the HOB elevation within the unit. The duration of the study was very brief to evaluate compliance and nursing satisfaction with the device. A follow-up study to evaluate sustaining compliance over time and the impact on decreasing VAP will be particularly valuable in moving forward with this type of device.

This study suggests that there are innovative, cost-effective methods to accomplish success and ease in maintaining HOB elevation. Although there are beds with built-in angle indicators, not all ICUs have the funding to replace the beds currently in use. Homegrown, simple to read, readily accessible devices, and satisfactory support from the nursing staff will likely improve compliance. Continued observation, data collection, and feedback using this type of device will be essential to maintain consistency over time.

C. A. Schorr, RN, MSN

Determinants of long-term survival after intensive care
Williams TA, Dobb GJ, Finn JC, et al (Univ of Western Australia, Perth, Australia)
Crit Care Med 36:1523-1530, 2008

Objective.—To identify prognostic determinants of long-term survival for patients treated in intensive care units (ICUs) who survived to hospital discharge.

Design.—An ICU clinical cohort linked to state-wide hospital records and death registers.

Setting and Patients.—Adult patients admitted to a 22-bed ICU at a major teaching hospital in Perth, Western Australia, between 1987 and 2002 who survived to hospital discharge (n = 19,921) were followed-up until December 31, 2003.

Measurements.—The main outcome measures are crude and adjusted survival.

Main Results.—The risk of death in the first year after hospital discharge was high for patients who survived the ICU compared with the general population (standardized mortality rate [SMR] at 1 yr = 2.90, 95% confidence interval [CI] 2.73–3.08) and remained higher than the general population for every year during 15 yrs of follow up (SMR at 15 yrs = 2.01, 95% CI 1.64–2.46). Factors that were independently associated with survival during the first year were older age (hazard ratio [HR] = 4.09; 95% CI 3.20–5.23), severe comorbidity (HR = 5.23; 95% CI 4.25–6.43), ICU diagnostic group (HR range 2.20 to 8.95), new malignancy (HR = 4.60; 95% CI 3.68–5.76), high acute physiology score on admission (HR = 1.55; 95% CI 1.23–1.96), and peak number of organ failures (HR = 1.51; 95% CI 1.11–2.04). All of these factors were independently associated with subsequent survival for those patients who were alive 1 yr after discharge from the hospital with the addition of male gender (HR = 1.17; 95% CI 1.10–1.25) and prolonged length of stay in ICU (HR = 1.42; 95% CI 1.29–1.55).

Conclusions.—Patients who survived an admission to the ICU have worse survival than the general population for at least 15 yrs. The factors that determine long-term survival include age, comorbidity, and primary diagnosis. Severity of illness was also associated with long-term survival and this suggests that an episode of critical illness, or its treatment, may shorten life-expectancy (Fig 2).

▶ There has been a dramatic increase in the number of critical care beds in the United States over the last 20 years.[1] The appropriateness of admissions to intensive care units is being scrutinized because of the increase in medical dollars being spent on critically ill patients.[2] This article is important because it attempts to define the prognostic indicators of long-term survival of patients discharged from intensive care units. The strengths of the study are its prospective nature, the size of the database analyzed, and the length of time the patients were tracked. The authors should be commended about their long-term follow-

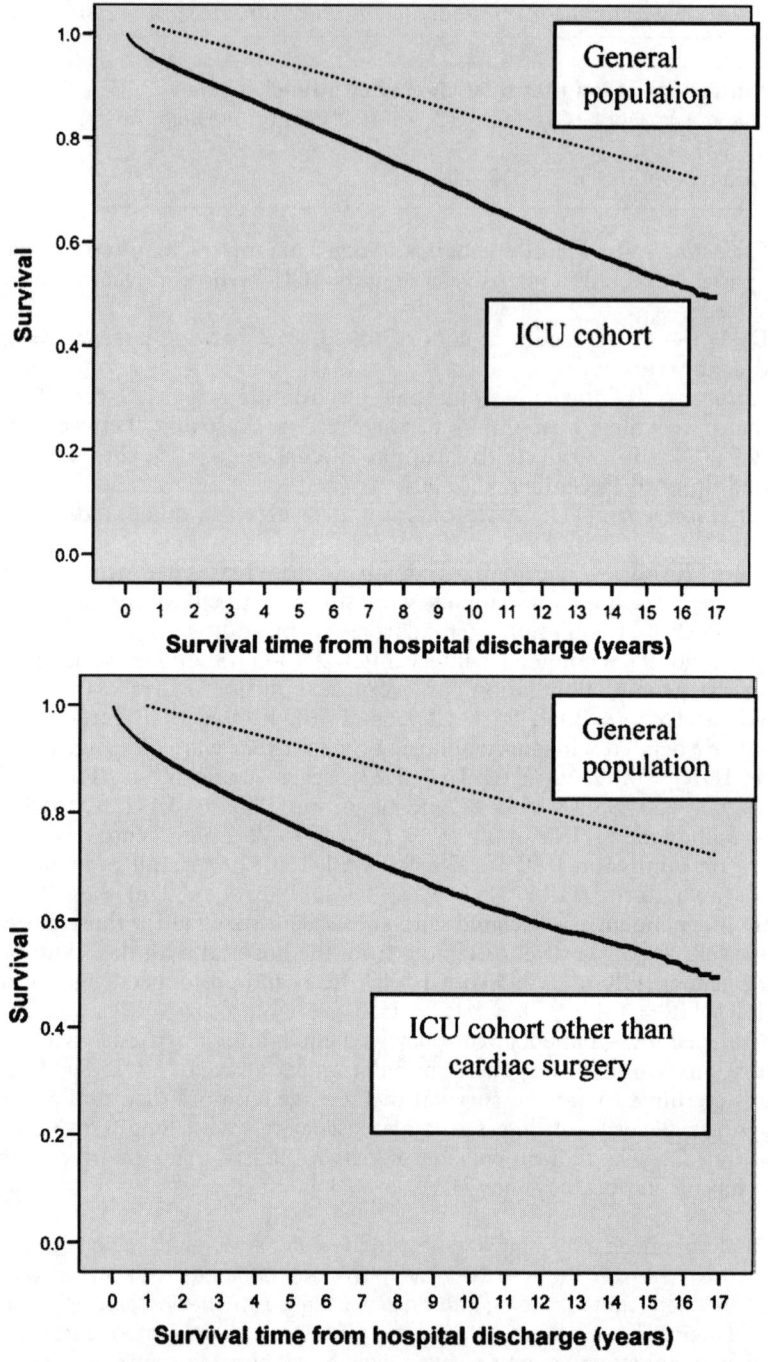

FIGURE 2.—Kaplan-Meier survival curve for patients discharged from the hospital after intensive care unit (*ICU*) admission compared with age, gender, and era-matched Australian general population. *Top*, all patients; *Bottom*, patients other than cardiac surgery. (Reprinted from Williams TA, Dobb GJ, Finn JC, et al. Determinants of long-term survival after intensive care. *Crit Care Med.* 2008;36:1523-1530, with permission from the Society of Critical Care Medicine.)

up, which is unique and likely not replicable in the United States. Patients had an increase risk of death in the first year after discharge from the intensive care unit and the increased mortality trend persisted during the 15 years of follow-up (Fig 2). Age, comorbidities, the type of illness, and the severity of physiologic abnormalities all impacted patient's survival. The authors concluded that an "episode" of critical illness may decrease patient's life expectancy. The heterogeneous nature of their patient population makes the reader question this conclusion as the trauma, elective surgical, and cardiac patients included in their study are generally not as ill as general medical patients. For example, almost half of their patients (44%) were postoperative cardiac surgery survivors. Another limitation was that their cohort did not include patients who actually died after admission into the intensive care unit, thus leaving an important group out of their analysis. Their study provides further reason for researchers to explore the long-term physiologic effects of critical illness. The epidemiological inferences derived from their study may help intensivists decide whether a patient qualifies for admission to an intensive care unit. The definitive association between age and other comorbid conditions upon long-term survival may cause intensivists to question the admission of a given patient to the intensive care unit when resources are limited.

N. Puri, MD
C. Bekes, MD

References

1. Ross C, Simini B, Brazzi L, et al. Variable costs of ICU patients: a multicenter prospective study. *Intensive Care Med.* 2006;32:454-552.
2. Hennessy D, Juzwishin K, Yergens D, Noseworthy T, Doig C. Outcomes of elderly survivors of intensive care: a review of the literature. *Chest.* 2005;127:1764-1774.

The views of patients and relatives of what makes a good intensivist: a European survey
CoBaTrICE Collaboration (Univ Hosp, Berne, Switzerland)
Intensive Care Med 33:1913-1920, 2007

Objective.—This study examined the views of adult patients and relatives about desirable characteristics of specialists in intensive care medicine (ICM) to incorporate these into an international competency-based training programme, CoBaTrICE.

Design.—Convenience sample of patients and relatives administered after discharge from 70 participating ICUs in eight European countries (1,398 evaluable responses). The structured questionnaire included 21 characteristics of medical competence categorised as 'medical knowledge and skills', 'communication with patients', and 'communication with relatives'. It was available in the national languages of the countries involved. Questions were rated by respondents for importance using a four-point Likert scale. Responses to open questions were also invited.

TABLE 3.—Ranking of Statements For Importance By Country. For Each Country The Rank For Each Item is Given As Number (1 = highest rank, 21 = lowest rank). The Items Are Shown In This Table In Sequence, As Defined By Rank Of The Total Sample (*SP* Spain, *IT* Italy, *CR* Czech Republic, *PL* Poland, *SW* Switzerland, *NL* The Netherlands, *DK* Denmark, *UK* United Kingdom)

	South		East		Central			West	
	SP	IT	CR	PL	SW	NL	DK	UK	All
Be decisive when action is needed	4	4	1	1	1	1	1	1	1
Up-to-date knowledge about illness and treatment	1	2	3	3	4	2	4	2	2
Handle crises calmly	5	3	2	5	6	3	2	5	3
Carry out practical procedures skilfully	11	7	5	4	5	4	7	4	4
Do everything possible to control pain	7	11	7	2	7	5	12	3	5
Explain in ways patients can understand	3	5	10	9	3	8	6	7	6
Treat patients as individuals	6	1	8	11	2	9	10	6	7
Work well as member of a team	2	6	4	14	11	6	3	10	8
Give bad news in a caring way	10	9	9	12	12	14	8	8	9
Do not talk as if patients were not there	15	10	11	8	10	7	5	13	10
Listen to patients	8	12	12	16	9	11	11	9	11
Inform patients about future care	12	14	15	6	8	10	14	11	12
Be courteous and polite	9	8	6	7	17	17	15	16	13
Discuss fears and anxieties with patients	13	13	13	10	13	12	16	12	14
Give the relatives an opportunity to ask questions	14	15	14	13	15	15	9	14	15
Give patients the opportunity to ask questions	16	16	16	15	14	13	13	15	16
Involve relatives in decisions about care and treatment	18	17	21	18	18	19	17	17	17
Involve patients in decisions about care and treatment	19	21	17	21	19	16	19	19	18
Give patients full information even when this is upsetting	21	18	19	19	16	18	18	18	19
Find out what relatives think and feel	17	19	20	20	20	21	20	20	20
Do not give information that is upsetting	20	20	18	17	21	20	21	21	21

For interpretation of the references to color in this Table legend, the reader is referred to the web version of this article. (Reprinted from CoBaTrICE Collaboration, The views of patients and relatives of what makes a good intensivist: a European survey. *Intensive Care Med.* 2007;33:1913-1920, with kind permission from Springer Science+Business Media: Intensive Care Medicine.)

Results.—Most characteristics were highly rated, with priority given to medical knowledge and skills. Women were more likely to emphasise communication skills. There were no consistent regional differences. Free-text responses welcomed the opportunity to participate.

Conclusions.—Patients and relatives with experience of intensive care in different European countries share similar views on the importance of knowledge, skills, decision making and communication in the training of intensive care specialists. These generic patient-centred components of training have been incorporated into the international competency-based ICM training programme, CoBaTrICE (Table 3).

▶ CoBaTrICE[1] is a competency-based training program in intensive care medicine developed by an international partnership of training organizations. The purpose of this program is to develop core competencies for specialists training in intensive care medicine.

Expectations of intensive care patients and their relatives differ both quantitatively and qualitatively from those receiving care in hospital wards. Clear and timely information provided in a compassionate manner is seen by patients and relatives as part of a positive ICU experience.[2] Patients and their relatives are in a unique position to provide an insight into the desirable characteristics and competencies of intensivists. Incorporating these attributes into the training of intensive care specialists will improve patient satisfaction and reduce the burden of bereavement among relatives.

In this study, a self-completion survey was conducted in 8 European countries to develop a general view of what patients and relatives consider being the most important qualities for an intensivist. The three general themes explored were (1) medical knowledge and skills, (2) communication with patients, and (3) communication with relatives.

The top 5 desirable attributes all belonged to the theme "medical knowledge and skills" (Table 3). Survey participants rated quality of communication to be more important than involvement in the process of decision-making. The results were consistent across different countries and regions despite cultural and social differences. This suggests that what patients and relatives regard as desirable characteristics in an intensivist is relatively universal. The findings of this study lend support to the idea of an international standardized, competency based training program for specialists in intensive care medicine.

M. K. Athar, MD
C. Bekes, MD

References

1. CoBaTrICE Collaboration, Bion JF, Barrett H. Development of core competencies for an international training programme in intensive care medicine. *Intensive Care Med.* 2006;32:1371-1383.
2. Buchman TG, Ray SE, Wax ML, Cassell J, Rich D, Niemczycki MA. Families' perceptions of surgical intensive care. *J Am Coll Card.* 2003;196:977-983.

Changes in Intensive Care Unit Performance Measures Associated With Opening a Dedicated Thoracic Surgical Progressive Care Unit
Keegan MT, Brown DR, Thieke MP, et al (Mayo Clinic, Rochester, MN)
J Cardiothorac Vasc Anesth 22:347-353, 2008

Objective.—To determine the effect of the introduction of a specialty-specific progressive care unit (PCU) on the intensive care unit (ICU) to which relatively low-acuity patients had previously been admitted.

Design.—Retrospective cohort study.
Setting.—The thoracic (noncardiac) surgical ICU of a tertiary referral institution.
Patients.—Four thousand fifty-three patients admitted to the ICU after thoracic surgery between October 1994 and December 2003.
Interventions.—None.
Measurements and Results.—The institutional Acute Physiology and Chronic Health Evaluation (APACHE) III database was searched to compare the number of admissions, severity of illness, mortality, and other aspects of care for periods before and after the introduction of the PCU. Patients in the post-PCU group were more severely ill by APACHE criteria. The ICU mortality rates for the periods before and after the introduction of the PCU were 1.14% (32/2,801 patients) and 7.27% (91/1,252 patients), respectively. The performance of the ICU appeared to be worse in the period after the opening of the PCU. The ICU- and hospital-customized standardized mortality ratio increased from 0.68 (95% confidence interval [CI], 0.47-0.96) in the pre-PCU group to 1.20 (95% CI, 0.96-1.47) in the post-PCU group and from 0.83 (95% CI, 0.66-1.03) to 1.24 (95% CI, 1.05-1.46).
Conclusions.—The introduction of a nonintensivist-directed PCU to care for thoracic surgical patients had a significant impact on the parent ICU. Of concern is that outcome and quality measures appeared to worsen and ICU readmission rate increased.

▶ Improving care and management of the critically ill patient, while reducing ICU length of stay and overall costs, may have created the groundwork for step-down/intermediate care unit development in some hospitals. Keegan et al point out the importance of preparation to determine changes impacting the success of the new unit and appraisal of the home unit's performance.

The authors report their anticipated changes, including a significant increase in patient acuity, more direct transfers from the operating room, and more patients with mechanical ventilation needs. Unanticipated changes after opening the PCU for thoracic surgical patients consisted of a greater ICU and hospital standardized mortality ratio for the "parent" ICU. Several causes for these unforeseen outcomes were identified including the service led team (thoracic surgical vs intensivist) on the PCU and the delay in transferring patients to the ICU. The authors also found a higher number of readmissions with an associated increased mortality.

Opening a critical care step-down unit may allow for more ICU admissions, but may also produce worse outcomes for the home ICU. Using the current available scoring systems to measure acuity may not truly reflect causes for worsening performance and a higher observed than expected mortality ratio specifically for readmissions. Hospital administrators planning for a new critical care step-down unit may consider factors including the transitioning team covering the unit, nursing experience, level of treatment required, origin on admission, and implications of pre-PCU length of stay when evaluating the effectiveness of the step-down/intermediate care unit as well as the home unit's performance.

C. A. Schorr, RN, MSN

Using the medical record to evaluate the quality of end-of-life care in the intensive care unit
Glavan BJ, Engelberg RA, Downey L, et al (Univ of Washington, Seattle)
Crit Care Med 36:1138-1146, 2008

Rationale.—We investigated whether proposed "quality markers" within the medical record are associated with family assessment of the quality of dying and death in the intensive care unit (ICU).

Objective.—To identify chart-based markers that could be used as measures for improving the quality of end-of-life care.

Design.—A multicenter study conducting standardized chart abstraction and surveying families of patients who died in the ICU or within 24 hrs of being transferred from an ICU.

Setting.—ICUs at ten hospitals in the northwest United States.

Patients.—Overall, 356 patients who died in the ICU or within 24 hrs of transfer from an ICU.

Measurements.—The 22-item family assessed Quality of Dying and Death (QODD-22) questionnaire and a single item rating of the overall quality of dying and death (QODD-1).

Analysis.—The associations of chart-based quality markers with QODD scores were tested using Mann-Whitney U tests, Kruskal-Wallis tests, or Spearman's rank-correlation coefficients as appropriate.

Results.—Higher QODD-22 scores were associated with documentation of a living will ($p = .03$), absence of cardiopulmonary resuscitation performed in the last hour of life ($p = .01$), withdrawal of tube feeding ($p = .04$), family presence at time of death ($p = .02$), and discussion of the patient's wish to withdraw life support during a family conference ($p < .001$). Additional correlates with a higher QODD-1 score included use of standardized comfort care orders and occurrence of a family conference ($p \leq .05$).

Conclusions.—We identified chart-based variables associated with higher QODD scores. These QODD scores could serve as targets for measuring and improving the quality of end-of-life care in the ICU.

▶ Meeting the needs of patients and families during end of life is an evolving quality concern in the critical care environment. Sudden awareness of critical illness and end-of-life issues find patients and their loved ones relying closely on clinicians to provide an informative, supportive, and comforting environment. The manner in which clinicians communicate illness severity, as well as death and dying, may have a significant impact on patient/family satisfaction and quality of care. In this study, Glavan et al set out to determine if chart-based markers in the medical record provide a good resource of potential predictors of the quality of the dying and death score (QODD), which were correlated with surveys completed by families of patients who died in the ICU or within 24 hours of being transferred from the ICU.

This multicenter study included 10 hospitals in western Washington representing teaching, nonteaching, community, and university-affiliated county hospitals conducted over a 2-year period. A demonstrated reliable and valid questionnaire, the QODD-22 questionnaire including 22 questions initially derived from a 31-item QODD, was used in this study. An additional single item summary question (QODD-1) was also sent to the patients' family to assess the patient's experience. It is not surprising that cardiopulmonary resuscitation (CPR) within the last hour of life was associated with a lower score, whereas documentation presence of a living will and the patient's wish to withdraw life support were associated with higher scores. Limitations of the study include the use of a retrospective chart review design with family reports to represent patient satisfaction at the end of life. Additionally, the study was restricted to a specific geographic location in the United States reducing the variability of diverse racial and ethnic backgrounds.

Bundling care has been successful in decreasing ventilator-associated pneumonia, central line-related blood stream infections, and decreasing mortality in severe sepsis. Developing an end-of-life care bundle, with a measurable set of time-based quality indicators, which may be easily retrieved from the patient chart, may assist clinicians in improving quality and satisfaction for patients and families in death and dying. Communicating clinical information to the patient and family, providing emotional support, pain management, and addressing spiritual needs are important measures to evaluate quality of care at end of life in the ICU. A method to identify predictable quality markers in the medical record for future quality improvement may be necessary to guide improving end-of-life care in our own critical care units.

C. A. Schorr, RN, MSN

Growth in adult prolonged acute mechanical ventilation: Implications for healthcare delivery
Zilberberg MD, de Wit M, Pirone JR, et al (Univ of Massachusetts, Amherst; Virginia Commonwealth Univ, Richmond; Washington Hosp Ctr, Washington, DC)
Crit Care Med 36:1451-1455, 2008

Objective.—Patients requiring prolonged acute mechanical ventilation (PAMV, defined as mechanical ventilation ≥96 hrs) have hospital survival rates similar to those requiring <96 hrs of mechanical ventilation and consume about two thirds of hospital resources devoted to mechanical ventilation care. Because of this disproportionate resource utilization and the shifting U.S. demographics, we projected the expected volume of adult PAMV cases through year 2020.

Design.—We used data from the National Inpatient Sample/Health Care Utilization Project of the Agency for Healthcare Research and

Quality from 2000 to 2005 to calculate historic annual age-adjusted PAMV incidence rates using estimated population statistics from the U.S. Census Bureau. To predict future growth by age group, we fit linear regression models to the historic incidence rate changes. Age-adjusted estimates were computed using population projections obtained from the U.S. Census Bureau.

Setting.—U.S. hospitals.

Patients.—Nationally representative sample of U.S. hospital discharges with PAMV (code 96.72 from the *International Classification of Diseases, Ninth Revision*).

Interventions.—None.

Measurements and Main Results.—Historic annualized increase in PAMV was ~5.5%, compared with ~1% per annum growth in both U.S. population and hospital admissions. The fastest annualized growth was observed among 44–65 (7.9%) followed by 18–44 (4.7%), ≥85 (4.6%), and 65–84 (3.4%) age groups. Factoring in both age-specific growth in PAMV population and overall U.S. adult population changes, we project PAMV to more than double from approximately 250,000 cases in 2000 to 605,898 cases by year 2020.

Conclusions.—Patients undergoing PAMV are a large and resource-intensive population whose increase outpaces growth in the general U.S. population and in overall hospital volume. Policy makers must factor this projected rapid growth in frequency of PAMV into future resource and work force planning. Given the resource-intensive nature of these patients, strategies need to be developed to optimize their care and to increase efficiency of healthcare delivery to this large and growing population.

▶ At a time when we face current and future shortages of critical care nurses and physicians, the last thing we want to learn is that there is a rapidly growing group of patients who require a high level of critical care resources. This report alerts us to the growing number of patients who require prolonged mechanical ventilation and challenge us to develop a strategy to improve our resource use and efficiency in managing these patients. At the current rate of growth, we may even need to consider whether or not we can afford to offer prolonged ventilatory support to everyone or every surrogate decision maker who wants to access this form of support. Fortunately, this issue is being considered brought up by various agencies that are developing strategies to guide resource utilization in the setting of mass casualty situations.[1,2-5]

R. A. Balk, MD

References

1. Devereaux A, Christian MD, Dichter JR, et al. Summary of suggestions from the Task Force for Mass Critical Care Summit, January 26-27, 2007. *Chest.* 2008;133: 1S-7S.
2. Christian MD, Devereaux AV, Dichter JR, Geiling JA, Rubinson L. Definitive care for the critically ill during a disaster: current capabilities and limitations. *Chest.* 2008;133:8S-17S.

3. Rubinson L, Hick JL, Hanfling DG, et al. Definitive care for the critically ill during a disaster: a framework for optimizing critical care surge capacity. *Chest.* 2008; 133:18S-31S.
4. Rubinson L, Hick JL, Curtis JR, et al. Definitive care for the critically ill during a disaster: medical resources for surge capacity. *Chest.* 2008;133:32S-50S.
5. Devereaux AV, Dichter JR, Christian MD, et al. Definitive care for the critically ill during a disaster: a framework for allocation of scarce resources in mass critical care. *Chest.* 2008;133:51S-66S.

A prospective study of primary surrogate decision makers' knowledge of intensive care

Rodriguez RM, Navarrete E, Schwaber J, et al (Univ of California San Francisco School of Medicine)
Crit Care Med 36:1633-1636, 2008

Objectives.—We sought to determine 1) primary surrogate decision makers' knowledge of their family members' intensive care and resuscitation status; 2) whether characteristics such as low education level and lack of English language fluency were associated with poor knowledge of intensive care; 3) surrogates' ratings of intensive care unit team communication; and 4) barriers to communication.

Design.—Prospective study.

Setting.—Medical intensive care units of a county hospital located in an urban area.

Subjects.—Primary surrogate decision makers of all adults admitted >48 hrs from August 2005 to April 2006, enrolled sequentially.

Interventions.—Using a structured instrument consisting of visual analog scales, Likert-type questions, and an objective assessment of knowledge of family member's current intensive care, we interviewed primary surrogate decision makers after they had at least one bedside patient visit.

Measurements and Main Results.—Of eligible primary surrogate decision makers, 81 were enrolled; 96% had spoken to hospital staff. On a scale in which 0 indicated the worst possible communication and 10 indicated the best possible communication, primary surrogate decision makers' mean (SD) ratings were 8.6 (2.3) for nurses and 7.8 (2.8) for doctors. Forty-seven percent of primary surrogate decision makers met the predetermined criteria for good understanding with no significant difference between college-educated (44%) and non-college-educated (50%) primary surrogate decision makers; more non-English-speaking primary surrogate decision makers (63%), however, had poor understanding than English speakers (40%) (mean difference in proportions 23%, 95% confidence interval 1% to 46%). Seventy-three percent (95% confidence interval 61–82) of primary surrogate decision makers correctly identified their family members' resuscitation orders (do-not-resuscitate, limited resuscitation, or full code). The primary reasons cited for poor communication/understanding were as follows: not given enough time (21%), explanations too complicated (16%), and too emotionally upset (5%).

Conclusions.—Although most primary surrogate decision makers reported good understanding and excellent staff communication, almost half had poor understanding on objective testing; non-English speakers were more likely to have poor understanding.

▶ Recent clinical guidelines have emphasized the need for patient-centered critical care. These guidelines emphasize the need for patients' wishes as communicated by them or their primary surrogate decision makers (PSDM) to be central to the care the patient receives. Available evidence suggests that clinicians are deficient with regard to communicating to families of critically ill patients and that PSDMs do not have a good grasp of the issues involved in the care of their loved ones. Against this backdrop, the study by Dr Rodriguez and others aimed to assess PSDM's comprehension of their family member's current intensive care and their ratings of intensive care unit (ICU) team communication, among other objectives.

Their findings are not surprising and are largely consistent with our previous body of knowledge on the subject. However, some of their reported observations raise questions that deserve to be addressed.

How does one measure adequacy of communication? PSDMs cited insufficient time with staff and excessive technical information as the most important reasons for failure to understand providers. Yet during objective testing, college education and increased reported time spent in discussions with ICU staff was not associated with better understanding. Although many factors may be responsible for these apparent incongruencies, one consideration may be deficiencies in our assessment tools. A similar survey adapted for their clinicians would most likely yield very different observations, as also would third-party reviews of video recordings of the clinician-PSDM interactions. Responses to questionnaires are a composite of information provided, cognition, retention, and recall and are highly subject to a recall bias. Whether acknowledged or not, critical illness in a loved one is a highly emotional event and influences cognition, retention, and recall of information provided. Simple questionnaires, although practical, may not suffice as tools to correctly measure clinician communication critical care settings.

Secondly, although shared decision-making is a good idea, the question remains, how much information is enough? Critical care clinicians with years of training and clinical experience still grapple daily with the very decisions we want PSDMs to participate in an informed manner. Too much information is just as dangerous as too little information, frequently gets processed by the brain as a blur, and can lead to a paralysis of analysis. Although the principle of shared decision-making seems to be omnipresent in today's critical care units, it may be difficult to closely adhere to this principle. Dr Misak, drawing on her experience as an ICU patient with septic shock, acute respiratory distress syndrome (ARDS), and multiple organ failure has narrated her experience where she was actively involved in making her care decisions although she knew she clearly lacked the capacity for correct judgment being in a psychological and emotional haze and was confused even though she seemed okay to her clinicians.[1] Franklin and Rosenbloom[2] pointed out, that the stakes are higher in critical care medicine: an irrational decision taken by a critically ill patient is likely to be catastrophic. The same holds for a PSDM.

As expressed by Dr Gawande, "Our contemporary medical credo has made us exquisitely attuned to the requirements of patient autonomy. But there are times—and they are more frequent than we readily admit—when a doctor has to steer patients to do what's right for themselves."[3]

How can we communicate effectively with patients and families? How can we confirm that they fully understand the decisions they are facing? These questions should be addressed rather urgently to form a framework with which these study results can be interpreted and also further studies can be carried out.

O. Okorie, MD
C. Bekes, MD

References

1. Misak C. ICU psychosis and patient autonomy: some thoughts from the inside. *J Med Philos.* 2005;30:411-430.
2. Franklin C, Rosenbloom B. Proposing a new standard to establish medical competence for the purpose of critical care intervention. *Critical Care Medicine.* 2000; 28:3035-3038.
3. Gawande A. *Complications: A surgeon?s notes on an imperfect science.* New York: Henry Holt; 2002. p.216.

Occurrence and outcome of fever in critically ill adults

Laupland KB, Shahpori R, Kirkpatrick AW, et al (Univ of Calgary, Canada)
Crit Care Med 36:1531-1535, 2008

Objective.—Although fever is common in the critically ill, only a small number of studies have specifically investigated its epidemiology in the intensive care unit (ICU). The objective of this study was to describe the occurrence of fever in the critically ill and assess its effect on ICU outcome.

Design.—Retrospective cohort. Fever was defined by temperature ≥38.3°C and high fever by ≥39.5°C.

Setting.—Calgary Health Region during 2000–2006.

Patients.—All adults (≥18 yrs) admitted to ICUs.

Interventions.—None.

Measurements and Main Results.—A total of 24,204 ICU admission episodes occurred among 20,466 patients; 35% were classified as medical, 33% as cardiac surgical, 16% as other surgical, and 15% as trauma/neurologic. The cumulative incidence of fever and high fever was 44% and 8% and the incidence density was 24.3 and 2.7 per 100 days of ICU admission, respectively. The incidence density of fever was higher in trauma/neuro patients, males, younger patients, and was lower in those with admission Acute Physiology and Chronic Health Evaluation II scores ≥25. Seventeen percent and 31% of patients with fever and high fever had associated positive cultures. Resolution of fever and high fever occurred in 27% and 53% of patients before ICU discharge and prolonged fever and high fever lasting for 5 or more days in the ICU occurred in 18% and 11% of febrile patients, respectively. Although the presence of fever was not associated with increased ICU mortality (13% vs. 12%; $p = .08$), high fever was associated with significantly increased risk for death (20.3% vs. 12%, $p < .0001$). After controlling for confounding factors using multivariable logistic regression models, the influence of fever on the ICU mortality varied significantly according to its timing of onset, degree, and main admission category.

Conclusions.—Fever is common in patients admitted to the ICU and its occurrence and impact on outcome varies among defined patient populations.

▶ Infectious and noninfectious causes of fever in critically ill patients are common, often prompting further work-up and initiation of therapies including antibiotics. Determining the cause of the fever can place the patient at risk for increased invasive and noninvasive testing leading to added medical costs. Laupland et al studied the occurrence, causes, and outcome effects of fever in a large number of patients in Canada within various types of ICUs. The authors reported the ability to track physiologic validated data at a minimum of every hour for each patient providing a significant amount of information. The value of this data allows the investigators to distinctively describe outcomes based on admission classification. The findings show medical patients had more culture-associated fever compared with surgical, trauma/neurologic with the lowest in the cardiac surgical patient group. Culture negative and those not having cultures may have caused a low estimate of infections recorded in this study. All diagnostic categories found that fever incidence density progressively decreased with advanced age and high fever ($\geq 39.5°C$) was associated with significantly increased risk for death. Limitations of this study include the variable number of temperatures measured for each patient and the inability to evaluate the use of antipyretics and cooling devices to reduce fever and their effects in maintaining normothermia. Determining a rational approach to managing critically ill patients with fever and a protocolized approach to treatment may be of benefit for further investigation.

C. A. Schorr, RN, MSN

Mortality after discharge from the intensive care unit during the early weekend period: a population-based cohort study in Denmark
Obel N, Schierbeck J, Pedersen L, et al (Odense Univ Hosp, Denmark; Aarhus Univ Hosp, Denmark; et al)
Acta Anaesthesiol Scand 51:1225-1230, 2007

Background.—As a result of a shortage of intensive care capacity, patients may be discharged prematurely early during weekends which may lead to an increased mortality and risk of readmission to intensive care units (ICU). We examined whether discharge from the ICU during the first part of the weekend was associated with an increased mortality and readmission to the ICU.

Methods.—The study was conducted at a university clinic of internal medicine and included all patients admitted for the first time to the ICU, and discharged alive in the period 1 January 2001 to 31 December 2005. Patients were divided in those discharged between 00.00 h Friday and 24.00 h Saturday (weekend group) and those discharged Sunday to Thursday (non-weekend group). The main outcome was time from discharge from the ICU to the combined endpoint death or re-admission to ICU which ever came first. We used Kaplan–Meier analysis and Cox's proportional-hazards regression to compute survival curves and risk ratio estimates.

Results.—There were 228 patients in the weekend group and 555 patients in the non-weekend group. Crude and adjusted 28-day risk ratio of the combined endpoint was 1.50 [95% confidence interval (CI): 1.15–1.97] and 1.43 (1.09–1.87) in the weekend group. Although an increased risk of death was observed in the weekend group immediately after discharge from the ICU, the difference in mortality between the two groups had disappeared after 2 years.

Conclusion.—Medical patients discharged from the ICU early in the weekends seem to have an increased mortality and risk of readmission to the ICU.

▶ As clinicians and potential consumers of health care, should we be concerned that the day of the week and time of ICU discharge may have a negative impact on patient outcomes? In many institutions, medical staff coverage in ICU is generally decreased on the weekend. The effect of limited medical staff on weekends may lead to earlier discharge from the ICU to accommodate the reduction in ICU capacity and/or coverage. This article examined the effect of early weekend (between 00.00 Friday and 24.00 Saturday) discharge on mortality and readmissions for first time ICU patients admitted to a tertiary hospital in Denmark. The primary outcome was the 28-day risk of the combined endpoint of time from ICU discharge until death or readmission. In this study, medical patients in the weekend group had a greater risk of dying or readmission to the ICU compared with the nonweekend group. The results of this single center study in a heterogeneous patient group may not be applicable to all ICUs. However, this study does raise questions about the decisions clinicians are faced with everyday, prompting premature discharge of patients to a lower level care based on staffing or hospital overcrowding rather than clinical stability.

The results of this study give new meaning to rise and shine, when it comes to early weekend discharges. Evaluating timing of ICU discharges may uncover markers to avoid premature discharge from the ICU. A study in 2002 reported late ICU discharges and high discharge—Therapeutic Intervention Scoring System (TISS) scores being associated with increased mortality.[1] Additional research into use of the TISS scoring system and the use of an intermediate care unit for early discharges may provide additional information to assist clinicians in providing ample care with limited resources.

C. A. Schorr, RN, MSN

Reference

1. Beck DH, McQuillan P, Smith GB. Waiting for the break of dawn? The effects of discharge time, discharge TISS scores and discharge facility on hospital mortality after intensive care. *Intensive Care Med.* 2002;28:1287-1293.

Miscellaneous

Costs of Intravenous Adverse Drug Events in Academic and Nonacademic Intensive Care Units
Nuckols TK, Paddock SM, Bower AG, et al (The RAND Corporation, Santa Monica, CA; Amgen, Inc., Thousand Oaks, CA; et al)
Med Care 46:17-24, 2008

Background.—Adverse drug events (ADEs), particularly those involving intravenous medications (IV-ADEs), are common among intensive care unit (ICU) patients and may increase hospitalization costs. Precise cost estimates have not been reported for academic ICUs, and no studies have included nonacademic ICUs.

Objectives.—To estimate increases in costs and length of stay after IV-ADEs at an academic and a nonacademic hospital.

Research Design.—This study reviewed medical records to identify IV-ADEs, and then, using a nested case-control design with propensity-score matching, assessed differences in costs and length of stay between cases and controls.

Subjects.—A total of 4604 adult ICU patients in 3 ICUs at an academic hospital and 2 ICUs at a nonacademic hospital in 2003 and 2004.

Measures.—Increased cost and length of stay associated with IV-ADEs.

Results.—Three hundred ninety-seven IV-ADEs were identified: 79% temporary physical injuries, 0% permanent physical injuries, 20% interventions to sustain life, and 2% in-hospital deaths. In the academic ICUs, patients with IV-ADEs had $6647 greater costs ($P < 0.0001$) and 4.8-day longer stays ($P = 0.0003$) compared with controls. In the nonacademic ICUs, IV-ADEs were not associated with greater costs ($188, $P = 0.4236$) or lengths of stay (-0.3 days, $P = 0.8016$). Cost and length-of-stay differences between the hospitals were statistically significant ($P = 0.0012$). However, there were no differences in IV-ADE severity or preventability, and the characteristics of patients experiencing IV-ADEs differed only modestly.

Conclusions.—IV-ADEs substantially increased hospitalization costs and length of stay in ICUs at an academic hospital but not at a nonacademic hospital, likely because of differences in practices after IV-ADEs occurred (Table 2).

▶ The highest rate of adverse drug events (ADEs) in hospitals occur in medical intensive care units.[1] Yet, a paucity of data exist about the costs of ADEs in intensive care units (ICUs). Nuckols et al attempt to compare the financial implications of these mistakes on the length of stay (LOS) in both an academic and a nonacademic medical center (see Table 2). The inclusion

TABLE 2.—Postevent Costs and Length of Stay of Cases Vs. Controls Within Each Hospital

	Academic Hospital					Nonacademic Hospital				
	Cases	Controls	Difference (Increment)	Change	P	Cases	Controls	Difference (Increment)	Change	P
Total postevent costs, mean (SD)*	$19,176 ($20,062)	$12,529 ($13,215)	$6647 ($22,507)	53%	<0.0001	$17,528 ($22,296)	$17,340 ($21,949)	$188 ($28,885)	1%	0.4236
Postevent daily costs, mean (SD)†	$1156 ($660)	$1326 ($1272)	−$170 ($1285)	−13%	0.5622	$1547 ($1361)	$1697 ($1803)	−$150 ($2061)	−9%	0.6966
Postevent length of stay, in days, mean (SD)‡	16.0 (14.7)	11.3 (11.5)	4.8 (17.8)	42%	0.0003	10.2 (10.4)	10.5 (11.4)	−0.3 d (14.1)	−3%	0.8016
Total no. participants	139	139				194	194			

*Total postevent costs = total hospitalization costs incurred on or after the day of the IV-ADE.
†Postevent daily costs = average cost incurred per hospital day on or after the day of the IV-ADE.
‡Postevent length of stay = length of stay in hospital including and after the day of the IV-ADE.
(Reprinted from Nuckols TK, Paddock SM, Bower AG, et al. Costs of intravenous adverse drug events in academic and nonacademic intensive care units. *Med Care.* 2008;46:17-24.)

of a nonacademic institution is noteworthy as data about the costs of ADEs in these institutions are scant. The difference in hospital costs and LOS between these institutions is important as it raises the question; why do patients with ADEs have increased LOS in academic centers? Is nausea or transient hypotension related to opiate overdose an adequate reason to be kept in the ICU for observation? It is possible that the differences in the LOS among institutions may be more reflective of the weaknesses rather than the strengths of this study. The hospital populations were compared with a propensity score that has inherent limitations, and originally this study was designed to see if smart intravenous (IV) pumps reduced ADEs. The authors also acknowledge that reviewing medical records to pick up an ADE is less than ideal. It is not clear if the morbidity, which occurred in the nonacademic institution, was because of ADEs or the control's baseline illness as their Acute Physiology and Chronic Health Evaluation (APACHE)-II score 24 hours before the event was comparatively elevated. This study has important implications as more research needs to be done in both nonacademic hospital centers and in a wider variety of academic centers about ADEs. Both hospitals in this study had limited minority populations, and clinicians may wonder how ADEs would affect the LOS in hospitals with traditionally larger minority and indigent populations. If the authors' conclusions are correct then academic centers may need to reexamine their practice concerning medical errors. This study forces practitioners to examine their own response to medical errors and makes one realize that observing patients unnecessarily may only be contributing to spiraling medical costs.

N. Puri, MD
C. Bekes, MD

Reference

1. Kopp BJ, Erstad BL, Allen ME, et al. Medication errors and adverse drug events in an intensive care unit: direct observation approach for detection. *Crit Care Med.* 2006;34:415-425.

Family Satisfaction in the ICU: Differences Between Families of Survivors and Nonsurvivors
Wall RJ, Curtis JR, Cooke CR, et al (Univ of Washington, Seattle, WA)
Chest 132:1425-1433, 2007

Background.—We previously noted that the families of patients dying in the ICU reported higher satisfaction with their ICU experience than the families of survivors. However, the reasons for this finding were unclear. In the current study, we sought to confirm these findings and identify specific aspects of care that were rated more highly by the family members of patients dying in the ICU compared to family members of ICU survivors.

Methods.—A total of 539 family members with a patient in the ICU were surveyed. Family satisfaction was measured using the 24-item family satisfaction in the ICU questionnaire. Ordinal logistic regression identified which components of family satisfaction were associated with the patient's outcome (ie, whether the patient lived or died).

Results.—A total of 51% of respondents had a loved one die in the ICU. Overall, the families of patients dying in the ICU were more satisfied with their ICU experience than were families of ICU survivors, and the largest differences were noted for care aspects directly affecting family members. Significant differences were found for inclusion in decision making, communication, emotional support, respect and compassion shown to family, and consideration of family needs (p < 0.01).

Conclusions.—The families of patients dying in the ICU were more satisfied with their ICU experience than were the families of ICU survivors. The reasons for this difference were higher ratings on family-centered aspects of care. These findings suggest that efforts to improve the support of ICU family members should focus not only on the families of dying patients but also on the families of patients who survive their ICU stay.

▶ The abilities to communicate with patients and families and deliver compassionate care distinguish true ICU professionals from mere technicians. In this survey, from a study of 539 families of ICU patients, the authors report that families of nonsurvivors were more satisfied with their experience compared with the families of survivors. Their survey revealed that, of the 24 items aspects of ICU care evaluated, families of nonsurvivors were significantly more satisfied with 12 of them. Of these, many were aspects of care that were considered family centered, involving communication and respect for family needs.

Why would this be the case? Many possible explanations could account for ICU professionals devoting more time to family centered needs when caring for the dying, including their own family experiences and attitudes toward death. This study, although representative of only 1 patient population and ICU staff, reminds us that all families of ICU patients require and deserve good communication from staff, respect for their needs, and family centered care.

T. Lonergan, MD
C. Bekes, MD

Patient-initiated device removal in intensive care units: A national prevalence study
Mion LC, Minnick AF, Leipzig RM, et al (Metro-Health Med Ctr, Cleveland, OH; Vanderbilt Univ School of Nursing, Nashville, TN; Mount Sinai School of Medicine, NY, et al)
Crit Care Med 35:2714-2720, 2007

Objective.—Information is needed about patient-initiated device removal to guide quality initiatives addressing regulations aimed at minimizing physical restraint use. Research objectives were to determine the prevalence of device removal, describe patient contexts, examine unit-level adjusted risk factors, and describe consequences.

Design.—Prospective prevalence.

Setting.—Total of 49 adult intensive care units (ICUs) from a random sample of 39 hospitals in five states.

Methods.—Data were collected daily for 49,482 patient-days by trained nurses and included unit census, ventilator days, restraint days, and days accounted for by men and by elderly. For each device removal episode, data were collected on demographic and clinical variables.

Results.—Patients removed 1,623 devices on 1,097 occasions: overall rate, 22.1 episodes/1000 patient-days; range, 0–102.4. Surgical ICUs had lower rates (16.1 episodes) than general (23.6 episodes) and medical (23.4 episodes) ICUs. ICUs with fewer resources had fewer all-type device removal relative to ICUs with greater resources (relative risk, 0.76; 95% confidence interval, 0.66–0.87) but higher self-extubation rates (relative risk, 1.27; 95% confidence interval, 1.07–1.52). Men accounted for 57% of the episodes, 44% were restrained at the time, and 30% had not received any sedation, narcotic, or psychotropic drug in the previous 24 hrs. There was no association between rates of device removal with restraint rates, proportion of men, or elderly. Self-extubation rates were inversely associated with ventilator days ($r_s = -0.31$, $p = .03$). Patient harm occurred in 250 (23%) episodes; ten incurred major harm. No deaths occurred. Reinsertion rates varied by device: 23.5% of surgical drains to 88.9% of monitor leads. Additional resources (e.g., radiography) were used in 58% of the episodes.

Conclusion.—Device removal by ICU patients is common, resulting in harm in one fourth of patients and significant resource expenditure. Further examination of patient-, unit-, and practitioner-level variables may help explain variation in rates and provide direction for further targeted interventions.

▶ Patient-initiated premature removal of invasive devices in the critical care environment is not without risk and may lead to potentially detrimental outcomes. Maintaining patient safety while assuring compliance with the federal regulations for the use of physical restraints can produce additional unforeseen consequences. In this study, Mion and colleagues report that patient-initiated device removal is not uncommon but varies among ICUs and types of ICUs. In this study, ICUs with more resources had lower self-extubation rates but higher overall removal when minor and major devices were included. The degree of harm accounted for in this study was often minor, with no deaths reported.

This is a well-designed study to describe a variety of patient variables and outcomes associated with premature device removal. The 49 ICUs in this study represent various types of ICU throughout 6 metropolitan regions of the United States, making the results of this study a potential tool for benchmarking descriptions and outcomes associated with patient-initiated device removal. Limitations in the data collection process may underestimate the prevalence of patient-initiated removal in this study. Established preset times for data collection and having to rely on staff to complete a notification card for those patients experiencing premature removal of a device could have resulted in missed events. Another study used a card, completed by the staff, to record premature device removal. The role of a card-based reporting system increased patient safety event reporting significantly compared with preintervention Web-based reporting. My institution has adopted an anonymous reporting system to capture events and near events such as premature device removal. However, the number of events reported varies from month to month. Patient-initiated device removal is primarily captured during retrospective chart review when entering data into our quality/performance improvement database. Therefore, caution should be used when reporting premature device removal based on staff reporting alone, as it may underestimate overall device removal.

Assuring compliance with regulatory agencies may be accomplished while preventing patients from harm because of premature device removal. Evaluating patients for delirium, decreasing sedation, assessing daily for weaning from mechanical ventilation, with the use of associated protocols for analgesia and/or sedation may decrease the frequency of patient-initiated premature device removal in the ICU.

C. A. Schorr, RN, MSN

Attitudes towards and evaluation of medical emergency teams: A survey of trainees in intensive care medicine

Jacques T, Harrison GA, McLaws M-L (Univ of New South Wales, Sydney)
Anaesth Intensive Care 36:90-95, 2008

A survey was conducted to explore the perception of intensive care registrars on the impact of activities outside the intensive care unit (ICU), particularly in medical emergency teams, on their training and the care of patients.

An anonymous mail-out survey was sent to 356 trainees registered with the Joint Faculty of Intensive Care Medicine, half of whom were determined to be involved in ICU duties. No patients were involved and respondents participated voluntarily. The main outcome measures were barriers and predictors of satisfaction with ICU training.

One-hundred-and-thirty-six (38%) trainees responded. Seventy-eight percent had participated in a medical emergency team, of whom 99% of respondents stated the medical emergency team included an ICU registrar but rarely (3%) an ICU consultant. Sixty-six percent of respondents reported that medical emergency team involvement had a positive effect on training but 77% reported little or no supervision of team duties. While trainees did not believe they spent too much time performing medical emergency team duties, the time spent on medical emergency teams at night, when ICU staffing levels are at their lowest, was the same as during the day. Serious concern was expressed about the negative impact of medical emergency team activities on their ability to care for ICU patients and the additional stress on ICU medical and nursing staff.

Overall, ICU trainees regarded participation in a medical emergency team as positive on training and on patient care in wards, but other results have resource implications for the provision of clinical emergency response systems, care of patients in ICUs and the training of the future intensive care workforce (Table 3).

▶ This article examines the impact of medical emergency teams (MET) on trainees in critical care medicine in Australia and New Zealand. Questionnaires were sent to trainees in intensive care medicine. Thirty-eight percent of the original questionnaires were returned and 76% of the estimated number of trainees engaged in ICU activities responded. Table 3 shows the percentage of time the trainees committed to MET duties.

Most of the trainees felt that the MET duties enhanced the quality of their training and that they were well trained to handle the scenarios they encountered. They did, however, feel that the use of the MET teams left an easy "out" for the floor team to relinquish care of the sick patient. Many of the calls took over 20 minutes of time, thus taking resources from the ICU to the floor. Seventy-one percent of respondents felt that the MET team accelerated the end-of-life discussions.

Although it clearly seems that there should be an easily activated system to get emergency care for a patient who is not doing well, we need to be careful how we allocate our already scarce medical resources. In June of 2006, the Institute for Healthcare Improvement (IHI) announced its Save 100 000 Lives Campaign, which included the implementation of the rapid response teams (equivalent to the MET in this article). Although Don Berwick and the IHI are to be commended for bringing a patient safety focus to the forefront, we have not used evidence-based medicine to support some of the recommendations that were made. As Auerbach[1] reviewed in his article on improving care, we find that interventions that appear to be promising on the basis of preliminary data are often found to have little or no benefit in the improvement of

TABLE 3.—Percentage of Time Committed to Duties Over Seven Days During ICU in-Hours and Out-of-Hours

%ICU Training Time Spent	MET Duties In-Hours % (n)	MET Duties Out of Hours % [95% CI] (n)	Non-MET Out of Hours % [95% CI] (n)
≤25%	30 (33)	39 (41)	81 (88)
26%-50%	30 (33)	15 (16)	18 (20)
51-75%	13 (14)	7 (8)	0(0)
76-100%	27 (29)	39 (41)	1 (1)
Total	100 (109)	100 (106)	100 (109)

(Reprinted from Jacques T, Harrison GA, McLaws M-L, et al. Attitudes towards and evaluation of medical emergency teams: a survey of trainees in intensive care medicine. *Anaesth Intensive Care*. 2008;36:90-95, with permission from the Australian Society of Anaesthetists.)

outcome. In the case of rapid response teams, they come with both direct and indirect costs. In the MET article, teams were spending a great deal of time outside the ICU. The impact on the quality of care has not been examined. Data to date have shown mixed outcomes with some studies reporting improvement but many others have not. The IHI claims that the lives saved have surpassed the goal of 100 000. Wachter and Pronovost[2] question the validity of that number and urge the use of rigorous processes to prioritize and implement quality and safety interventions.

We need rigorous testing and studies to examine the benefits of improvements in quality or safety just as we would with any other intervention in medicine. MET or rapid response teams have not yet met that rigorous testing despite the fact that we have spent a large amount of money and personnel resources on this endeavor.

A. Spevetz, MD
C. Bekes, MD

References

1. Tovey G, Stokes M. A survey of the use of 2D ultrasound guidance for insertion of central venous catheters by UK consultant paediatric anaesthetists. *Eur J Anaesthesiol.* 2007;24:71-75.
2. Watcher RM, Pronovost PJ. The 100,000 lives campaign: a scientific and policy review. *Jt Comm J Qual Patient Saf.* 2006;32:621-627.

Costs of adverse events in intensive care units
Kaushal R, Bates DW, Franz C, et al (Harvard Medical School, Boston, MA; Eastern Research Group, Lexington, MA)
Critical Care Medicine 35:2479-2483, 2007

Context.—Iatrogenic injuries are very common in critically ill adults. However, the financial implications of these events are incompletely understood.

Objective.—To determine the costs of adverse events in patients in the medical intensive care unit and in the cardiac intensive care unit.

Design, Setting, and Patients.—We performed a matched case-control analysis on data collected during a prospective 1-yr observation study (July 2002 to June 2003) of medical intensive care unit and cardiac intensive care unit patients at an academic, tertiary care urban hospital. A total of 108 cases were matched with 375 controls in our study.

Main Outcome Measures.—Costs of care and lengths of stay were determined from hospital billing systems for patients in the medical and cardiac intensive care units. We then determined the incremental costs and lengths of stay for patients with adverse events compared with patients without events while in the intensive care unit. Costs were truncated for patients with a second adverse event on a subsequent day during the intensive care unit stay.

Results.—For 56 medical intensive care unit patients, the cost of an adverse event was $3,961 ($p = .010$) and the increase in length of stay was 0.77 days ($p = .048$). This extrapolated to annual costs of $853,000 for adverse events in the medical intensive care unit. Similarly, for 52 cardiac intensive care unit patients, the cost of an adverse event was $3,857 ($p = .023$), corresponding to $630,000 in annual costs. On average, patients with events in the cardiac intensive care unit had an increase of 1.08 days in length of stay ($p = .003$).

Conclusions.—Patients who require intensive care are especially at risk for adverse events, and the associated costs with such events are substantial. The costs of adverse events may justify further investment in prevention strategies.

▶ The authors quantify only additional costs that accrued during a patient's ICU stay, and it is interesting to note that for the general medical patients, the total hospital costs were not significantly different than controls. Although the authors state that they classified adverse events as either avoidable or unavoidable during their data collection, this distinction plays no role in their analysis. This is in keeping with their stated goal to quantify the costs of all adverse events in an ICU population. But, if as the authors argue, this study is to "further justify investments in quality improvement and patient safety strategies," an analysis of the costs of avoidable adverse events would be more relevant. In the end, there are many reasons to develop strategies to limit adverse events in the ICU, including cost, patient safety and quality of life, and risk management.

T. Lonergan, MD
C. Bekes, MD

Impact of 2 different levels of performance feedback on compliance with infection control process measures in 2 intensive care units

Assanasen S, Edmond M, Bearman G, et al (Univ Med Ctr, Richmond, VA)
Am J Infect Control 36:407-413, 2008

Background.—Performance monitoring and feedback of infection control process measures is an important tool for improving guideline adherence. Different feedback strategies may lead to distinctive outcomes.

Objectives.—Our objective was to determine the relative impact of 2 different levels of feedback on compliance in an intensive care unit (ICU) setting.

Methods.—Proportion of head of bed (HOB) elevation, hand hygiene (HH) compliance, and proportion of femoral catheter (FC) to all central venous catheter-days were observed in a medical ICU and a surgical ICU. After a 3-month baseline observation phase (phase 1; P1), we provided quarterly feedback on these process measures and major health care-associated infections (HAIs) to unit leaders from July 2004 to June

2005 (P2). From July 2005 to June 2006 (P3), feedback parameters were also provided to unit leaders and to all staff via 48 × 72-inch color posters in ICU personnel-only areas. At the end of the study, a survey was performed to assess the influence of the posters and HH observations.

Results.—The analysis of IC process measures included 6948 HOB elevation observations, 1576 HH opportunities, and 16,591 catheter-days. In P2, the overall compliance with HOB elevation and the proportion of FC use significantly improved from 51% to 88% ($P < .001$) and 13% to 7% ($P < .001$), respectively. No significant difference in HH compliance was observed during this phase (40% vs 47%, respectively; $P = .28$). Comparing P3 with P2, HH compliance significantly improved from 47% to 71% ($P < .001$), and there was a slight improvement in HOB elevation rate from 88% to 93% ($P < .001$). There was no significant change in FC use in P3. There were 53 survey respondents. Sixty percent reported that the poster information changed their practices. Nearly all respondents (92%) knew that their HH behavior was being observed; however, 61% claimed that HH compliance was not influenced by observation.

Conclusion.—Feedback of infection control process measures and major HAIs to unit leadership significantly improved compliance with HOB elevation rate and FC use but not HH. Multilevel feedback significantly improved HH compliance and delivered a satisfactory level of compliance with HOB and FC use in both ICUs during the study period.

▶ Audit and feedback are crucial in keeping leadership and staff informed regarding process performance compliance. The mechanism for effective feedback promoting behavior change and performance improvement is a multifaceted process. This study was designed to evaluate the impact of 2 different levels of performance feedback strategies. There were 3 phases in this study: a 3-month observation (phase 1) followed by quarterly feedback on process measures and health care–associated infections (phase 2) and the use of large posters displayed in ICU personnel areas, email reports, and communication with unit leadership provided multilevel feedback in the last stage (phase 3). The results of this study found significant improvement in compliance with hand hygiene in phase 3, and high-level compliance with head-of-bed (HOB) elevation in both phase 2 and 3 and significant improvement in proportion of femoral catheter use in phase 2. A survey conducted at the end of this study assessed the influence of the posters and the observation of hand hygiene. There were only 53 surveys completed with 60% of the respondents reporting that the poster information changed their practice.

In a similar study published in 2006, feedback and process measures decreased the use of femoral catheters and increased compliance with HOB elevation, although no significant improvement was observed in hand hygiene.[1] Using a variety of methods to provide feedback is needed to maintain a captive audience. I have used large posters, similar to the format used in this study, to report quarterly performance measures for our severe sepsis patient population. After 3.5 years, the posters remain intact in 8 key areas of the hospital, with quarterly updates posted to reflect new data. Initially this feedback method was effective. New bright posters attracted the attention of the staff. However, after 2 years the poster seemed to blend in as wallpaper with little attention to the quarterly changes in performance. Altering the color of the poster and/or compliance graphs can bring new attention to current interventions and results. Innovative methods to provide feedback in verbal, written, or display form enables sharing of information while framing problem areas as new opportunities for improvement. Providing feedback allows clinicians to alter behavior and make adjustments to improve process improvement. Inability to deliver feedback will most likely lead to process change failure.

C. A. Schorr, RN, MSN

Reference

1. Behre M, Edmond MD, Bearman G. Measurement and feedback of infection control process measures in the intensive care unit: impact on compliance. *Am J Infect Control.* 2006;34:537-539.

Validation of Surgical Intensive Care-Infection Registry: A Medical Informatics System for Intensive Care Unit Research, Quality of Care Improvement, and Daily Patient Care
Golob Jr. JF, Fadlalla AMA, Kan JA, et al (Reserve Univ School of Medicine Cleveland, OH; Cleveland State Univ, OH)
J Am Coll Surg 207:164-173, 2008

Background.—We developed a prototype electronic clinical information system called the Surgical Intensive Care-Infection Registry (SIC-IR) to prospectively study infectious complications and monitor quality of care improvement programs in the surgical and trauma intensive care unit. The objective of this study was to validate SIC-IR as a successful health information technology with an accurate clinical data repository.

Study Design.—Using the DeLone and McLean Model of Information Systems Success as a framework, we evaluated SIC-IR in a 3-month prospective crossover study of physician use in one of our two surgical and trauma intensive care units (SIC-IR unit versus non SIC-IR unit). Three simultaneous research methodologies were used: a user survey study, a pair of time-motion studies, and an accuracy study of SIC-IR's clinical data repository.

Results.—The SIC-IR user survey results were positive for system reliability, graphic user interface, efficiency, and overall benefit to patient care. There was a significant decrease in prerounding time of nearly 4 minutes per patient on the SIC-IR unit compared with the non SIC-IR unit. The SIC-IR documentation and data archiving was accurate 74% to 100% of the time depending on the data entry method used. This accuracy was significantly improved compared with normal hand-written documentation on the non SIC-IR unit.

Conclusions.—SIC-IR proved to be a useful application both at individual user and organizational levels and will serve as an accurate tool to conduct prospective research and monitor quality of care improvement programs.

▶ Inconsistent, missing, or incorrect chart documentation may cause delayed or inappropriate treatment leading to increased complications and poor outcomes. Improving accuracy and efficiency of information provided during ICU rounds might decrease the chance of error, ensure the patient is getting the most appropriate timely care, and build confidence among the team. The use of an electronic clinical information system to increase clinician accuracy and efficiency may serve as an invaluable resource in the ICU. This study evaluated the investigator-developed electronic clinical information system, Surgical Intensive Care-Infection Registry (SIC-IR), as a resource to provide a relational database for research, quality improvement, and daily patient care.

The study evaluated the system's accuracy, quality, and the impact on individuals and the organization. The tool was initially developed as a research tool and subsequently proved to be a valuable clinical application tool. In this study, non SIC-IR documentation of antibiotic indication, antibiotic day of treatment, and treatment stop date were significantly lower compared with the SIC-IR group. When applying the completeness and correctness for culture results, the SIC-IR had 100% accuracy and the non SIC-IR unit notes were 20% accurate. Based on the survey results, the residents believed that the system decreased their busy work and improved the care they delivered to the critically ill.

Minimizing noneducational work for residents, although improving accuracy and completeness in documenting daily progress notes, is very useful. An electronic tool that facilitates consistency in patient management from shift-to-shift and week-to-week is invaluable. The daily hand-off report may help decrease inaccurate or omitted patient information when transferring care from one clinician to another. Movement toward interface capability, data transfer, and electronic documentation will help decrease error and facilitate safe and efficient patient care.

C. A. Schorr, RN, BSN

13 Pharmacology/Sedation-Analgesia

A randomized trial of protocol-directed sedation management for mechanical ventilation in an Australian intensive care unit
Bucknall TK, Manias E, Presneill JJ (Deakin Univ, Victoria, Australia; Univ of Melbourne, Victoria, Australia)
Crit Care Med 36:1444-1450, 2008

Objective.—To compare protocol-directed sedation management with traditional non-protocol-directed practice in mechanically ventilated patients.
Design.—Randomized, controlled trial.
Setting.—General intensive care unit (24 beds) in an Australian metropolitan teaching hospital.
Patients.—Adult, mechanically ventilated patients (n = 312).
Interventions.—Patients were randomly assigned to receive sedation directed by formal guidelines (protocol group, n = 153) or usual local clinical practice (control, n = 159).
Measurements and Main Results.—The median (95% confidence interval) duration of ventilation was 79 hrs (56–93 hrs) for patients in the protocol group compared with 58 hrs (44–78 hrs) for patients who received control care ($p = .20$). Lengths of stay (median [range]) in the intensive care unit (94 [2–1106] hrs vs. 88 [14–962] hrs, $p = .58$) and hospital (13 [1–113] days vs. 13 [1–365] days, $p = .97$) were similar, as were the proportions of subjects receiving a tracheostomy (17% vs. 15%, $p = .64$) or undergoing unplanned self-extubation (1.3% vs. 0.6%, $p = .61$). Death in the intensive care unit occurred in 32 (21%) patients in the protocol group and 32 (20%) control subjects ($p = .89$), with a similar overall proportion of deaths in hospital (25% vs. 22%, $p = .51$). A Cox proportional hazards model, after adjustment for age, gender, Acute Physiology and Chronic Health Evaluation II score, diagnostic category, and doses of commonly used drugs, estimated that protocol sedation management was associated with a 22% decrease (95% confidence interval 40% decrease to 2% increase, $p = .07$) in the occurrence of successful weaning from mechanical ventilation.
Conclusions.—This randomized trial provided no evidence of a substantial reduction in the duration of mechanical ventilation or length of stay, in either the intensive care unit or the hospital, with the use of

protocol-directed sedation compared with usual local management. Qualified high-intensity nurse staffing and routine Australian intensive care unit nursing responsibility for many aspects of ventilatory practice may explain the contrast between these findings and some recent North American studies.

▶ Protocols can improve care under many, if not, most circumstances. This should not, however, be interpreted to mean that they will always improve care. For example, if one's local practice is maximized from an outcomes perspective, then a protocol is unlikely to demonstrate improvement. In addition, protocols may fail to demonstrate improvement secondary to being too complex or based on incorrect evidence or unknown confounders in a local environment. Finally, compliance with an optimized protocol is required for it to be associated with a subsequent improvement in outcomes. Finally, some protocols are used to improve process and not outcomes; thus, a demonstration of their equality to standard practice is useful. This study failed to show a benefit of an implemented protocol for several of these stated limitations, including the Hawthorne effect, as the same nurses utilized standard and protocolized approaches and could voice their suggestions for therapeutic options to the care providers. Finally, other aspects of care can negate the effects of a protocol. For example, in this study more patients in the protocol arm received paralytics.

T. Dorman, MD

The effects of sedation on gastric emptying and intra-gastric meal distribution in critical illness

Nguyen NQ, Chapman MJ, Fraser RJ, et al (Royal Adelaide Hosp, Australia)
Intensive Care Med 34:454-460, 2008

Objective.—To evaluate the effects of sedation with morphine and midazolam (M&M) versus propofol on gastric emptying in critically ill patients.

Design.—Descriptive study.

Setting.—Mixed medical and surgical intensive care unit.

Patients.—Thirty-six unselected, mechanically ventilated, critically ill patients.

Interventions.—Gastric scintigraphic data were analysed retrospectively according to whether patients were receiving M&M ($n = 20$; 14M, 6F) or propofol ($n = 16$; 7M, 9F). Measurements were performed over 4 h after administration of 100 ml of Ensure®, labelled with 20 MBq Tc ^{99m}.

Measurements and Results.—Gastric half-emptying time ($t_{1/2}$) and total and regional (proximal and distal stomach) meal retention (%) were assessed. The median $t_{1/2}$ of patients receiving M&M (153 (IQR: 72–434) min) was significantly longer than that of patients receiving propofol (58 (34–166) min, $p = 0.02$). Total gastric retention was greater in patients receiving M&M compared to those receiving propofol ($p < 0.01$). Proximal ($p = 0.02$) but not distal ($p = 0.80$) gastric retention was greater in patients who received M&M. Patients who received M&M were more likely to have ≥ 5% meal retention at 240 min than those treated with propofol (95% (19/20) vs. 56% (9/16); $p=0.01$). Changes in blood glucose concentrations during the study were similar in the two groups.

Conclusions.—In critical illness, patients receiving M&M for sedation are more likely to have slow gastric emptying, and proximal meal retention than those receiving propofol. The apparent beneficial effects of propofol-based sedation need confirmation by a prospective randomised controlled study.

▶ Enteral feeding in a critically ill patient is a complicated venture. Altered gastrointestinal motility and delayed gastric emptying are commonly encountered. It is difficult to identify a single etiology for this physiologic disruption, as there are multiple factors that likely contribute. This study by Dr Nguyen et al addresses an important aspect of intensive care medicine that is commonly overlooked with regard to its impact on enteral nutrition in this setting. This study retrospectively evaluated 2 sedation regimens and their impact on gastric emptying. Overall gastric retention was higher in the group given morphine and midazolam, as compared with those given propofol. Delay in proximal emptying of the stomach in the morphine and midazolam group likely accounted for the overall higher incidence of gastric retention. The design of this study did not afford a control arm, thereby limiting the potential use of the results. The analysis was retrospective and involved a small number of patients. However, it does offer some intriguing information. One of the most common complications in critically ill patients is aspiration pneumonia. The data gleaned from this study suggest that the choice of sedative medication may lower the percentage of gastric retention. Theoretically, this may decrease the risk of aspiration in this setting. Ultimately, this may alter tangible objectives such as length of intensive care stay, morbidity rates, and overall hospital costs. The results of these sought after questions, however, will require prospective studies involving larger numbers of critically ill subjects.

C. Deitch, MD

Prevalence and Risk Factors for Development of Delirium in Surgical and Trauma Intensive Care Unit Patients

Pandharipande P, Cotton BA, Shintani A, et al (Vanderbilt Univ School of Medicine, Nashville, TN)
J Trauma 65:34-41, 2008

Background.—Although known to be an independent predictor of poor outcomes in medical intensive care unit (ICU) patients, limited data exist regarding the prevalence of and risk factors for delirium among surgical (SICU) and trauma ICU (TICU) patients. The purpose of this study was to analyze the prevalence of and risk factors for delirium in surgical and trauma ICU patients.

Methods.—SICU and TICU patients requiring mechanical ventilation (MV) >24 hours were prospectively evaluated for delirium using the Richmond Agitation Sedation Scale (RASS) and the Confusion Assessment Method for the ICU (CAM-ICU). Those with baseline dementia, intracranial injury, or ischemic/hemorrhagic strokes that would confound the evaluation of delirium were excluded. Markov models were used to analyze predictors for daily transition to delirium.

Results.—One hundred patients (46 SICU and 54 TICU) were enrolled. Prevalence of delirium was 73% in the SICU and 67% in the TICU. Multivariable analyses identified midazolam [OR 2.75 (CI 1.43–5.26, $p = 0.002$)] exposure as the strongest independent risk factor for transitioning to delirium. Opiate exposure showed an inconsistent message such that fentanyl was a risk factor for delirium in the SICU ($p = 0.007$) but not in the TICU ($p = 0.936$), whereas morphine exposure was associated with a lower risk of delirium (SICU, $p = 0.069$; TICU $p = 0.024$).

Conclusion.—Approximately 7 of 10 SICU and TICU patients experience delirium. In keeping with other recent data on benzodiazepines, exposure to midazolam is an independent and potentially modifiable risk factor for the transitioning to delirium.

▶ This important study reveals the significant incidence of disordered mentation in a surgical patient population without identified predisposing factors. I have no doubt that the authors are correct in their statement that delirium is a significant and underappreciated problem for the surgeon.

However, I have several reservations about this report. There is no standardization of medication administration. Although the authors report common use of a set of agents consistent with guidelines published in Critical Care Medicine in 2002, the preponderance of fentanyl and midazolam as agents used and as agents associated with delirium leads me to cast some doubt on these results.[1] In addition, delirium assessment takes place once daily. How does this conform to drug administration? Is there a consistent drug holiday policy? When do holidays occur? In addition, the authors indicate that confounding factors such as substance abuse and brain injury are excluded in this study population. How can I be sure of this when in the trauma population, for example, I am not given a Glasgow Coma Score? Because this is only an observational trial, systematic administration of medications in balanced amounts does not take place. Morphine, which is ubiquitous in my intensive care unit, is underrepresented here.

Although fentanyl and midazolam perform poorly in this study, I was intrigued to see a recent French trial with a titration protocol for the identical agents where patient synchrony with mechanical ventilation was improved if midazolam and fentanyl were given in a protocol setting rather than at physician discretion.[2,3]

Fentanyl and midazolam titration was not tightly controlled in the Vanderbilt study. In what appears to be a successful French protocol, titration of agents is strictly done. Although I do not deny the observations of the Vanderbilt group, I prefer interventional trials with accepted agents using controlled algorithms as popularized by the Vanderbilt investigators in other reports.[4]

D. J. Dries, MSE, MD

References

1. Jacobi J, Fraser GL, Coursin DB, et al. Clinical practice guidelines for the sustained use of sedatives and analgesics in the critically ill adult. *Crit Care Med.* 2002;30:119-141.
2. De Jonghe B, Bastuji-Garin S, Fangio P, et al. Sedation algorithm in critically ill patients without acute brain injury. *Crit Care Med.* 2005;33:120-127.
3. De Jonghe B, Cook D, Griffith L, et al. Adaptation to the Intensive Care Environment (ATICE): Development and validation of a new sedation assessment instrument. *Crit Care Med.* 2003;31:2344-2354.
4. Ely EW, Baker AM, Dunagan DP, et al. Effect on the duration of mechanical ventilation of identifying patients capable of breathing spontaneously. *N Engl J Med.* 1996;335:1864-1869.

Subject Index

A

Abciximab
 emergency administration for acute ischemic stroke, 221
Acid-base disorders
 central venous base deficit versus arterial base deficit as predictor of survival in acute trauma, 192
Activated protein C
 for acute lung injury, 13
Acute coronary syndromes
 emergency cardiac CT for suspected, 49
 red blood cell transfusion for
  impact on clinical outcomes, 53
  utility and outcomes, 78
Acute kidney injury
 (see also Acute renal failure)
 continuous renal replacement therapy for, amino acid requirements during, 181
 as predictor of outcomes in critically ill patients, 182
 severe, 5-year outcomes, 187
Acute lung injury (ALI)
 activated protein C for, 13
 mechanical ventilation in
  bedside open lung biopsy during, yield and safety, 5
  strategy using low tidal volumes, recruitment maneuvers, and high positive end-expiratory pressure, 17
 mortality rates over time, 12
 positive end-expiratory pressure setting in adults with, 6
Acute myocardial infarction (see Myocardial infarction)
Acute renal failure
 (see also Acute kidney injury)
 in burn injuries, 97
 intra-abdominal hypertension and, 184
Acute respiratory distress syndrome (ARDS)
 after pulmonary resection, extrapulmonary ventilation for, 3
 angiotensin-converting enzyme insertion/deletion polymorphism as predictor of susceptibility and outcome in, 10
 biomarker evidence of myocardial cell injury and mortality in, 8
 lung ultrasound in diagnosis of, 37
 mechanical ventilation in
  bedside open lung biopsy during, yield and safety, 5
  low tidal volume, barriers to, 20
  strategy using low tidal volumes, recruitment maneuvers, and high positive end-expiratory pressure, 17
 mortality rates over time, 12
 positive end-expiratory pressure setting in adults with, 6
 prone positioning in
  after cardiac surgery, feasibility, safety, and efficacy, 16
  right ventricular pressure during, 2
 recruitment maneuvers in, cytokine release following, 1
 risk factors for development in patients receiving mechanical ventilation for more than 48 h, 19
Adrenal cortex
 hormone response as outcome predictor in acute critical illness, 167
Adrenal insufficiency
 in severe burn injuries, risk factors associated with, 176
Adverse drug events
 intravenous, costs in academic and nonacademic ICUs, 267
ALI (see Acute lung injury)
Amino acids
 requirements during continuous renal replacement therapy for acute kidney injury, 181
Amiodarone
 for prevention of atrial fibrillation after coronary artery bypass surgery, cost effectiveness of, 137
Angiography
 CT pulmonary, versus ventilation-perfusion scan for detection of pulmonary embolism, 67
Angioplasty
 primary, effectiveness versus thrombolysis for myocardial infarction and its relationship to time delay, 51
Angiotensin-converting enzyme insertion/deletion polymorphism
 pneumonia risk and outcome and, 113
 as predictor of susceptibility and outcome in sepsis and ARDS, 10
Apolipoprotein CI
 correlation of preoperative levels with proinflammatory response in endotoxemia following elective cardiac surgery, 143
Applanation tonometry
 for radial artery pulse contour analysis, 81

ARDS (*see* Acute respiratory distress syndrome)
Arginine vasopressin
  in septic shock, effect of body mass on hemodynamic response, 85
Arterial catheters
  (*see also* Pulmonary artery catheter)
  heparinized solution versus saline solution for maintenance of, 84
Arterial gas embolism
  non-diving related, hyperbaric therapy for, 225
Atrial fibrillation
  amiodarone for prevention after coronary artery bypass surgery, cost effectiveness of, 137

B

B-type natriuretic peptide
  changes in level during spontaneous breathing trial, for improved predictive value, 22
  timing of measurement and treatment delay in acute decompensated heart failure, 48
Base deficit
  central venous versus arterial, as predictor of survival in acute trauma, 192
  as early predictor of morbidity and mortality in burns, 94
Beta-blockers
  in isolated blunt head injury, 226
Bladder pressure
  for correction of the effect of expiratory muscle activity on central venous pressure, 89
Blast injury
  in civilian setting, diagnosis of traumatic brain injury in, 195
Blood glucose
  bedside capillary measurements in critically ill patients, accuracy of, 169, 171
  hyperglycemia as predictor of in-hospital mortality in elderly patients without diabetes in a sub-intensive care unit, 175
Bloodstream infections
  after coronary artery bypass surgery, mortality associated with, 125
  after subarachnoid hemorrhage, 231
  catheter-associated, chlorhexidine bathing for reduction in, 107
  fungal
    in burn injuries, 96
    nosocomial, in ICU patients, 110

number of blood cultures needed for detection of, 122
  in previously hospitalized patients, 134
  real-time PCR for quantitative detection of *S. aureus* and *E. faecalis* DNA in blood in, 123
  timing of specimen collection for blood cultures in febrile patients with, 125
Body mass index
  functional outcomes in acute burns and, 99
Brain tissue oxygen tension
  following traumatic brain injury, 213
Bronchoalveolar lavage
  bilateral, for diagnosis of ventilator-associated pneumonia, 108
Burns
  acute renal failure in, 97
  adrenal insufficiency in, risk factors associated with, 176
  base deficit and lactate as early predictors of morbidity and mortality, 94
  body mass index and function outcomes in, 99
  comparison of premortem clinical diagnosis and autopsy findings in, 100
  fungal cultures in, 96
  heparin treatment for, 95
  inhaled heparin/N-acetylcystine for inhalation injury, 105
  intensive insulin protocol for, safety and efficacy, 103
  lightning injuries, 103
  shock resuscitation in, practice guidelines, 101

C

C-reactive protein
  high-sensitivity, correlation with delayed ischemic neurologic deficits after subarachnoid hemorrhage, 233
CABG (*see* Coronary artery bypass surgery)
Candida infections
  empirical fluconazole versus placebo for prevention in ICU patients, 129
  incidence, management, and outcome in ICU patients, 110
Cardiac arrest
  due to acute myocardial infarction, mild therapeutic hypothermia with primary PCI for, 55
  due to ventricular and non-ventricular fibrillation, therapeutic hypothermia for, 56

Subject Index / 287

ICU admission after, health care costs, long-term survival, and quality of life following, 61
in-hospital
  debriefing for improvement in performance and outcomes, 75
  delayed time to defibrillation after, 59
  simulation-based training for improved quality of care during team responses to, 245
  survival during nights and weekends, 58, 246
out-of-hospital, minimally interrupted cardiac resuscitation for, 72
prognosis in trauma patients, 74
Cardiac biomarkers
  mortality in ARDS and, 8
Cardiac output monitoring
  continuous and intermittent, pulmonary artery catheter versus lithium dilution technique for, 83
  noninvasive, using applanation tonometry-derived radial artery pulse contour analysis, 81
  pulse contour method for, effects of vasodilation on, 90
Cardiac surgery
  (see also Coronary artery bypass surgery)
  effects of quality improvement program on mortality after, 144
  preoperative apolipoprotein CI levels and proinflammatory response in endotoxemia following, 143
  respiratory failure after, predictors and early and late outcomes, 140
  stroke after, pulse pressure as an age-independent predictor of, 148
Cardiopulmonary bypass
  effect of mannitol on renal function following, in patients with established renal dysfunction, 141
  preoperative apolipoprotein CI levels and proinflammatory response in endotoxemia following, 143
Cardiopulmonary resuscitation
  for in-hospital cardiac arrest, debriefing for improvement in performance and outcomes, 75
  minimally interrupted by emergency medical services for out-of-hospital cardiac arrest, 72
  vasopressin with epinephrine versus epinephrine alone in, 77
Central venous base deficit
  versus arterial base deficit, as predictor of survival in acute trauma, 192

Central venous catheters
  NICE guidelines for ultrasound guidance, effect of implementation on complication rates, 87
Central venous pressure
  use of bladder pressure to correct for effect of expiratory muscle activity on, 89
Cerebral infarction
  posttraumatic, incidence, outcome, and risk factors, 211
Cerebral salt wasting
  versus inappropriate antidiuretic hormone secretion as cause of hyponatremia in acute neurological disease, 220
Chest physiotherapy
  during mechanical ventilation, impact on duration and outcome, 28
Chest radiographs
  daily routine versus on-demand in critically ill mechanically ventilated patients, 24
  effect on number and impact of CT and ultrasound studies in critically ill patients, 34
  indications for, in ICU patients, 35
Chlorhexidine
  bathing, for reduction in catheter-associated bloodstream infections, 107
Chronic obstructive pulmonary disease
  acute exacerbations, characteristics and long-term outcome, 38
Coagulopathy
  after trauma, hypoperfusion and, 204
Computed tomography (CT)
  emergency cardiac, for suspected acute coronary syndrome, 49
  pulmonary angiography, versus ventilation-perfusion scan for detection of pulmonary embolism, 67
  for pulmonary embolism detection in ICU patients, 63
Continuous positive airway pressure (CPAP)
  versus noninvasive intermittent positive-pressure ventilation for acute cardiogenic pulmonary edema, 47
  versus proportional assist ventilation for acute cardiogenic pulmonary edema, 45
Coronary artery bypass surgery (CABG)
  amiodarone for prevention of atrial fibrillation following, cost effectiveness of, 137

mortality associated with bloodstream infection after, 125
off-pump versus on-pump, oxygenation and release of inflammatory mediators after, 146
respiratory failure after, predictors and early and late outcomes, 140

Craniectomy
decompressive for severe traumatic brain injury, outcome after, 238

Cytokines
release following recruitment maneuvers, 1

Cytomegalovirus (CMV)
reactivation in critically ill immunocompetent patients, 131

D

Delirium
prevalence and risk factors for development in surgical and trauma ICU patients, 281
recognition and labeling of symptoms by intensivists, 229

Dexmedetomidine
versus lorazepam for sedation during mechanical ventilation, effect on acute brain dysfunction, 217

Dialysis
short-term, risk of nosocomial infection with femoral versus jugular venous catheterization for, 128

E

End-of-life care, in the ICU
family member satisfaction with decision making, 249
quality evaluation of, 259

Endotracheal tubes
polyurethane cuffed, for prevention of early postoperative pneumonia after cardiac surgery, 117
silver-coated, incidence of ventilator-associated pneumonia and, 115

Epinephrine
with vasopressin versus epinephrine alone in cardiopulmonary resuscitation, 77

Esophageal perforations
pathogenesis, diagnosis, and management options, 177

Etomidate
duration of adrenal inhibition following single dose in critically ill patients, 30

Extracorporeal membrane oxygenation (ECMO)
in severe Hantavirus cardiopulmonary syndrome, 15

Extrapulmonary ventilation
for severe ARDS after pulmonary resection, 3

F

Femoral shaft fractures
impact of initial stabilization method in patients with multiple injuries at risk for complications, 207

Fever
occurrence and outcome in critically ill adults, 264

Fluconazole
empirical, versus placebo for prevention of candidiasis in ICU patients, 129

Fluid resuscitation
in burn injuries, practice guidelines, 101
hypertonic resuscitation of hypovolemic shock after blunt trauma, 193

Fondaparinux
for ST-segment elevation myocardial infarction, in patients not receiving reperfusion treatment, 43

Fresh frozen plasma transfusion
infection in critically ill surgical patients and, 120

Fungal infections
in burn injuries, 96
empirical fluconazole versus placebo for prevention of candiduria/candidemia in ICU patients, 129
nosocomial candidemia and candiduria in ICU patients, 110

G

Gastric emptying
effects of sedation with morphine and midazolam versus propofol on, 280

H

Heart failure
acute decompensated, timing of B-natriuretic peptide levels and treatment delay in, 48
advanced low-output, sodium nitroprusside for, 69

Hemodialysis
short-term, risk of nosocomial infection with femoral versus jugular venous catheterization for, 128

Hemodynamic monitoring
  bedside transpulmonary, for goal-directed fluid management following subarachnoid hemorrhage, 214
Heparin
  in burn injury, 95
  solution, versus saline solution for maintenance of arterial catheters, 84
Heparin/N-acetylcystine
  inhaled, for inhalation injury, 105
High-frequency ventilation
  feasibility of frequencies up to 15Hz in ARDS, 9
Humidification
  during mechanical ventilation, impact on clinical outcomes, 26
Hydrocortisone
  for septic shock, 156
Hyperbaric therapy
  for non-diving related arterial gas embolism, 225
Hyperglycemia
  as predictor of in-hospital mortality in elderly patients without diabetes in a sub-intensive care unit, 175
Hyponatremia
  in acute neurological disease, cerebral salt wasting versus inappropriate antidiuretic hormone secretion as cause of, 220
Hypothermia, therapeutic
  with immediate PCI after out-of-hospital cardiac arrest due myocardial infarction, 55
  for ventricular and non-ventricular fibrillation cardiac arrest, early predictors of outcome, 56

I

Infection control process
  measures in ICU, impact of 2 different levels of performance feedback on compliance with, 275
Inferior vena cava filters, retrievable
  bedside placement guided by intravascular ultrasound in the critically injured, 66
  factors influencing successful removal, 65
Inflammatory adhesion molecules
  correlation with delayed ischemic neurologic deficits after subarachnoid hemorrhage, 233
Inhalation injury
  inhaled heparin/N-acetylcystine for, 105
Insulin
  early versus late intravenous administration in critically ill patients, 173
  intensive protocol in a burn-trauma ICU, safety and efficacy, 103
Intensive care medicine
  patients' and relatives' views of desirable characteristics of specialists in, 255
  residents' attitudes towards and evaluation of emergency medical teams, 272
Intensive care unit (ICU)
  adverse events in, costs of, 274
  changes in performance measures following opening of a dedicated thoracic surgical progressive care unit, 257
  determinants of long-term survival after treatment in, 253
  end-of-life care in
    family member satisfaction with decision making for, 249
    quality evaluation of, 259
  infection control process measures in, impact of 2 different levels of performance feedback on compliance with, 275
  intravenous adverse drug events in academic and nonacademic, costs of, 267
  mortality after discharge during the early weekend period, 265
  patient-initiated premature device removal in, 270
  primary surrogate decision maker's knowledge of family member's care in, 262
  satisfaction with experience, differences between families of survivors and nonsurvivors, 269
  validation of Surgical Intensive Care-Infection Registry, 277
Intra-abdominal hypertension
  acute renal failure and, 184
Intracranial pressure
  dose–response relationship of mannitol and, 223

L

Lactate
  as early predictor of morbidity and mortality in burns, 94
Left ventricular hypokinesia
  global, incidence in septic shock, 164
Lightning injuries

review, 103
Lithium dilution technique
  versus pulmonary artery catheter for continuous and intermittent cardiac output measurement, 83
Lung biopsy
  bedside open during mechanical ventilation in ALI/ARDS, yield and safety, 5
Lung ultrasonography
  in diagnosis of acute respiratory failure, 37

M

Mannitol
  dose–response relationship to intracranial pressure, 223
  effect on renal function after cardiopulmonary bypass in patients with established renal dysfunction, 141
  equiosmolar solution versus hypertonic saline, effect on intraoperative brain relaxation and electrolyte balance, 228
Mechanical ventilation
  for ALI/ARDS
    bedside open lung biopsy in, yield and safety, 5
    low tidal volume, barriers to, 20
    positive end-expiratory pressure settings in, 6
    strategy using low tidal volumes, recruitment maneuvers, and high positive end-expiratory pressure, 17
    very high-frequency oscillatory, feasibility of, 9
  chest physiotherapy during, impact on duration and outcome, 28
  daily routine chest radiographs versus restrictive use in, 24
  device to increase compliance in maintaining 30-degree head-of-bed elevation during, 251
  noninvasive (see Noninvasive ventilation)
  passive humidification during, impact on clinical outcomes, 26
  prolonged in adults, implications for healthcare delivery, 260
  protocol-direction sedation management for, 279
  relationship between arterial PO_2 and mixed venous PO_2 in response to changes in positive end-expiratory pressure, 18

risk factors for development of ARDS, 19
sedation with dexmedetomidine versus lorazepam in, effect on acute brain dysfunction, 217
weaning
  changes in B-type natriuretic peptide during spontaneous breathing trial, for improved predictive value, 22
  paired sedation and weaning protocol, efficacy and safety, 27
Methicillin-resistant *Staphylococcus aureus* (MRSA)
  emergence of the USA300 strain in a burn-trauma unit, 93
Methylprednisolone
  high-dose in acute spinal cord injury, early complications of, 242
Myasthenic crisis
  noninvasive ventilation in, 224
Myocardial infarction
  effectiveness of primary angioplasty versus thrombolysis and its relationship to time delay, 51
  red blood cell transfusion for, impact on clinical outcomes, 53
  ST-segment elevation
    citywide protocol for primary PCI in, 41
    fondaparinux for, in patients not receiving reperfusion treatment, 43
    out-of-hospital cardiac arrest due to, mild therapeutic hypothermia with immediate PCI for, 55

N

Negative pressure wound therapy
  clinical effectiveness and safety, 150
Noninvasive ventilation
  for acute cardiogenic pulmonary edema
    continuous positive airway pressure versus noninvasive intermittent positive-pressure ventilation, 47
    continuous positive airway pressure versus proportional assist ventilation, 45
  in myasthenic crisis, 224

O

Obesity
  functional outcomes in acute burns and, 99

P

Percutaneous coronary intervention (PCI)
  citywide protocol for, in ST-segment elevation myocardial infarction, 41

with mild therapeutic hypothermia, after out-of-hospital cardiac arrest due to ST-segment myocardial infarction, 55
Pneumonia
  after subarachnoid hemorrhage, 231
  angiotensin-converting enzyme insertion/deletion polymorphism and risk/outcome of, 113
  community-acquired
    tool for prediction of need for intensive respiratory or vasopressor support, 114
  community-acquired, outcomes after admission to ward versus ICU, 111
  postoperative, polyurethane cuffed endotracheal tubes for prevention of, 117
Positive end-expiratory pressure (PEEP)
  relationship between arterial PO_2 and mixed venous PO_2 in response to changes in, 18
  setting in adults with ALI or ARDS, 6
Post-traumatic stress disorder
  pain shortly after traumatic injury as predictor of, 197
Procalcitonin
  for shortening of antibiotic treatment duration in sepsis, 158
Prone positioning, for ARDS
  after cardiac surgery, feasibility, safety, and efficacy, 16
  right ventricular pressure and, 2
Pseudomonas aeruginosa bacteremia
  community-onset, clinical significance and predictors of, 132
Pulmonary artery catheter
  versus lithium dilution technique for continuous and intermittent cardiac output measurement, 83
Pulmonary edema, acute cardiogenic
  continuous positive airway pressure versus noninvasive intermittent positive-pressure ventilation for, 47
  continuous positive airway pressure versus proportional assist ventilation for, 45
Pulmonary embolism
  clinicians' knowledge of appropriate evaluation for, 64
  CT for detection in ICU patients, 63
  CT pulmonary angiography versus ventilation-perfusion scan for detection of, 67
  hospital volume and patient outcomes in, 62
  retrievable inferior vena cava filters for prevention of
    bedside placement guided by intravascular ultrasound in the critically injured, 66
    factors influencing successful removal, 65
Pulse contour method
  for cardiac output measurement, effects of vasodilation on, 90
Pulse pressure
  as an age-independent predictor of stroke after cardiac surgery, 148

R

Radial artery pulse
  applanation tonometry-derived contour analysis, 81
Recruitment maneuvers
  cytokine release following, 1
Red blood cell transfusions
  for acute myocardial infarction
    impact on clinical outcomes, 53
    utility and outcomes, 78
  in closed head injury, mortality and, 241
  duration of blood storage and complications from, after cardiac surgery, 119
  guidelines for reducing use in the ICU, 151
  in ischemic heart disease, 78
  leukoreduced products for, infectious complications in trauma and, 200
  massive in combat-related trauma, ratio of blood products transfused and mortality following, 189
  mortality rates in sepsis and, 165
Renal dysfunction (*see* Acute kidney injury; Acute renal failure)
Renal replacement therapy
  continuous for acute kidney injury, amino acid requirements during, 181
Respiratory failure
  after cardiac surgery, predictors and early and late outcomes, 139

S

Sedation
  with morphine and midazolam versus propofol, effect on gastric emptying and intra-gastric meal distribution, 280

protocol-directed management in mechanical ventilation, 279
Seizures
  focal motor, induction by alerting stimuli in critically ill patients, 234
  nonconvulsive electrographic after traumatic brain injury, effect on intracranial pressure and microdialysis lactate/pyruvate ratio, 216
  outcomes of status epilepticus in critically ill patients, 240
Sepsis/septic shock
  angiotensin-converting enzyme insertion/deletion polymorphism as predictor of susceptibility and outcome in, 10
  arginine vasopressin during, effect of body mass on hemodynamic response to, 85
  early, cardiac morphological and functional changes during, 160, 162
  global left ventricular hypokinesia in, incidence of, 164
  hydrocortisone therapy for, 156
  isolated and reversible impairment of ventricular relaxation in, 153
  liberal versus conservative vasopressor use for maintenance of mean arterial blood pressure in, 154
  procalcitonin for shortening of antibiotic treatment duration in, 158
  red blood cell transfusions and mortality in, 165
Shock
  hypovolemic after blunt trauma, hypertonic resuscitation of, 193
Sodium nitroprusside
  for advanced low-output heart failure, 69
Spinal cord injury
  high-dose methylprednisolone for, early complications of, 242
Status epilepticus
  outcomes in critically ill patients, 240
Stevens-Johnson syndrome
  effect of treatment on mortality, 98
Stroke
  acute ischemic
    aggressive blood pressure–lowering treatment before intravenous tissue plasminogen activator therapy for, 236
    classification instrument using CT or MR angiography, 235
    emergency administration of abciximab for, 221

after cardiac surgery, pulse pressure as an age-independent predictor of, 148
Subarachnoid hemorrhage
  goal-directed fluid management by bedside transpulmonary hemodynamic monitoring following, 214
  nosocomial infectious complications after, 231
  serum inflammatory adhesion molecules and high-sensitivity C-reactive protein levels after, correlation with delayed ischemic neurologic deficits, 233
Syndrome of inappropriate antidiuretic hormone secretion (SIADH)
  versus cerebral salt wasting as cause of hyponatremia in acute neurological disease, 220

T

Tissue plasminogen activator (tPA)
  for acute ischemic stroke, aggressive blood pressure–lowering treatment before, 236
Toxic epidermal necrolysis
  effect of treatment on mortality, 98
Tracheal tube cuff
  monitoring pressures in the ICU, 32
Tracheostomy
  current practice on timing, correction of coagulation disorders, and perioperative management, 31
Trauma
  acute coagulopathy of, hypoperfusion and, 204
  autopsy following, perceived value among trauma medical directors and coroners, 202
  blast injury in a civilian setting, diagnosis of traumatic brain injury in, 195
  blunt, hypertonic resuscitation of hypovolemic shock after, 193
  blunt splenic, healing patterns following, 205
  brain (see Traumatic brain injury)
  central venous and arterial base deficit as predictor of survival in, 192
  combat-related, ratio of blood products transfused and mortality following massive transfusions for, 189
  high-dose methylprednisolone in acute spinal cord injury, early complications of, 242

Subject Index / 293

impact of initial stabilization method for femoral shaft fracture in patients with multiple injuries at risk for complications, 207
leukoreduced red blood cell products in, infectious complications and use of, 200
major, quality of life 2 to 7 years after, 190
mortality prediction model based on the anatomic injury scale, 199
pain after, as risk factor for post-traumatic stress disorder, 197
prognosis of cardiac arrest in, 74
Traumatic brain injury
in blast injury in a civilian setting, diagnosis of, 195
brain tissue oxygen tension following, 213
cerebral infarction following, incidence, outcome, and risk factors, 211
with closed head injury, effect of anemia and blood transfusions on mortality in, 241
decompressive craniectomy for, outcome after, 238
isolated blunt, beta-blockers for, 226
nonconvulsive electrographic seizures after, effect on intracranial pressure and microdialysis lactate/pyruvate ratio, 216

U

Ultrasonography
for central venous catheter placement, effect of implementation of NICE guidelines on complication rates, 87
for evaluation of central veins in the ICU, 82

intravascular, for bedside placement of removable vena cava filters, 66
lung, in diagnosis of acute respiratory failure, 37

V

Vascular access
risk of nosocomial infection with femoral versus jugular venous catheterization for short-term dialysis, 128
Vasopressin
with epinephrine versus epinephrine alone in cardiopulmonary resuscitation, 77
Vasopressors
liberal versus conservative use for maintenance of mean arterial blood pressure during resuscitation of septic shock, 154
Venous thromboembolism
(*see also* Pulmonary embolism)
postoperative, clinical presentation and time-course, 68
Ventilator-associated pneumonia
bilateral bronchoalveolar lavage for diagnosis, 108
silver-coated endotracheal tubes and incidence of, 115
Ventricular relaxation
isolated and reversible, in septic shock, 153

W

Wound therapy
negative pressure versus conventional, clinical effectiveness and safety, 150

Author Index

A

Abrahams Z, 69
Adams HP Jr, 221
Aegerter P, 110
Afessa B, 115
Afzal R, 43
Agniel D, 125
Ajiki M, 214
Alaniz C, 181
Albright KC, 236
Aleem RF, 99
Alibhai SMH, 229
Aminian A, 220
Andel D, 94
Anderson DR, 67
Anderson M, 238
Annane D, 156
Anzueto A, 115
Arbelot C, 153
Arcelus JI, 68
Aronson D, 53
Arora V, 75
Assanasen S, 275
Asseburg C, 51
Aujesky D, 62

B

Badia JR, 3
Bajwa EK, 8
Balke L, 5
Ballard J, 96
Barrantes F, 182
Bates DW, 274
Bauer SR, 85
Baumann HJ, 5
Bearman G, 275
Bele N, 240
Benjo A, 148
Bennett MH, 225
Berbée JFP, 143
Berkius J, 38
Best D, 141
Binnekade JM, 34
Bleasdale SC, 107
Bobrow BJ, 72
Bochicchio GV, 195
Bollaert P-E, 45
Bonstein L, 53
Borgman MA, 189
Bougnoux M-E, 110
Bouhemad B, 153
Bourbeau P, 125
Bower AG, 267

Boyce PD, 8
Brimioulle S, 220
Brodaty D, 16
Brohi K, 204
Broux C, 30
Brower RG, 9
Brown DR, 257
Btaiche IF, 181
Bucknall TK, 279
Bulger EM, 193
Buzas JS, 199

C

Caille V, 2, 164
Callahan A, 169
Camp SL, 144
Cancio LC, 101
Caprini JA, 68
Castillo JG, 139
Cha SS, 85
Chan PS, 59
Chan R, 251
Chang S-C, 134
Chanzy E, 77
Chapman MJ, 280
Charles PGP, 114
Charron C, 2, 164
Chen S-Y, 134
Cheong HS, 132
Cheung CZ, 229
Chiarandini P, 83
Chien J-Y, 22
Christensen TD, 137
Cipolle MD, 238
Claassen J, 234
Clark LL, 72
Clavel M, 160, 162
Clec'h C, 24
Cochran A, 103
Cohen MJ, 204
Compton F, 81
Cook DJ, 17
Cooke CR, 269
Costa MG, 83
Cotton BA, 281
Critchell CD, 169
Curtis JR, 249, 269

D

Dalfino L, 184
Dann EJ, 53
David J-S, 74, 77, 226
Davis L, 103

Dean D, 202
Dean L, 120
de Cagny B, 82
Del Cotillo M, 84
Della Rocca G, 83
Deneer VHM, 113
Dennison CR, 20
Depuydt P, 117
Desachy A, 171
de Wit M, 260
De Wolf A, 117
Didwania A, 245
Dietl CA, 15
Dimopoulou I, 167
Dimsdale JE, 197
Dionne R, 41
Dobb GJ, 253
Dodd JD, 49
Doig GS, 61
Donadio I, 184
Dongelmans DA, 31
Downey L, 259
Duane TM, 241
Dunkman WJ, 120

E

Edelman L, 96
Edelson DP, 75
Edmond M, 275
Edwards JE Jr, 129
Effron MB, 221
Endeman H, 113
Engelberg RA, 259
Ernst NE, 108
Etchecopar-Chevreuil C,
    160, 162
Ewy GA, 72

F

Fadlalla AMA, 277
Fagot J-P, 98
Farrell RT, 99
Faucher LD, 65
Faure P, 30
Feihl F, 56
Feinglass J, 245
Feissel M, 45
Fernandez A, 231
Fessler HE, 9
Filsoufi F, 139
Fine D, 148
Finn JC, 253

Fischer R, 187
Flores C, 10
Francis GS, 69
François B, 160, 162
Franz C, 274
Fraser RJ, 280
Friese RS, 200
Frontera JA, 231
Fuchs BD, 27

G

Gamelli RL, 99
Ganter MT, 204
Geng M, 62
Gerber DR, 78
Ghazali AD, 171
Gibran NS, 101
Gierveld S, 123
Girard TD, 27
Glance L, 199
Glavan BJ, 259
Golob JF Jr, 277
Gonzalez IM, 107
González-Castro A, 242
Goodacre S, 47
Graat ME, 34
Graf J, 61
Graf J-D, 158
Grandhi R, 241
Grané N, 84
Gray A, 47
Gregor S, 150
Gries CJ, 249
Groeneveld ABJ, 18
Gueugniaud P-Y, 74, 77
Guyatt GH, 17

H

Hacking MB, 87
Hager DN, 9
Hallevi H, 236
Hamdi A, 24
Hanson MD, 95
Harbarth S, 158
Harkins CL, 176
Harrison GA, 272
Hayes JR, 202
He J, 235
Hejblum G, 35
Hemmila MR, 151
Hermsen JL, 65
Herr DL, 217
Hirsch LJ, 234
Holt J, 105

Honiden S, 173
Howard JL, 238
Huang Y-CT, 22

I

Ibele AR, 65
Iglesias M, 3
Ilias I, 167
Im SA, 173
Inaba K, 226
Ioos V, 35

J

Jackson S-R, 108
Jacques T, 272
Januzzi JL, 8
Jia X, 19
Jurkovich GJ, 193

K

Kac G, 110
Kahn SR, 67
Kakino S, 233
Kallinen O, 100
Kalva S, 49
Kamolz LP, 94
Kan JA, 277
Kang C-I, 132
Kaushal R, 274
Kazumata K, 214
Kealey GP, 93
Keegan MT, 257
Keh D, 156
Keir MJ, 64
Kelly E, 251
Kirby KA, 131
Kirkpatrick AW, 264
Kluge S, 5
Koch CG, 119
Kollef MH, 115
Kopterides P, 26
Krauss M, 125
Kress JP, 27
Kristiansen IS, 137
Kröner A, 34
Krumholz HM, 59
Kubo Y, 233
Kvåle R, 190
Kwolek C, 66

L

Lam SW, 85
Larkin GL, 58, 246
Latenser BA, 93
Laugesen H, 146
Laupland KB, 264
Leatherman JW, 89
Lee A, 122
Legedza A, 1
Legriel S, 240
Leipzig RM, 270
Le May MR, 41
Levin PD, 63
Levitt J, 13
Li L, 119
Licht A, 63
Lichtenstein DA, 37
Limaye AP, 131
Lin M-S, 22
Litzinger B, 75
Liu KD, 13
Llavoré M, 84
Llorca J, 242
Longhi L, 213
Lumpkins K, 195

M

Maegele M, 150
Maggio PM, 151
Magnotti LJ, 205
Maillet J-M, 16
Maisel AS, 48
Maisniemi K, 100
Malhotra A, 19
Mandrekar J, 224
Manias E, 279
Manley GT, 223
Mårdh C, 38
Martinez E, 3
Martin-Schild S, 236
Mattox KL, 177
Mayglothling J, 241
McArthur D, 216
McGwin G Jr, 176
McLaws M-L, 272
McManus JG, 103
McMullin N, 48
McQueen AS, 64
Meade MO, 17
Mégarbane B, 128
Mendez-Tellez PA, 20
Mercat A, 6
Mezière GA, 37

Miller C, 216
Minnick AF, 270
Mion LC, 270
Mirrett S, 122
Mirvis SE, 211
Mohammad RA, 181
Monreal M, 68
Mor MK, 62
Morandi A, 175
Morley J, 207
Morris LG, 32
Morris SE, 103, 105
Mortensen EM, 111
Morton MJ, 103
Mourvillier B, 240
Muangman S, 228
Mueller EW, 108
Mühlhoff C, 61
Mullens W, 69
Mustonen K-M, 97
Mutoh T, 214

N

Nathens AB, 193
Navarrete E, 262
Newby DE, 47
Nguyen NQ, 280
Nichol G, 59
Nicolas-Robin A, 153
Nishiyama T, 90
Nobre V, 158
Nolin T, 38
Norman SB, 197
Nuckols TK, 267

O

Obel N, 265
O'Connor J, 195
Oddo M, 56
Ogasawara K, 233
Oldgren J, 43
Olsen MA, 125
Orellana-Jimenez C, 220
Oremus M, 95
Ornato JP, 58, 246
Osler T, 199

P

Paddock SM, 267
Pagan F, 213

Palazzo MGA, 28
Palmer S, 51
Pandharipande P, 281
Pandharipande PP, 217
Pang T, 234
Pape H-C, 207
Parienti J-J, 128
Partanen TA, 100
Peacock WF, 48
Peberdy MA, 58, 246
Pedersen L, 265
Pena A, 49
Pérez-Méndez L, 10
Perkins JG, 189
Perron AD, 192
Peters RPH, 123
Pett SB, 15
Pham TN, 101
Phelan HA, 200
Phoa KN, 31
Pierau C, 55
Pirone JR, 260
Poelaert J, 117
Presneill JJ, 279
Pun BT, 217

Q

Qureshi AS, 89

R

Radke PW, 55
Rahmanian PB, 139
Rasmussen BS, 146
Rehman A, 154
Reiff DA, 176
Reller LB, 122
Restrepo MI, 111
Ribordy V, 56
Richard J-CM, 6
Riedel S, 125
Riou B, 74
Ritenour AE, 103
Rixen D, 207
Robinson M, 229
Roccaforte JD, 32
Rodger MA, 67
Rodriguez RM, 262
Roka J, 94
Rozet I, 228

Rubenfeld GD, 131
Rusterholtz T, 45

S

Sabatini T, 175
Saeed M, 19
Saffle J, 96
Saffle JR, 105
Sakr Y, 165
Samy Modeliar S, 82
Santanello S, 202
Sarani B, 120
Sarge T, 1
Sauerland S, 150
Savage SA, 205
Savarese V, 169
Schaefer J-H, 81
Schierbeck J, 265
Schiffl H, 187
Schippers EF, 143
Schmelzer TM, 192
Schmidt JM, 231
Schneck J, 98
Schneider AJ, 18
Schultz A, 173
Schuster MG, 129
Schwaber J, 262
Sekula P, 98
Seneviratne J, 224
Sessler DI, 119
Sevestre M-A, 82
Shahpori R, 264
Shapiro RS, 89
Sheppard SV, 141
Shintani A, 281
Sibbald WJ, 63
Siempos II, 26
Simon P, 24
Sleiman I, 175
Smith MNA, 141
Smythe JF, 87
So DY, 41
Sobel JD, 129
Sollid J, 146
Sorani MD, 223
Spaniolas K, 66
Sperry JL, 200
Spinella PC, 189
Sprung CL, 156, 165
Stamou SC, 144
Stamoulis K, 167
Stein DM, 211
Stein MB, 197
Stiegel RM, 144

Suberviola B, 242
Subramanian S, 154
Swartz B, 125

T

Talmor D, 1
Tawil I, 211
Teixeira PGR, 226
Templeton M, 28
Thieke MP, 257
Thierry S, 16
Thirion M, 128
Thomason MH, 192
Thompson RE, 148
Tian J, 182
Tontisirin N, 228
Torner J, 221
Torres-Mozqueda F, 235
Trick WE, 107
Trytko BE, 225
Tullo L, 184

U

Ulvik A, 190

V

Valeriani V, 213
Van Agtmael MA, 123
van de Garde EMW, 113
van Disseldorp IM, 143
Vardakas KZ, 26
Vazquez R, 182
Veelo DP, 31
Velez JA, 111
Velmahos GC, 66
Vergel YB, 51
Vespa PM, 216
Vibert J-F, 35
Vieillard-Baron A, 2, 164
Vielle B, 6
Villar J, 10
Vincent J-L, 12, 165
Vinclair M, 30
Vuagnat AC, 171
Vuola J, 97

W

Wall MJ Jr, 177
Wall RJ, 249, 269
Wallentin L, 43
Wang W, 20
Wayne DB, 245
Wendy WL, 151
Wentzel-Larsen T, 190
Wernly JA, 15
Whitby M, 114
Whitlock R, 95

Wi YM, 132
Wibbenmeyer LA, 93
Wigmore TJ, 87
Wijdicks EFM, 224
Williams TA, 253
Williams Z, 251
Wittrock M, 81
Wolfe R, 114
Wolfrum S, 55
Worthy S, 64
Wu GH-M, 134
Wu JT, 177

Y

Yamashita K, 90
Yeh IB, 235
Yilmaz M, 154
Yokoyama T, 90

Z

Zambon M, 12
Zarzaur BL, 205
Zebis LR, 137
Zhuo H, 13
Zilberberg MD, 260
Zoumalan RA, 32